£21.99.

Implementing Change in Health Systems

Market Reforms in the United Kingdom,
Sweden and the Netherlands

Implementing Change in Health Systems

Market Reforms in the United Kingdom, Sweden, and the Netherlands

Michael I. Harrison

SAGE Publications
London • Thousand Oaks • New Delhi

SAGE Publications Ltd
1 Olivers Yard
London EC1Y1SP

SAGE Publications Inc
2455 Teller Road
Thousand Oaks, California 91320

SAGE Publications India Pvt Ltd
B-42, Panchsheel Enclave
Post Box 4109
New Delhi 100 017

British Library Cataloguing in Publication data

A catalogue record for this book is available
from the British Library

ISBN 0 7619 6175 5
     0 7619 6176 3

Library of Congress control number available

Typeset by C&M Digitals (P) Ltd, Chennai, India
Printed in India at Gopsons Paper Ltd, Noida

Contents

Preface

Do health systems become more efficient, less subject to cost escalation, and more responsive to patient needs when there is competition among insurers and providers and these organizations adopt modern business practices? During the 1990s in Europe and elsewhere, many policymakers and analysts enthusiastically cited the examples of the United States, the United Kingdom, Sweden, and the Netherlands as evidence that markets could deliver these benefits. I began my research in reaction to this wave of enthusiasm. I wanted to know what had actually happened in the nations that were so often mentioned as leaders in market reform. I also wanted to know whether other countries could reasonably follow the example of these prominent nations. I decided to concentrate on European leaders in market reform, since the United States differed from most advanced industrial nations in its level of health expenditure, its reliance on for-profit insurers and providers, and its lack of national health insurance. This book reports how I recast the deceptively simple questions that motivated my study, what I learned about market reforms, and how I came to understand the processes of policy implementation and health system change.

I could not have carried out this research without the help and cooperation of many health researchers, managers, and practitioners. Chief among them were the people who gave generously of their time in interviews. Unfortunately, most must remain anonymous. I particularly appreciate the hospitality and assistance of the professional and administrative staff of the Swedish hospital that is called Brookside in this book. Listing the many other people who helped me in my work does not do justice to the full extent of their logistical support, sharing of valuable information, encouragement, collegiality, and international friendship. For help in Sweden I owe thanks to Lennart Kohler, Johan Calltorp, John Ovretveit, Rose Wesley-Lindahl and other members of the staff of the Nordic School of Public Health; Tobjörn Malm and the staff of the Western Stockholm Medical Services District; Sven-Eric Bergman, Leif Borgert, Per Olof Brogren, and Olle Saemond. For help in the Netherlands, thanks to Eirk Konen and the staff of the National Hospital Institute; Bert Hermans, Harm Lieverdink, Aad de Roo, and Rafael Smit. In the United Kingdom, thanks are due to Stephen Harrison, David Hunter and the staff of the Nuffield Institute for Health at the University of Leeds; Chris Ham and Jonathan Shapiro at the Health Services Management Centre of the University of Birmingham; John Appleby and Neil Goodwin.

Other colleagues to whom I am grateful for help and encouragement on one or more phases of the project include Jeorg Althammer, Christa Altenstetter, Mats Brommels, Reinhard Busse, David Chinitz, Brad Kirkman-Liff, Denis Kodner, Donald Light, Anita Pfaff, Martin Pfaff, Bruce Rosen, Friedrich Wilhelm Schwartz, Mordechai Shani, Richard Saltman, Arie Shirom, and Andrew Twaddle. Special mention is due to the people who commented on draft chapters and earlier, related papers and reports: Sven-Eric Bergman, David Hunter, Stephen Harrison, Johan Calltorp, Erik Konnen, Hava Etzioni-Halevi, Harm Lieverdink, Nicholas Mays, Debra Stone, and Ilan Talmud.

I wrote portions of this study during a stay as a Visiting Scholar at the Institute for Health Policy at Brandeis University. Thanks to Stanley Wallack, Stuart Altman, Christine Bishop, Grant Ritter, and other institute members for their cooperation and help. I also worked on the study while I was a Visiting Scholar at Georgetown University's Graduate Institute for Public Policy and its Institute for Health Care Research and Policy. Thanks to Judy Feder and the institute staff for their hospitality and support. Thanks also to Irene Fraser and the staff of the Center for Delivery, Organization, and Markets at the Agency for Healthcare Research and Quality for supporting my work on the final stages of manuscript preparation. I appreciate the help of the following people who provided research assistance on various stages of the project: Aviv Barhom, Jane Cohen, Joseph Elias, Tracy Hartman, Shirly Hering, Merav Kinan, Edna Mirziof, Ednah Smolin, and Ronit Yitshaki Hagai.

The research was supported by grants from the Israel National Institute for Health Policy, the Schnitzer Fund of Bar-Ilan University, and the Medical Research and Development Fund for Health Services (Sheba Medical Center, Tel Ha Shomer, Israel), which provided a publication grant. Support for travel and sabbatical leave came from Bar-Ilan University. The book's contents do not represent the views of the funding organizations. Nor do they represent the views of the Agency for Healthcare Research and Policy in Washington, DC, where I am currently a Senior Research Scientist.

I want to acknowledge the encouragement of my son Natan and my late father, Milton Harrison. My deepest debt is to my wife Jo-Ann, who saw me through a decade of research on Europe with the same combination of encouragement, guidance, and generous tolerance that she has offered ever since our days together in graduate school, when we first began to learn how to live and work together.

DEDICATION

In memory of my parents, Milton and Joan Harrison.

1

Health System Reform and Policy Implementation

During the last 25 years, the governments of nearly every industrialized nation considered making major structural and institutional changes in their health systems. Many nations implemented these ambitious reforms. In Europe and Scandinavia, three main periods of reform stand out, even though there were many differences among the reforms and much diversity within national policies. Each period is distinguished by the primary objectives for reform and the distinctive mechanisms through which policymakers sought to attain their objectives. Reforms in the first period, which began in the late 1970s and early 1980s, aimed mainly at containing the costs of health care and making it more efficient. Policymakers sought to attain these objectives by imposing budget ceilings on health care providers and introducing other forms of governmental regulation of health expenditures and services. During the second period of reform, which began in the late 1980s and peaked during the 1990s, policymakers put new emphasis on making service providers more directly accountable for the quality and costs of their services and more responsive to patients' needs and priorities. While continuing and even intensifying their regulatory steps toward cost containment, policymakers gave prominence to a new mechanism for containing costs and revitalizing publicly-funded health care: development of market-like processes that would provide incentives for statutory insurers and providers to become more efficient, reduce charges, and improve quality.[1]

This book's central concern is the implementation in Europe of these market reforms.[2] Despite important variations (Jacobs, 1998), all the prominent market reforms in Europe sought to foster competition among health care providers, among insurers, or both (Paton, 2000). Both types of government-supervised competition are referred to as *managed* or *regulated competition* and as *quasi-markets* (Bartlett et al., 1998a; Enthoven, 1978, 1993; Light, 2001; van de Ven,

1990).[3] These terms indicate that governmental regulation was required to foster fair competition. Thus during market reforms, governments explicitly or implicitly set the rules under which competition could occur and continued to regulate emerging market-like relations among health providers and funding agencies. Regulation was also needed to help governments in countries with strong social democratic traditions resolve a basic dilemma: Market-like conditions might sharpen inequalities in health finance and access to health care and thereby undermine the national commitment to solidarity – universal and equal access to comprehensive services, regardless of ability to pay. Continuing government action was needed to preserve solidarity from erosion by market forces.

In addition to fostering managed competition, market reforms often introduced practices and standards from the world of business into health care management and finance. In keeping with this trend, many European countries experimented with decentralized budgeting and management, managerial control over service production and costs, assessment of efficiency through input-output comparisons, and stimulation of service production through arrangements that linked payments to service volume (Saltman and Figueras, 1997).

By the mid 1990s, health system reform entered a third period as national priorities and policies became more diverse and paid more attention to ways to improve public health and wellness, as opposed to just reorganizing medical services. Without abandoning the policy goals of previous reforms, decision-makers renewed their attention to social and economic determinants of health and access to care. They also sought to reinforce the rights of citizens to health care and their responsibilities for improving their own health. During this period, policymakers recognized that market forces alone could not bring about the sought-for changes in their health systems. Instead, they sought to combine regulatory and market forces. In this way they hoped to progress toward an increasingly diverse set of health policy goals and foster cooperation among the many agencies and sectors in the health system and in related social services.

The first objective of this book is to analyze how market reform of health care was implemented in the United Kingdom (UK), Sweden, and the Netherlands – three nations that pioneered the introduction of managed competition in Europe and served as exemplars for policymakers and analysts across the globe (Organization for Economic Cooperation and Development (OECD), 1992; Saltman and von Otter, 1992). To understand the reforms in each country, I examine their background, content, political and socio-economic context, implementation processes, and outcomes.

The book's second objective is to assess the potential contribution of market reform to the efficiency and quality of publicly funded and publicly regulated health systems. This assessment of market reforms in health can contribute to the continuing debate about the merits of market-oriented reform (e.g., 'Tougher than...,' 2001; Evans, 1997; Rice, 1998; Rice et al., 2000) and to evaluation of the merits and effects of an even broader movement known as the New Public Management (Hood, 1991; Jones et al., 1997). This term encompasses a diverse set of approaches that favor introducing business and market concepts into the public sector, along with a variety of other steps toward reforming government agencies (e.g., Osborne and Gaebler, 1992; Osborne and Plastrik, 2000). A third objective for this book is the development of a new analytical framework for investigating implementation of public policies. This framework contributes to policy research by combining divergent theoretical perspectives into a model that guides examination of implementation processes and their outcomes.

3

The first part of this chapter gives additional background on the three periods of health system reform. The second part reviews theory and research relevant to understanding policy implementation in health systems and other public systems. This review leads to construction of a new framework for investigating implementation of public policies. The discussion also helps explain why health providers – and especially hospitals and hospital physicians – pose the greatest challenges to health system reform. This section concludes by presenting the research questions addressed in Chapters 2 through 8. The third part of the chapter describes the logic and methods of the research. The fourth compares major features of the health systems in each of the countries studied in depth.

TWO DECADES OF HEALTH SYSTEM REFORM

The origins of the last two decades of European and American health care reforms lie in the late 1960s and 1970s. At that time, health care gradually ceased to be defined as the purely technical province of physicians and governmental administrators. Instead health care entered an increasingly contested and volatile political arena (Starr and Immergut, 1987). Policymakers and analysts, along with the public at large, became more skeptical and critical of the technical authority and reliability of physicians and health administrators. Conflicting claims on the health system by divergent constituencies and interest groups generated much debate over objectives, spending patterns, and structures in health care.

During the 1970s and 1980s these debates converged around two related themes. The first concentrated on total national health expenditures, most of which were government-funded. Health expenditures as a proportion of total domestic expenditures (i.e., GDP) grew very rapidly during the 1960s, increasing by 30.7%[4] As Figure 1.1 shows, rapid growth in health expenditures continued throughout the 1970s (+35%). Expenditure increases became more moderate in the 1980s (+7.2%) and the 1990s (+3.3%)[5] The expenditure patterns of the UK, Sweden, and the Netherlands are discussed in the last section of this chapter.

Among the main causes of rapid growth in health care expenditures were growing public demand for care and rising expectations about care quality and accessibility (e.g. World Health Organization, 1985). In addition, ever more sophisticated and complex technologies, most of which were located in modern acute-care hospitals, created powerful forces for growth in costs (Evans, 1983; Newhouse, 1993).[6] Cost growth also reflected the rising number and proportion of older people, who rely very heavily on both ambulatory and hospital care (Federation of Swedish County Councils, 1993; Saltman and Figureras, 1997).

At the same time that health costs rose throughout the West, political and economic developments weakened the capacity and commitment of governments

4

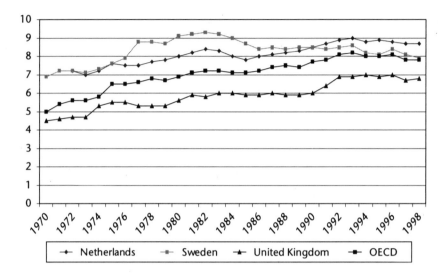

Figure 1.1   *Total health expenditures as per cent of gross domestic product*

to pay for most health care (Abel-Smith, 1992). The recession that spread through most of Europe during the 1970s and early 1980s had a major impact on political support for health expenditures. Competition for public funds increased, as expenditures for unemployment relief and social services intensified the burden on public spending. Governments were hard pressed to raise taxes further in order to pay for labor-intensive services, such as health, welfare, and education. In many countries the recession was accompanied by growing debate over the wisdom of increasing government spending (Pen, 1987). Political pressure mounted for cuts in government spending, including social benefits, so as to reduce taxes, interest rates, and labor costs (e.g., Webber, 1992). Advocates of reductions in public spending argued that these cuts would create more jobs and enhance the competitiveness of local industries in the international marketplace. In the 1990s the Maastricht limitations on government debt in countries planning to introduce the new European currency added further urgency to reductions in government spending.

During the late 1970s and the 1980s, in response to these political, economic, and technical developments, consensus grew about the need to curtail growth in health costs. Policymakers debated a variety of ways to contain costs and make publicly-funded health care more efficient and accountable. Many European countries implemented cost-containment programs. These programs relied heavily on governmental control and regulation of health finance. Some countries – including the UK, the Netherlands, and Sweden – imposed tight restraints on health expenditures. Fiscal constraints, technological innovations like minimally invasive forms of surgery and diagnosis, and changing medical practices contributed to reductions in the length of hospital stays and a rapid growth in day surgery and outpatient care. Between 1980 and 1990 the average length of stay in acute hospital settings fell by 17% in OECD nations, from 10.8 to nine days (n=20). On the other hand, there was far less progress toward other goals for health system change as articulated by the World Health Organization (WHO, 1985), endorsed by the European Parliament and several nations, and advocated by many health policy analysts. These goals included redistributing resources toward primary care, extending preventive treatment, enhancing equality of access to care, integrating health sectors, and developing ways to compare the costs and benefits of alternative forms of care.

Health system reforms in the UK during this period drew heavily on the ideas of the New Public Management, which had grown in popularity throughout the English-speaking world (Ferlie et al., 1996). Adherents of this approach saw public bureaucracies as bloated, unresponsive to public needs, and lacking accountability. They argued that health organizations could be made more efficient and effective by downsizing and applying management techniques that were originally developed by manufacturing firms and mass retailers of goods and services. Introduction of these business techniques would yield tighter managerial control over health care practitioners (Harrison and Pollitt, 1994).

Although they experienced some success in their initial cost-containment efforts, toward the end of the 1980s and the start of the 1990s several European nations, including the three studied here, launched more ambitious structural and financial reforms of health care finance and delivery. Besides concern over health-care costs and the efficiency of health providers, this second wave of European health system reforms reflected growing doubts about the efficacy of medical practices and technologies; criticisms of the equity of current systems for financing and delivering health care; concerns about the quality of medical care; and changing beliefs about governmental involvement in the delivery of public services (OECD, 1992, 1994, 1995).

During the second period of reform, policymakers put new emphasis on introducing market mechanisms into national health systems and reducing direct government regulation. Besides aiming at economic objectives, the reforms in this period sought to provide patients with greater freedom to choose providers or insurers. Despite the new rhetoric, during this period governments did not typically reduce their regulation of the health system and in some cases even further centralized state control over providers and insurers.

In the UK and the Netherlands, and to a somewhat lesser degree in other European countries, this second period of reforms drew inspiration from neo-liberal economic theories and conservative political ideologies. European policymakers were also influenced by organizational changes occurring in the United States in health care and many public services. The American market reforms in health drew in particular on neo-liberal economic views as articulated by Dr. Paul Ellwood (1972), Professor Alan Enthoven (1978), and other health economists, along with advocates of the New Public Management. According to these pro-market analysts, whose ideas diffused throughout English-speaking nations, the Netherlands, and Sweden (Common, 1998), governmental planning and regulation were ineffective, and traditional public budgets created 'perverse incentives' for waste. In contrast, competition among publicly-owned agencies

6

or competition between public and private firms would create incentives for public services to become more efficient and hold down costs. Instead of hierarchical control by government, contracting between and within public agencies and outsourcing to private contractors would become the dominant means of coordinating the new public services (see McMaster, 1998 for a critique). To support their expectation that competition would increase organizational efficiency and help contain costs, advocates of market-based reform, like Enthoven, cited the efficiencies and cost reductions attained by health maintenance organizations in the United States.

Conservative politicians and analysts became especially vocal supporters of market reforms of the public sector. They favored private ownership of services and utilities. Where this step was impractical, the conservatives advocated private investment in capital development for public services, competitive tendering of services provided to public agencies, competition among public agencies, and separation of purchasers and providers of public services. Further support for privatization and for public-private partnerships came from prestigious and influential international agencies, including the World Bank, the International Monetary Fund, and the European Commission (Gaffney et al., 1999c). As they came to power during the 1970s and 1980s, the conservatives sold state-owned industries and agencies to private investors, sought to downsize government organizations, reduced social benefits, and introduced private ownership and market forces into many areas that were formerly dominated by public bureaucracies – including health, education, social services, and transportation (Altensteler and Haywood, 1991; Bartlett et al., 1998b; Kavanagh and Seldon, 1989).

Rather than privatizing most services, the market reforms in health care in Western Europe and Scandinavia, along with those in several other advanced industrial countries, mainly promoted competition within two sectors: (1) publicly financed *providers*; and (2) *insurers or public payers*.[7] Nations including the UK, Sweden, New Zealand, Singapore, and Korea restructured their health systems to foster competition among public providers of care – hospitals and physicians that were owned by the state or strictly regulated by it. Italy, Spain, the Netherlands, and Israel introduced less comprehensive forms of provider competition. Competition between private and public providers was also encouraged (Fougere, 2001; Cabiedes and Guillen, 2001; Harrison and Shalom, 2002; Hsaio, 1994). The Netherlands, Germany, Israel, Chile, and the Philippines were among the countries that sought to generate competition among payers – not-for-profit insurers and health maintenance organizations, public agencies responsible for contracting with health care providers, or a mix of not-for-profit and for-profit payers (Brown and Amelung, 1999; Gres et al., 2002; Gross and Harrison, 2001; Hsaio, 1994).

The third period of reform was marked by a growing list of ambitious goals for health policy, disenchantment with market reform, and reliance on an eclectic and rapidly shifting mix of market and regulatory mechanisms. While acknowledging the need for efficiency gains and cost control, politicians, managers, providers, and policy analysts increasingly focused their debates on problems that did not seem amenable to market solutions and could even be aggravated by competition among health providers. Among the old and new issues on this crowded policy agenda were assuring quality of care, improving the health and wellbeing of entire populations and communities, involving patients and citizens in decisions about health care delivery and funding, and reducing socio-economic and regional differences in access to care. There was also increasing interest in assuring the cost-effectiveness of care and setting priorities and objective criteria for health service delivery and funding (WHO, 1998; Honigsbaum et al., 1995). The latter two goals led to activity in areas like evidence-based medicine, medical technology assessment, clinical guidelines, and managed care (Perleth et al., 2001; Fairfield et al., 1997). Another concern that emerged in the Netherlands, and to a lesser degree elsewhere, was encouragement of individual responsibility for health and wellbeing.

This new policy agenda both reflected and intensified a growing lack of optimism about the prospects for competitive reform. In the second half of the 1990s, national politicians increasingly worried that reliance on market forces would intensify unemployment without solving other problems facing the health system. Moreover, they now aimed to foster cooperation and coordination among the health system actors, who had been further divided by market incentives. Policymakers also encouraged health agencies to cooperate with social services, like housing and welfare. Despite the pullbacks from competitive reform, decision makers did not lose enthusiasm for other types of business-like reform. Nor did they aim to revert to planning and tight governmental control over the health system.

Instead, policymakers now seek an appropriate combination of market and governmental forces in health care, as they do in economics and social services. As a result 'a set of third ways' ('Crumbs from...', 1999) are emerging in different countries and even within single nations. In health, these new arrangements continue to rely on contracting in health financing and delivery. The emerging systems combine private and semi-autonomous public providers of health care; public and private funding; state regulation of insurers; and state, managerial, and professional regulation of health providers. The architects of these new programs, along with many other actors in the health system, are struggling to find ways to coordinate and integrate the increasingly complex set of organizations responsible for health care funding and provision.

IMPLEMENTING POLICIES FOR HEALTH SYSTEM REFORM

This study mainly focuses on implementation of health system reforms, rather than on the initial stages of health policymaking – which include issue definition, building agendas for governmental action; and policy formulation (Kenis and Schneider, 1991, p. 43).[8] Implementation starts after the formulation of a policy initiative in a piece of legislation or an official policy document and encompasses the development of operational programs by national, regional, and local governments, along with actions by many other types of organizations and groups that are affected by government policies. Distinguishing policy implementation from formulation helps raise questions about what happens to policies *in practice* after they are formulated by central governmental agencies and how interaction among diverse policy actors shape policy outcomes.

8

Framing Policy Implementation

This part of the chapter proposes a new way of viewing implementation of health policies, as well as other types of public policy. This approach uses a four-fold framework that synthesizes divergent streams of research on implementation and planned change in systems and organizations. The framework, and the model derived from it, guide the analysis in subsequent chapters of implementation processes and outcomes and should also prove useful for research on other types of policy implementation.

A growing number of researchers call for a synthesis of the diverse approaches to implementation research (e.g., Lazin, 1995; O' Toole, 1986; Sabatier, 1986, 1991). Moreover, several have effectively combined divergent theoretical perspectives in their empirical studies (e.g., Cauthen and Amenta, 1996; Dohler, 1991; Grin and van de Graaf, 1996; Spillane, 1998). To date, no one has developed a model of policy implementation that reflects a wide range of research and theory, and yet remains simple enough to be useful in implementation research.[9]

The framework proposed here combines the classic, 'top-down', administrative approach to implementation, with a 'bottom-up', bargaining perspective, an interpretive perspective, and an institutional view. By bringing together disparate themes in the literature on implementation and organizational change, this framework yields more nuanced and non-intuitive understandings of implementation processes and outcomes than do analyses based on just one or two theoretical perspectives. Besides contributing to research, the new framework may help policymakers and managers anticipate and deal with the complexities of planned change.

Alternative theories and research approaches provide distinctive analytical *frames*. Framing refers to the way that theories, models, and research techniques draw attention to certain phenomenon, while diverting attention from others (Schon and Rein, 1994). Frames also build in assumptions about the ways that social processes operate. Multiple framing can help researchers, consultants, and policymakers move beyond the concepts and frames they take for granted and use routinely. By choosing a limited number of frames, each of which adds analytical power to the set, investigators avoid the burden of trying to work with too many concepts and findings at once. This approach to framing has been applied in the past to theory and diagnosis in organizational and management studies (Bolman and Deal, 1991; Morgan, 1986; Harrison and Shirom,1999). Frame combination draws insights from social constructionist and post-modernist thinking about organizations and management (e.g., Astley and Zammuto, 1992; Chia, 1995), while avoiding the linguistic and philosophical pitfalls that often characterize post-modernist writing.

Four theoretical frames capture much of the variation within past research and theorizing on implementation.[10] The first frame views implementation as *administration* – specifying national mandates and programs, moving them down the administrative hierarchy, and diffusing them to allied organizations. This 'top-down' view of implementation reflects the popular assumption that governmental bureaucracies are instruments for policy implementation. Government officials are supposed to translate national policies into workable programs and use their authority to assure that these programs are implemented by officials at lower levels in the hierarchy and by managers of organizations subject to governmental regulation and funding. From the administrative standpoint, policies are successfully implemented when programs derived from them are enacted and policy objectives are achieved.

The administrative frame provides a useful starting point for investigating implementation of national policies that are clearly stated by national or regional governmental actors in laws or policy documents (Sabatier, 1986). Researchers can follow implementation of the original policy as it moves down to lower levels of government and out to related organizations and agencies. By tracing these developments over a decade or more (Sabatier, 1991), it is sometimes possible to discern significant deviations from national policy thrusts and uncover the processes that produced these emergent policy changes. Analyses guided by this perspective have uncovered recurring sources of implementation failure – including bureaucratic inflexibility and communication barriers. (Mayntz, 1979; Kenis and Schneider, 1991; Hall, 1991) and the difficulties of coordinating the actions of divergent and even conflicting groups at many administrative and governmental levels (Pressman and Wildavsky, 1973). Implementation can also be blocked by first-line professionals, who staff the operating core (Mintzberg, 1979) of organizations responsible for program implementation and exercise much control over delivery of the organizations' primary services (Lipsky, 1980; Prottas, 1979). Finally, uncontrollable external developments, such as electoral outcomes and economic trends, can divert program implementation and harm program outcomes.

For all these reasons, implementation and outcomes of national and regional polices and programs in the human services cannot be assured by the choice of substantively appropriate policies, precise planning and programming, or investment of substantial resources in the programs. In the final analysis, the implementation and outcomes of human-service programs depend overwhelmingly on *local* contexts, processes, and human-resource conditions. Chief among these are the capacity of local leaders and activists to mobilize support for programs, adapt the change program to local conditions, and direct implementation (Levin and Ferman, 1985; Pettigrew et al., 1992).

Despite its contributions, the administrative view of implementation suffers from serious limitations. In particular it fails to recognize that interest groups defend and promote their interests whenever opportunities arise during the policy process (Hill, 1981). Furthermore, the administrative frame creates an artificial distinction between interest group politics and implementation, which supposedly involves politically neutral forms of administrative behavior. An additional difficulty is that by narrowly defining the consequences of implementation in terms of the outcomes envisioned by advocates of national policies and programs, the administrative frame diverts attention from other important and often unintended consequences of national policies and programs.

The second frame views implementation as *bargaining* and coalition formation among divergent policy actors (Barrett & Fudge, 1981; Elmore, 1979–80; Rathwell, 1998; Walt, 1998). Bargaining occurs among national, regional, and local actors and between actors at different levels. For example, national representatives of an interest group like hospital physicians may negotiate with their local constituencies within hospitals, while also negotiating with representatives of other national organizations and state officials.

The bargaining perspective leads to consideration of a broad range of paths for policy implementations and a wide range of implementation outcomes. From the bargaining perspective, policymaking occurs during all policy phases, including implementation (Hill, 1995). Policy change results from negotiations, realignments, and power shifts among policy actors, as well as from changes in the actors' interests and goals (Light, 1991). These dynamic forces can produce emergent policies that were not originally envisioned by policymakers. Policy implementation can trigger political and structural realignments among actors, as well as being influenced by these alignments.

The bargaining frame provides a valuable complement to the administrative frame. By combining the two perspectives, investigators can forge a modified top-down method of analysis (Lazin, 1995; Sabatier, 1986). As they trace the fate of national policies, researchers using this method treat multiple national governmental actors, lower-level governmental actors, allied agencies, and independent interest groups as active political players in the policy process. Lower-level actors react to moves by higher-level bodies, proactively press for policy change, and enact policy through their own actions and daily practices.

The most influential actors in policy bargaining are groups and organizations that maintain horizontal ties within policy networks (Dowding, 1995; Marin & Mayntz, 1991). Collective actors in European health-policy networks typically include legislators, governmental administrators and ministers, elected officials and administrators at regional levels (e.g., state or county council), members of city governments, researchers and policy-analysts, insurers, patient groups, employers' and business associations, providers' associations (such as hospital associations), (non-medical) labor unions, and members of occupations working in and around medical organizations – physicians, nurses, other paramedical occupations, administrators, and service employees. Members of medical occupations are often represented by national unions and by professional associations.

Rather than focusing on formal properties of policy networks (e.g., Knoke et al., 1996), investigators using a bargaining frame look at exchanges *among* networks and relations *inside* them to see how negotiations take place among actors and how alliances shift over time (Dowding, 1995). Participants in networks are partially autonomous and vary greatly in their power (Pfeffer, 1981) and their involvement in policymaking (Cohen et al., 1972; Kenis and Schneider, 1991). Among the factors that affect actors' involvement are: the phase in the policy-making process; substantive issues at stake; administrative level (e.g., regional versus local); timing and visibility of policy negotiations; and the actors' degree of organization and mobilization (Jenkins, 1983).

Some policy networks develop into tightly integrated and enduring 'policy communities', that dominate policymaking within a sector for many years. Other 'issue networks', which are shorter-lived and less integrated, form around specific policy questions and practices (Marsh and Rhodes, 1992). When policy networks become well integrated and endure over time, their members can exercise decisive influence over policy development and block state approval or implementation of policies. For example, in Britain for several decades after World War II, elite physicians dominated the health policy network and resisted policy developments that ran counter to their conception of appropriate goals for public health care and the best ways to deliver care. Physician dominance of health policy prevailed until Prime Minister Thatcher's managerial revolution began to be felt in the late 1980s and early 1990s (Wistow, 1992).

Although the bargaining frame contributes greatly to our understanding of policy formation, it too suffers from weaknesses. Analysts employing a bargaining frame sometimes fail to acknowledge that policy agendas and actor interests are themselves products of negotiation and interpretation, not unchanging and unproblematic givens. Moreover, the bargaining perspective can lead analysts to treat policy actors' ideas and rhetoric as mere artifacts, or political tools. Yet rhetoric, in the sense of persuasive discourse (Nelson et al.,1987), and beliefs, help shape the ways that policy actors influence one another. An additional difficulty with the bargaining frame is that it ties the substance of policy directly to the interests and influence of particular collective actors. Yet policy sometimes endures despite changes in actors and their interests.

The third frame, which treats implementation as a process of *interpretation*, examines processes of social construction (Berger and Luckman, 1967) and negotiation of meanings (Silverman, 1970; Weick, 1979). This frame thus identifies important forces overlooked by the more instrumentally-oriented administrative and bargaining frames. The interpretive frame calls attention to the ways that policy actors, members of organizations affected by policies, and the public at large make sense and construct their understandings of key elements in policymaking. These elements include social, economic, and political conditions; actions by legislators and other policy actors; policy documents and other texts; and the actors' own interests, motives, and behavior (Grin & van de Graaf, 1996; Yanow, 1993). Many factors influence actors' interpretations of these elements in policymaking. Among the factors are prior cognitions, experience, and values; interactions (Morrione, 1985); political, social, organizational, and economic contexts (Walt, 1998); substantive policy information available to actors (Sabatier, 1991); and the actors' past experience with implementation of particular policies (Sabatier, 1986). Actor's interpretations, and even their public discourse, not only influence other actors, but also ultimately shape the way they view themselves and evaluate possibilities for action (Harrison, 1995b).

By emphasizing actors' understandings, priorities, and discourse, the interpretive perspective points to the possibility that policy implementation sometimes has symbolic consequences that do not show up immediately in quantitative

12

measures of policy outcomes or even in the observed behavior of system actors (Czarniawska-Joerges, 1989). Implementation processes can affect the ways that people talk and think about their tasks, organizations, and social institutions. Policy change and implementation can also sometimes produce lasting transformations in actors' beliefs, norms, and values.

From the interpretive perspective, national policy agendas, problems, issues, and solutions are socially constructed by politicians and governmental officials, other policy actors, the mass media, and the public at large (Edelman, 1988; Gamson, 1989; Gamson and Lasch, 1983). For example, policymakers only deal with conditions like hospital inefficiency, low quality care, and underfunding after these conditions have been *defined* as political problems requiring policy-related action. Policy solutions – like local control, user fees, competition among public providers, or privatization – often exist independently of particular issues and problems. When political interests, prevailing beliefs, and decision opportunities are supportive, policymakers define specific policy solutions as fitting particular problems (Kingdon, 1984; Cohen et al., 1972; Elmore and Sykes, 1992).

The interpretive frame places special emphasis on the rhetorical functions of public policies and programs (Edelman, 1964). When they present policies, programs, and administrative changes to others, advocates of such moves legitimate their proposals and enhance their own status. Change advocates thereby reinforce their reputations for being innovative, committed to vigorous action, and loyal to other widely shared values (Meyer and Rowan, 1977; Scott, 1995; Abrahamson, 1996). More generally programs of governmental reorganization symbolize and reinforce belief in the purposiveness of government, its commitment to progress, and the feasibility of effective leadership and meaningful administrative action (March and Olson, 1983). Rhetorical and symbolic activities like these are not mere epiphenomena. Instead, symbolic actions by governments and powerful managers can redefine peoples' expectations and assumptions about collective action and gradually lead to enduring change in beliefs, actions, and even social structures. For example, when government rhetoric leads public employees to expect to be rewarded on the basis of their performance, this rhetorical shift can produce *anticipatory* changes in employee behavior before changes in budgets and rewards take effect.

A further contribution of the interpretive frame is its focus on diversity in beliefs, perceptions, and values among policy actors (Barrett and Fudge, 1981; Spillane, 1998) and even among members of the same group or organization. Sometimes subgroups within organizations (Martin, 1992), occupational groups, networks of policy experts (Haas, 1992), and coalitions of actors (Sabatier, 1988), develop sets of shared assumptions and beliefs. These common interpretations sustain distinctive views about policy goals and priorities, external conditions requiring action, causal processes associated with policy intervention, and appropriate techniques for implementing policies. On the other hand, there is often ambiguity among groups of actors, or even within groups, about the meaning of shared symbols and events (Martin, 1992). This ambiguity can lead to frequent renegotiation about the nature of current challenges and problems and the appropriateness of possible courses of action.

Unfortunately, many important ideas and concepts within the interpretive frame remain at the level of insight, and the interpretive literature contains few clear guidelines for applying interpretive concepts in research. Moreover, only a small body of literature adopts an explicitly interpretive approach to policy research, and most of these studies concentrate on policy formulation more than on implementation. Some of the literature on interpretation within organizations poses an additional difficulty when it suggests that negotiation over meanings and norms is universal and continual. When applying the interpretive perspective to implementation, investigators need to bear in mind that powerful actors can often decisively shape collective definitions and define rules for inter-group relations (Bordieu, 1989, Lukes, 1974). Once such definitions are institutionalized, they become resistant to dissent and change.

The fourth frame looks at implementation in terms of the *institutional structuring* of political processes and organizational practices. This frame focuses on the ways that institutional rules, norms, and historical precedents create boundaries and constraints on the behavior of governmental and non-governmental actors. This approach, which is most closely identified with historical institutionalism (Immergut, 1998), emphasizes the ways that social and political institutions structure interactions among political stakeholders, favor some groups over others, and create categories for expressing group and collective concerns – such as equality and entitlements to medical care. Institutional arrangements shape both the substance and the processes of policymaking (Alford, 1975; Epsing-Andersen, 1994). Research informed by this frame shows how legal, political, economic, and organizational contexts define formal and informal rules for bargaining among policy actors, restrict alternative moves available to these actors, and shape shared beliefs and norms that guide policymaking (March and Olsen, 1989; Walt, 1998). This frame also draws attention to ways in which policy legacies (Weir and Skocpol, 1985), such as prior legislation and practice, can shape the formation and implementation of new policies (Heclo, 1974). From the vantage point of historical institutionalism, the most important consequences of policy implementation are the creation of precedents for future action and shifts in the institutional rules and arrangements governing collective action.

Institutional patterns help account for policy differences among nations. For example, there are important differences among Western countries in the power of the central government, the structure and power of the medical profession, and the constellation of relations between the state and the profession (Light, 1991; Wilsford, 1995; Tuohy, 1999b). These institutional variations help explain national differences in the development and implementation of health system reforms.

The fourth frame, with its focus on policy precedents and established institutions, provides a valuable supplement to the distinctive concerns of the other analytical frames. The institutional frame helps investigators explain differences among nations and national continuity in policymaking over many decades. In fact, institutional forces can be so strong that they sustain some policies in the face of the changes in key policy actors and the rise and fall of political coalitions (e.g., Gross and Harrison, 2001). A further contribution of the institutional frame is its ability to draw attention to ways that policymaking is embedded in social structures and norms that extend beyond the formal political system, like concepts and norms governing the professions (Abbott, 1988), and assumptions about entitlements to social welfare support (Epsing-Anderson, 1994). Unlike the bargaining and interpretive frames, the institutional frame provides limited help in explaining policy change, as opposed to continuity. Another difficulty involves lack of consensus and clear definitions of some of the central concepts and explanatory mechanisms underlying institutional analyses. Nonetheless, analysts have used the perspective to develop persuasive analyses of the ways that historical and institutional forces contribute to national differences in health policy (e.g., Dohler, 1991; Jacobs, 1998).

Combining Frames

In summary, as shown in Table 1.1, each frame focuses attention on different aspects of the policy implementation process and emphasizes different outcomes of implementation. Combining the perspectives embodied in each of the four frames can help researchers construct richer and more incisive explanations of policy implementation than those based on just one or two frames. Multi-frame analysis also contributes to explanations of historical change in policy and cross-national policy divergence. What is more, multiple frames illuminate possible consequences of policy implementation that might be overlooked if only one frame were used. In the long run, research based on a multi-frame approach holds promise for the development of integrative theories of policy implementation.

In the chapters that follow, I draw on all four frames, often without referring to them by name or making additional references to the literature from which the frames were derived. I start with a modified top-down approach, which combines administrative and bargaining perspectives. This synthetic approach assumes that national policy actors take the initiatives in formulating reform policies, but that other policy actors bargain with national actors and with one another at all stages of policymaking. This modified top-down view fits the analytical task at hand, because the reforms studied here typically found expression early in their development in official policy documents – like the British White Papers (e.g., Secretary of State for Health, 1989) – legislation, and formal governmental programs. The influence of the administrative frame will be evident in discussions of the ways in which reform policies changed direction or lost momentum as they moved down the administrative hierarchy. In Chapters 3, 5, and 7 the administrative frame will also guide comparisons between the declared objectives of policies and their actual outcomes. The bargaining frame, in turn, informs treatments in subsequent chapters of negotiations and coalitions among policy actors in each country – including state agencies and bodies. The bargaining frame also leads to assessments of the impact of implementation on the power of key policy actors and their alignments. In addition, drawing on the

Table 1.1   *Four frames for analyzing policy implementation*

	MAIN TOPICS	
FRAME	**Processes**	**Outcomes**
Administrative	Top-down transmission through hierarchy; coordination of local actors	Degree of implementation of original policies and programs; fit of outcomes to stated goals of national policymakers
Bargaining	Bargaining and coalition formation among key national, regional, local actors	Changes in actors' power; new coalitions and political arrangements
Interpretative	Sense-making and valuing by actors; discourse and rhetoric; divergence among actors' orientations (beliefs, norms, preferences, attitudes)	Effects of policies and programs on discourse, beliefs, norms, values
Institutional	Structuring of policymaking by social and political institutions; agenda and policy options affected by policy precedents	Policy precedents for future action; changes in institutions, especially those affecting implicit rules for policy formation and bargaining among actors

interpretive frame, the country studies consider the effects of policy actors' perceptions and beliefs about external conditions, reform programs, and the behavior of other actors. The interpretive approach also points to symbolic functions and outcomes of the reforms. Finally, the institutional frame illuminates ways that past policies and practices shaped recent health system reforms in each country and points to ways that social and political institutions constrained possibilities for action by the government and other policy players. The institutional frame also raises questions about whether policy implementation created new policy precedents and led to fundamental changes in the county's health system.

As a guide to this process of multiple framing, Figure 1.2 provides a graphic model of policy implementation as seen through all four analytic frames. Besides serving as a reference point for the analyses in the next six chapters, the model in Figure 1.2 may encourage applications of multi-frame analyses to other instances of policy implementation.

The *administrative* view becomes evident in the figure when we follow the entries on the outside sphere clockwise, starting from policy formulation. According to this view, governmental decisionmakers develop policies in response to conditions in and outside the health system; then they translate broad policies into programs for implementation. Implementation mainly centers on actions by governmental officials and health managers at the national, regional, and local levels. These actions are assumed to produce tangible

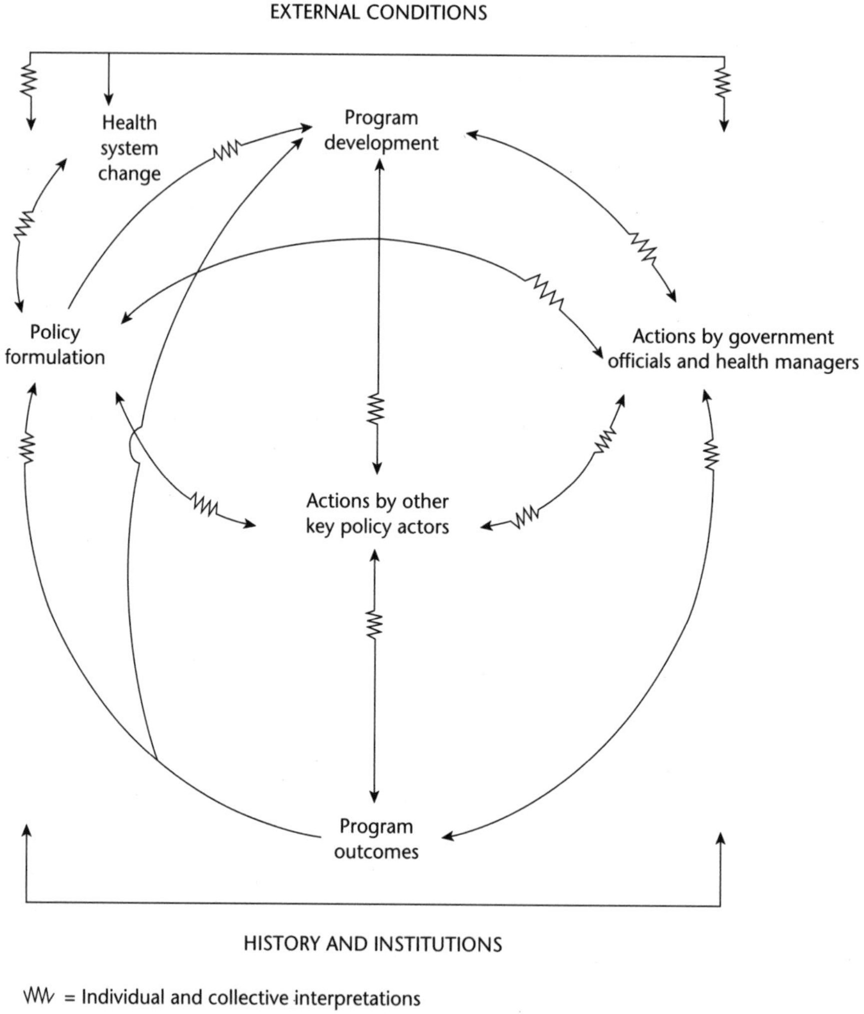

EXTERNAL CONDITIONS

Health
system
change

Program
development

Policy
formulation

Actions by government
officials and health managers

Actions by other
key policy actors

Program
outcomes

HISTORY AND INSTITUTIONS

WW = Individual and collective interpretations

Figure 1.2   *Model of policy implementation*

outcomes, which in turn provide feedback to policymakers about the success of
their original policies and the need for revisions of policies and programs. To
direct attention to *bargaining* among a wide range of policy actors, Figure 1.2
adds an entry for 'actions by other key policy actors' in the center of the sphere
and uses two directional arrows to show that these actors – as well as government officials and health managers – influence policy formulation and program
development and are influenced by them. For simplicity the figure does not
show the three or more levels of government and administration involved in the
implementation process or interactions between these levels. In practice, these

inter-level interactions affect administrative, bargaining, interpretive, and institutional aspects of implementation. Figure 1.2 portrays *interpretive processes* by showing that external developments and action vectors are 'filtered' by individual and collective interpretations. For example, the impact on policy formulation of external developments, such as consumerism and population ageing, depends on the ways that policymakers perceive, interpret, and evaluate these developments. The content of these cognitive and ideological filters can change during policy implementation, thereby adding additional sources of unpredictability and dynamism to implementation process. The *institutional* structuring of implementation – which interpenetrates the other elements shown in the model – is portrayed graphically as the historical and institutional 'foundation' for policy implementation and interactions among system actors.

The model in Figure 1.2 can also be used to call attention to the distinctive outcomes of implementation, as understood by each of the four theoretical perspectives (see Table 1.1). As the arrows directly linking program outcomes with policy formulation and program development suggest, the *administrative* view leads to evaluation of policies in terms of the fit between program outcomes and stated objectives for policies and programs. In contrast, the *bargaining* frame would focus attention on the center of the figure and on the entry in the 'two-o'clock' position – examining the consequences of all elements in the model for the power, alignments, and actions of policy actors. The *interpretive* frame would emphasize policy and program impacts on the various filters in the diagram – asking how policy implementation has changed the ways that people understand and judge external events, the actions of others, and their own actions. Finally, the *institutional* frame attends to ways in which policy implementation affect the historical foundations of future actions, by creating new precedents and altering institutions that shape policymaking.

So far this treatment of implementation research has been couched in terms that are general enough to apply to many types of policy. To make the discussion directly relevant to health system reforms, two additional components must be added: Examination of the crucial role played by general hospitals and their physicians in health system reforms and presentation of the fundamental institutional features of health care finance, delivery, and regulation in the countries under study. The discussion that follows addresses the first of these two topics.

Hospitals and Physicians – Key Players in Implementation

Much of the research reported in the chapters that follow concentrates on the ways that hospitals and their physicians influenced the implementation of reforms and were affected by them. This choice of research focus reflects the fundamental challenge that implementing change in hospitals poses for health system reform in Western nations.

There are four reasons why studies of market reforms in health care, along with examinations of other types of health system change, should pay special attention to hospitals and their physicians. First, the success of national programs for containing health costs ultimately depends on curtailing growth in hospital costs, which consume around 50% of public health expenditures in most industrialized nations.[11] Furthermore, in many countries, hospital costs have risen faster than the cost of living and the gross national product and have proved particularly resistant to control (Leichter, 1984; OECD, 2001). During the first period of European health reform, several countries, including Sweden and the UK, succeeded in curtailing their hospital costs by imposing tight budget ceilings and reducing hospital beds. But other nations, including the Netherlands and Germany, encountered greater difficulties in controlling overall hospital expenditures.

Second, during the first two decades after World War II, general hospitals and their physicians emerged as the dominant organizational and professional forces in health care in industrial nations. Many, and perhaps even most of the formative technological, professional, and organizational innovations in modern health care began in the hospital sector and then spread outward to ambulatory medicine. During this period, hospital physicians and their colleagues in schools of medicine diffused a powerful bio-medical paradigm that concentrated on technology-intensive diagnoses and intervention into disease. For years many health-policy analysts and agencies like the WHO contrasted this paradigm unfavorably to one that emphasizes prevention of disease, promotion of wellness, and attention to the inter-relations of social and health needs among subgroups and the entire population. Thus far, policymakers have made only limited progress toward supplanting the bio-medical intervention model.

Third, the market reforms of the early 1990s explicitly aimed at changing general hospitals and sought to redefine their role in the health system. Besides promoting hospital efficiency, these reforms sought to reduce hospital dominance. This change would come from strengthening the gatekeeping role of community physicians (Dixon et al., 1998), expanding community care, and relocating some forms of hospital care in the community. The reformers also tried to strengthen hospital quality assurance and make hospitals more responsive to the needs and preferences of patients.

Fourth, physicians, and particularly hospital specialists, can exercise substantial influence over the course of health system reforms, because they are powerful policy actors and hold major stakes in the content and implementation of the reforms (Harrison, 2002; Pettigrew et al., 1992; Saltman and de Roo, 1989; Shortell et al., 1990; Starr, 1982). As noted, in many countries, the physicians' national policy network influences the health-policy agenda, as well as affecting specific policy proposals. Elite hospital physicians also exercise much influence at the national and regional levels over areas like medical education, criteria for licensing of medical practitioners, and supervision and certification of health facilities. National physicians' organizations in some European countries have periodically waged highly visible campaigns to block or redirect policy initiatives and programs that seemed to threaten their members' earnings, employment opportunities, or professional autonomy. Physicians' organizations, along with unions representing other types of health professionals, often take an active role in national bargaining over wages and terms of employment. Since labor costs form a very large proportion of total health costs, the outcomes of these negotiations directly affect national health expenditures.

In Western Europe and Scandinavia there were few serious challenges to medical dominance until the 1980s. Despite recent inroads into their dominance, practicing physicians within hospitals and other European health care organizations continue to exercise much influence over care delivery (Freidson, 1985; Hafferty and McKinley, 1993). As they make decisions about diagnosis, referral, and treatment, physicians influence health care expenditures; direct the flow of patients to particular care sectors (hospitalization, outpatient clinics in hospitals, rehabilitation, community-based care, social care); determine the quality of doctor-patient interaction; and affect the clinical quality of care. Physicians also influence demand for health services by introducing new medical technologies, sub-specializations, and procedures, and by encouraging patients to take advantage of them. Much of the power that individual physicians and small groups of specialists wield through their medical activities comes from their control over information and their nearly exclusive knowledge about illnesses and their treatment. Because of their expertise and status, physicians also exercise influence over other health care professions and influence hospital strategies and policies (Young and Saltman, 1985).

To understand how physicians may influence reforms and be affected by them, it is useful to adopt a processual view of the professions. This approach treats the privileges enjoyed by an entire profession or an occupational subgroup as deriving from struggles to preserve and even expand their spheres of professional control (Abbott, 1988, Harrison, 1994; Starr, 1982) Changes in health care policies and programs, like those introduced by the reforms of the 1990s, provide opportunities for renegotiation of relations between occupations and between occupational subgroups (Harrison and Lieverdink, 2000; Light, 1988). These struggles occur at the level of the state, region, organization, and the work site (e.g., wards, clinics).

Control struggles affect four spheres of the physicians' professional control: [12]

- **Economic control** refers to professionals' ownership and control over the physical and technical facilities needed to produce their services. Economic control also refers to the degree to which professionals can set the terms of remuneration for their services and determine the conditions under which the services are delivered – for example, whom to treat and when.
- **Strategic control** concerns the ability to set or influence the goals, policies, and objectives of professional work.
- **Administrative control** deals with the ability to manage the organizational units in which professionals work and coordinate relations between units.
- **Operational control** (or clinical autonomy) entails the freedom to be guided by professional judgment and standards in professional practice, as opposed to being subject to controls by members of other occupations, such as management.

The European health system reforms of the 1990s threatened to intensify control by managers and government regulators over physicians in all four of these spheres – much as regulation, corporate control, and managed care practices had curtailed the power and control of physicians in the United States and to a lesser degree in Canada (Starr, 1982; Scott et al., 2000; Rappolt, 1997; Tuohy, 1999a). Hence, the reforms triggered struggles between physicians and managers and between physicians and government regulators. Less frequently, the reforms led to struggles and power realignments among sectors of the medical profession.

20

In summary, hospitals and physicians play key roles in implementation of reforms. They shape public perceptions and priorities for health care. Through their national bodies and representatives, physicians sometimes directly influence the formation of reform policies and programs. Physicians also indirectly influence government decisionmakers by leading officials to avoid steps that might generate conflict between the state and physicians' organizations. Once reforms are launched, physicians and hospital managers bargain actively over their implementation.

Research Questions

We have now examined the theoretical and research literature that helped guide the research reported in the next seven chapters. Here, in summary, are the main questions addressed in the chapters that follow:

1. **What forces affected implementation of market reforms?** This question derives from the broader study of forces affecting implementation of programs for changing complex systems.[13] In response to this research question, Chapters 2, 4, and 6 examine the historical and institutional background to the market reforms in the UK, Sweden, and the Netherlands. The chapters then trace interactions among policy actors and interpretations by them that affected the course of policy implementation. Also explored are contextual forces, like changes in the economy and developments in medical technology.

2. **What were the main outcomes of the market reforms?** To answer this question, Chapters 3, 5, and 7 examine administrative, bargaining, interpretive, and institutional outcomes of the main reform programs.

3. **Did the rapid rise and decline of political support for market reforms in health care reflect the dynamics of policy fashion?** This question arose from the observation that policymakers adopted market-reform policies quickly and uncritically. Decisionmakers and their constituencies soon became disenchanted with market reforms, once the proposed changes proved hard to implement. Many policies that aim at public-sector change travel a similar path of uncritical adoption, followed quickly by disillusion and growing enthusiasm for alternative policies. To account for this type of policy life cycle, Chapter 8 presents a model of policy fashion dynamics.

RESEARCH LOGIC AND METHODS

Cross-national comparisons in health policy and other policy areas can illuminate common tendencies among nations, suggest opportunities for improvement, point to promising change strategies and techniques, and raise issues deserving further study or planning. Still, unselective transplanting of policies, programs, and techniques from one country to another is very risky. The danger of overlooking differences in national history, culture, politics, economics, and social institutions is particularly great when comparative studies concentrate attention on just a few health system features or change mechanisms – such as competition among care providers or hospital payment systems (Glaser, 1987; Kimberly, Pouvourville et al., 1993). Divergences in national institutions, local political and economic conditions, and historic differences in health systems make it unlikely that broad policies or even specific innovations will be implemented in similar ways across nations and will have similar consequences. Comparisons between countries are more likely to be helpful to policymakers when the comparisons cover countries with important institutional similarities to the policymakers' own country.

The health systems of the three countries examined in this book share some common institutional and ideological traits with health systems in many other advanced industrial democracies. The UK, Sweden, and the Netherlands all developed social democratic institutions in health and welfare during the first few decades after World War II. Although there have been many changes in their health systems since then, all three continue to fund health services mainly from taxes or contributions to government-regulated insurance (see Table 1.2 on page 26). Despite growing inequalities in access to care, politicians and the public in all three countries still give high priority to preserving solidarity by assuring provision of universal care, payment according to ability, and equal access to care.

These broad similarities among European health institutions and values become clear when they are contrasted to those of the United States, where the national government only insures care for the indigent, the aged, and veterans. As a result, reliance on private funding is much greater than in most industrial nations. Fifty-nine percent of all health care expenditures in the United States came from private sources in 1987, and 55.5% did so in 1999; the OECD averages for these years were 28.2% and 25.8%. Rather than being defined as a social good, health care in the United States is 'essentially a private consumption good of which low-income families might be accorded a basic ration, but whose availability and quality should be allowed to vary with family income' (Reinhardt, 1994, p. 23). Instead of solidarity, the prevailing principles of the American health market are individualism, competition, and commercialism.

There are, of course, major differences between the health systems and policies of the UK, Sweden, and the Netherlands, and there are divergences between these countries and other advanced industrial nations. Such distinctive national features must be considered carefully when making cross-national generalizations or drawing policy implications from the practices of each country. To minimize the risk of overlooking critical national conditions, I first examined implementation of health system reforms within each country.[14] Only after completing in-depth country studies did I attempt to find common and contrasting tendencies among nations, like those presented in Chapter 8. To use a well-known distinction in comparative studies (Kohn, 1987), I first treated each country as an *object* of study and only treated it as a *context* for health system reform once the major features of the national systems were well understood.

The country studies reported here relied on several different data sources (see Appendix B). Chief among these were 104 semi-structured interviews that I conducted with physicians and nurses in hospitals and community care settings, hospital managers, managers in insurance companies and public purchasing bodies, representatives of professional associations and unions, researchers, and consultants. Interviews were clustered so as to provide details on particular hospitals, clinics, and purchasing bodies, as well as surveying broad developments. Although not representative of the full range or health system actors and agencies in each country, these interviews often provide insights into processes that are not well documented in the published research literature. In addition, the interviews add important details unavailable in published sources and richly illustrate many situations and conditions mentioned in the literature. I also analyzed documentary material and available statistical data.

Statistical data on health systems need to be used with caution, since coding categories are not always comparable between countries or across time within the same country. Furthermore, some crucial measures – like the official measure of hospital activity in the UK – suffer serious limitations of validity (see Chapter 3). An even greater difficulty is that there are no measures of the quality of care before and after the reforms in the OECD data for the 1990s or in other sources of national statistics.[15] Lack of data on patient characteristics (e.g., case mix) also makes performance data hard to interpret. Available statistics on hospital performance, for example, typically provide undifferentiated measures of volume – such as admissions, discharges, or consultations. These measures are then divided by expenditures or other appropriate denominators to produce 'efficiency' measures. Without quality and case-mix data, findings of gains in provider productivity are hard to interpret. Only if the quality of care is stable or is improving can production improvements legitimately be considered evidence of improved organizational efficiency.

Even well documented studies within a single country face serious challenges to valid inferences about macro-system and organizational processes and outcomes. At the same time that the medical systems underwent government-initiated reforms, they faced three major contextual and technological changes. First, gradual ageing of the population brought older and sicker people to hospitals and thereby posed new medical challenges and raised hospital costs. Second, new illnesses like AIDS, and medical problems like substance abuse, shifted patterns of illness within the population. These changes required restructuring of health services, redirection of existing resources, and further expenditures (Saltman and Figueras, 1997). Third, there were rapid developments in medical technologies (U.S. Congress, 1995). Many new medications and treatments raised costs, even as they opened up new treatment opportunities; other new technologies – like those supporting minimally invasive surgery and diagnosis – facilitated cost reductions through shifts from hospitalization to day surgery.

It is also hard to determine how specific government moves affected a health system, because the governments took divergent steps at almost the same time.

Over a very short period of time, each government studied introduced across-the-board constraints on health budgets, added funding to targeted programs and providers, made many regulatory changes, and created opportunities and incentives for market behavior. In an effort to disentangle the effects of such a wide spectrum of contextual, technological, and governmental forces, I compared trends in variables like hospital production over time and also made comparisons among organizations, municipalities, or nations. For example, trends in Stockholm, which implemented distinctive reform programs, were compared to developments in other parts of Sweden. In addition, I looked for qualitative evidence of causal linkages in interviews and documents. For example, hospital doctors reported during interviews that managers translated budget pressures into pressures on the doctors to reduce costs. Similarly in Sweden, nurses in general hospitals explained how their activities changed in the wake of a program that encouraged rapid transfer of elderly patients to municipal geriatric care.

23

MAIN FEATURES OF NATIONAL HEALTH CARE SYSTEMS IN THE UK, SWEDEN, AND THE NETHERLANDS

The reforms examined in depth in this book can best be understood when they are viewed against the backdrop of major institutional features of health finance, delivery, and regulation in each country prior to the market reorganizations.[16] Structures for handling health finance and delivery can be distinguished in terms of the ownership and goals of care delivery organizations (public; private, not-for-profit; and for-profit); the prevailing mix of public and private financing of care; and methods for paying providers (OECD, 1992). Regulatory systems are broadly distinguished by the mix of regulation through the market, hierarchical supervision, and professional self-regulation (Tuohy, 1999b).

Table 1.2 summarizes each health system's main features in 1987, on the eve of the market reforms.[17]

The UK finances care mainly through national tax revenues. Separate National Health Services (NHS) bureaucracies, in each of the states that make up the UK, supervise the state-owned hospitals, whose health professionals are NHS employees. Private practice within the NHS has existed since its founding (Mays and Keen, 1998), but the proportion of private funding within total health expenditure in the UK (15% in 1987) falls well below the OECD average (28%, n=24). Primary care physicians in the UK are self-employed entrepreneurs, who work under a national contract. Until 1990 they were supervised and paid by a separate national agency. Hospital specialists, although salaried, can also maintain private practices and hospitalize patients in private beds within state hospitals. Partly in response to tight NHS funding, expenditures for private, for-profit care grew rapidly during the 1980s (OECD, 1992, p. 116). In 1989 around 13% of the population had some form of private health insurance (Ham, 1992, p. 47).

24

Table 1.2   *Major health system features before the market reforms*

	Finance	Delivery	Regulation
United Kingdom	General taxation by national government; 15% from private sources[1]	*Hospitals*: public, salaried physicians & nurses; some private physicians (paid fee for service), some private beds in state & private hospitals *Primary care*: self-employed physicians own clinics & contract with national government (mix of capitation, fixed pay, fee for service)	Department of Health oversees National Health Service (NHS); NHS hierarchy oversees districts, which operate most general hospitals; separate government agency pays & supervises general practitioners. Managerial supervision of physicians grows in the 1980s, but they still retain much autonomy
Sweden	General taxation, mainly by county councils; 10% from private sources*	*Hospitals*: public, salaried physicians & nurses *Primary care*: public clinics with salaried staff. Patients do not choose physician	National regulation of county tax rates and fees to providers; national negotiation of staff pay; county operation of hospitals; municipal operation of clinics. Physicians retain autonomy over clinical activities, subject to budget constraints
Netherlands	Social insurance (income-related premium) for 2/3 of population; private for-profit insurance (risk-related premium) for wealthiest 1/3 of population; all covered by national exceptional medical insurance (income-based premium); 31% from private sources*	*Hospitals*: private, not-for-profit; most physicians are independent practitioners with rights to practice in a hospital, paid fee for service based on national fee scales *Primary care*: Self-employed physicians receive capitation for sickness fund patients and fee for service for privately insured; both subject to national regulation	Quasi-governmental bodies negotiate fees for hospitals, physicians, & other providers contracting with social insurance; Ministry of Health supervises providers & insurers. Ambulatory physicians subject to budget constraints; all physicians retain autonomy over practice

[1] Percent (rounded) in 1987 of total health expenditures coming from out-of-pocket payments, private insurance premiums, contributions by charities, health care provided by employer (OECD, 2001).

Sweden funds health care mainly through taxation and uses mostly public providers. However, until the mid-1990s, 23 county councils and three municipalities, rather than the national government, were responsible for raising most of the taxes and funding and delivering most care.[18] There was growth in the private sector during the 1980s, but private providers provided a small proportion of all care and were concentrated in the Stockholm area (Interviews, Rosenthal, 1992).

In contrast to the state-centered systems of Britain and Sweden, the health system in the Netherlands rests on corporatist institutions (Schut, 1995) and a combination of social and private insurance. The corporatist tradition expects organizations representing divergent parts of the society to play a formal role in mediating between citizens and government. Corporatism in the health sector led to reliance on private insurers and providers and representation in regulatory agencies of employers, health professions, providers, and insurers. Around two thirds of the Dutch population are covered by compulsory, statutory insurance. Income-related premiums are deducted from salaries and allocated on a capitation basis to not-for-profit sickness funds, which also receive government subsidies.[19] The other third of the population, who earn above a specified income level, purchase insurance policies from private, mostly for-profit firms, and pay risk-related premiums. These premiums include solidarity contributions to cover high-risk patients insured by the state. Catastrophic and long-term risks of the entire population are directly covered by a separate tax-supported, national insurance program. The fees paid to insurers and those paid by insurers to providers are negotiated in a series of quasi-governmental bodies in which insurers, providers, and government officials are represented. Charitable agencies own and run most of the hospitals in the Netherlands, while a smaller number are run by universities and municipalities. Unlike Sweden or the UK, most of Holland's hospital physicians are independent practitioners, who practice in a specialty group within a particular hospital. Until the mid-1990s these hospital specialists were directly reimbursed by insurers on a fee-for-service basis.

Some of the important differences among the countries in health expenditures, resource levels and resource utilization appear in Figure 1.1 on page 4 and Table 1.3 below. As Figure 1.1 shows, all of the countries studied, like Europe as a whole, experienced a rapid rise in health spending during the 1970s. During the 1980s the UK and Sweden succeeded in containing their expenditure growth, in contrast to Europe as a whole and to the United States.[20] The Netherlands contained expenditures in the first half of the 1980s but was unable to do so during the second half.[21] All three of the countries in this study made major reductions in their acute and non-acute hospital beds during the 1980s. Between 1980 and 1989, 20% of acute beds were eliminated in the UK, 15.7% in Sweden, and 15.4% in the Netherlands. Reduction of non-acute beds went even deeper. In the UK the reduction in public beds was accompanied by steep growth in private beds for geriatric patients and the mentally ill (Henscher and Edwards, 1999). During the 1990s health expenditures rose in the UK and the Netherlands, but expenditures declined somewhat in Sweden after 1994.[22]

Table 1.3   *Health expenditures, resources, and utilization, 1987*[1]

	UK	Sweden	Netherlands	OECD[2]	USA
Expenditures					
Total as % GDP	6.0	8.5	8.1	7.2	10.4
Per capita in $, PPP[3]	785	1271	1087	976	2012
Resources					
Practicing physicians/1000	1.4	2.8	2.4	2.4	2.3
Acute beds/1000	3.0	4.4	4.6	5.1	4.0
Utilization					
Acute, in-patient admissions/yr/1000	148[4]	170	104.1	151.7	130.6
Physician consultations per capita[5]	6.6	2.7	5.5	6.5	5.4
Avg. length of stay, acute hospitals	7.4	7.1	12.1	9.5	7.2

[1]Source: OECD (2001).
[2]The number of countries on which the OECD averages are based varies from 22 to 25.
[3]Purchasing power parities, see Chapter 1, footnote 24.
[4]Includes day patients.
[5]Ambulatory visits; excludes private visits for UK, excludes maternal and child care for Sweden and Netherlands.

The data in Table 1.3 refer to 1987, just before the start of the market reforms. Appendix C provides comparative data from the late 1990s. The table also shows how the countries under study compared to the OECD group of industrialized nations and the United States, which was sometimes cited as a model of efficiency in health care management.[23]

The spending patterns shown in Figure 1.1. and in Table 1.3 for the UK reflect it's long tradition of devoting a smaller proportion of its national resources to health care than most industrial nations.[24] As a result, in the UK the supply of health personnel and facilities per capita has long lagged behind that available in more munificent health systems of Northern Europe and Scandinavia, and even behind averages for the OECD as a whole.[25]

During the early 1980s Sweden and the Netherlands greatly exceeded European and OECD average expenditure levels and provided generous health resources to their citizens. The fact that both countries had fewer beds per capita in 1987 than the OECD average mainly reflects budgetary restraints imposed during the 1980s.

The data on health services utilization in the table also reflect important national differences. All three countries had reduced length of hospital stay in the 1980s, but the Netherlands had made far less progress in this direction than other OECD nations. The comparatively low level of consultations with physicians in Swedish ambulatory care probably reflects the practice of referring patients in primary care clinics to nurses and other paramedical personnel. Variations in hospital admission rates reflect many factors, including referral policies, availability of community-based services, and differences in the age distribution of the populations. In 1987, 17.7% of Sweden's population and 15.5%

of UK residents were over 65. In contrast, the Netherlands had a much younger population. With 12.4% of its population over 65, it was close to the OECD average (12.3%).

27

PLAN OF THE BOOK

This chapter has presented the theoretical and empirical background for the in-depth studies that follow. Chapters 2, 4, and 6 address the first research question by analyzing forces shaping the implementation of market reforms. Chapters 3, 5, and 7 respond to the second research question concerning the outcomes of market reforms. These chapters also describe policy developments that followed the market reforms. To facilitate comparisons among countries, the chapters use similar formats. Chapter 8 summarizes findings on the outcomes of the reforms and reflects on their policy implications. In response to the third research question, market reforms are analyzed as policy fashions. This chapter also proposes a decentralized, learning-focused approach to policy implementation, which offers an alternative to both market reform and centralized restructuring of health systems.

NOTES

1 In the United States market approaches were developed and discussed widely during the 1970s. A national bill in 1973 encouraged formation of health maintenance organizations (HMOs), but only in the early 1980s did important federal and state legislation and precedent-setting legal decisions create the basis for managed competition among HMOs. Thereafter, market approaches became an important force in health care (Scott et al., 2000).

2 Throughout this book, the term Europe will be used to include Scandinavia and the United Kingdom.

3 For readability, I usually substitute the term 'market' for the term 'quasi-market', although the latter is technically more precise.

4 The growth between 1960 and 1970 was calculated for the 16 countries for which data are available in both years. Comparisons like this one, which appear throughout this book, give the percentage of growth or decline over the stated period, *not* the numerical increment in the annual figures. Unless indicated otherwise, all statistical data in this book are derived from the database of the Organization for Economic Cooperation and Development (OECD, 2001).

5 Figure 1.1 and the percentages reported for periods between 1970 and 1999 are based on 23 countries reporting data for the entire period, except that data for Australia and Denmark are missing for the year 1970, and those for the Netherlands that are missing for 1971 and 1972. Australia was included in the 1970 OECD average by using the mid-point between its reported figures for 1969 and 1971. The 1999 data are from OECD (2002).

6 Recent research by Wennberg and his colleagues (2002) provides evidence that the supply of hospital services and physicians drives demand for technology-intensive services, with no evident improvement in quality (see also Kolata, 2002).

7 Countries in Central and Eastern Europe and in the former Soviet Union pursued a variety of routes to reform including privatization and quasi-market reform. See Saltman and Figueras (1997).

8 Throughout this book the term *policy* refers inclusively to statements of political intention and direction and more concrete laws, plans, and programs for action (see Mayntz, 1979). Policies thus encompass *goals*, like containing costs or enhancing equality of access to services; *strategies*, such as fostering competition among providers; and *programs* which are specific actions intended to further policy objectives, for example a funding program designed to help primary-care clinics provide services that were previously available mainly in hospitals.

9 Models contribute to empirical analysis and theory development by focusing on a limited set of system or organizational features and emphasizing particularly important relations among them. Since models are largely heuristic, they can be retained, modified, or abandoned in keeping with their usefulness, rather than being subject to direct tests of validity.

10 For analytical clarity, I stress the distinctive contributions of each theoretical frame, not areas of overlap and complimentarity among them. Examples of overlapping ideas include emphasis on the state and its subcomponents as key policy actors. This view is held both by scholars who stress the institutional structuring of policy formation (e.g., Weir and Skopcol, 1985) and many analysts who use a bargaining frame. There is also overlap between the historical-interpretive perspective used by social constructionists (e.g., Berger and Luckman, 1967) and some neo-institutional theories of organizations (e.g., Scott, 1995).

11 In 1997, among 20 OECD nations for which data were available, the average proportion of public health expenditures devoted to inpatient care was 49.8%. Countries spending less than 45% were the UK (31.2%), Japan, Germany, the Czech Republic, Turkey, and Luxembourg.

12 The concept of control encompasses the idea of professional jurisdiction (Abbott, 1988) and that of autonomy, which often only refers to control over practice (e.g., Hall, 1968). See Harrison (1994) for comparisons between the categories in the typology of control and those used by other authors. In the chapters that follow the terms operational control, clinical control, and clinical autonomy are used interchangeably.

13 For comparative discussions see Walt (1998), Rathwell (1998), and Harrison (1999).

14 In-depth examination of health system reform in Germany (Harrison, 1995a; Harrison, 2002) and Israel (Gross and Harrison, 2001; Harrison, and Shalom, 2002) also sharpened my view of common and distinctive features of Dutch, Swedish, and British health policy.

15 Quality of care is notoriously difficult to measure. It is multi-dimensional (Banta, 2000/2001), and correlations between its divergent dimensions are often low or even negative.

16 For comparisons among health systems and reforms in many countries, consult the publications and website of the WHO, European Observatory on Health Care Systems (http://www.who.dk/observatory); Saltman and Figueras (1997); and publications of the OECD (e.g., OECD, 1992, 1994).

17 In the discussion that follows, the present tense refers to features that still characterize these countries, while the past tense refers to features that changed after 1987.

18 The three cities that operated like county councils until the mid-1990s are grouped together with the 23 county councils in the remainder of this book. During the mid-1990s mergers took place among county councils in Western *Sweden*, and two regions were created. By the end of the 1990s health finance and administration were handled by 18 county councils, two new regions, and Stockholm County Council.

19 In 1987, 62% of the population were covered by compulsory insurance, another 6% had compulsory public employees' insurance, and 32% held private insurance (OECD, 1992).

20 Some of the drop shown for Sweden's health expenditures from 1980 to 1990 reflected the fact that after 1985 care for the mentally retarded was no longer classified as health expenditure (Gertham and Jonsson, 1994).

21 Expenditures rose from 7.3% of GDP in 1985 to eight per cent in 1990 (OECD, 2002).

22 In the early 1990s OECD reporting did not reflect the fact that expenditures for geriatric care disappeared from Sweden's health accounts in 1992 when responsibility for home care and nursing homes shifted from the counties to the municipalities in 1992 (see Chapter 3). The 2001 and 2002 OECD data sets correct for this artifact. There are other, smaller artifacts scattered throughout the OECD data, so they should be interpreted with caution.

23 Less frequently acknowledged by commentators who were impressed by efficiency in American health care was the fact that the United States spends far more on health than other industrial nations but falls below the OECD averages on important health indicators (Anderson and Hussey 2001). One explanation for this apparent paradox is that only 83% of Americans have any kind of health insurance, and coverage is often less than comprehensive.

24 Table 1.3 uses Purchasing Power Parities (PPPs) (see www.OECD.org/std/ppp). These are currency conversion rates that eliminate the differences in price levels between countries in the process of conversion. If the UK's expenditures were calculated using conventional exchange rates, the expenditure gap between Britain and the United States would appear even larger.

25 The UK has had a lower ratio of physicians to people since 1960, the earliest year reported by the OECD. By the mid 1970s the UK had fallen below the OECD average for beds and physicians per person.

2

Market Reforms in the United Kingdom

The market reforms of Britain's National Health System (NHS) were among the most ambitious and influential reorganizations of national health systems undertaken by Western governments during the last few decades. By introducing contracting between public purchasers of health care and health-service providers, these reforms created possibilities for public providers to compete on price and quality. The government also effectively privatized portions of the health services and related social services. At the same time, the central Government tightened fiscal and operational control over hospitals and public purchasers and strengthened managerial control over physicians and nurses.

This chapter examines the background and implementation of these reforms, with special emphasis on two processes that were crucial to the formation of a quasi-market for health services in the United Kingdom: *contracting* by public purchasers and *management* of acute hospitals. The chapter starts by reviewing the original reform policies and programs, along with subsequent policy initiatives. Then, drawing on administrative, bargaining, and interpretive perspectives on implementation, it examines why organizational processes that were crucial to market-like exchange and management failed to develop as anticipated. Chapter 3 examines outcomes of the market reforms in terms of all four of the implementation frames. There follows an assessment of the 'New NHS' policies introduced by the Labour Government after 1997.

BACKGROUND

From its inception in 1948 until the 1980s, the NHS enjoyed a solid reputation among its citizens and health-systems analysts for providing all residents with publicly funded, comprehensive health services, which were free at point of delivery. What is more, by enforcing tight global budget ceilings on the NHS-owned hospitals, the government kept total health expenditures below those of most other European nations (Leichter, 1989; OECD, 1992).

During the 1980s the NHS experienced serious fiscal difficulties and became the target of sharp criticism (Klein, 1989). As the Conservative government enforced tight budgets and hospital cutbacks, Conservative politicians and many other commentators and analysts attacked the NHS for being inefficient, inequitable, and ineffective. NHS administrators, members of the political opposition in Parliament, and many health-policy researchers countered that most of the NHS' weaknesses derived from 'resource starvation' (Webster, 1993, p. 16).

In the spirit of the New Public Management, Conservative politicians and many other commentators and analysts traced the NHS' weaknesses to its lack of effective performance assessment and its failure to make NHS managers and health professionals accountable for costs, efficiency, and quality of services (Day and Klein, 1989). In keeping with this view, in the mid-1980s, the government introduced the General Management reforms, which sought to run the NHS more like a traditional business. Rather than deriving from systematic planning and consultation among policy actors, the General Management reforms, like the Internal Market Reforms that followed them, began with a set of simple, yet persuasive, 'bright ideas' that gradually became guiding principles of government policy (Harrison and Wood, 1999).[1] The cumulative effect of General Management and other reforms of the 1980s period was tighter governmental control over public services, municipal government, and the self-regulating professions (Jenkins, 1995; Brazier et al., 1993).[2] In its search for a way to assure the accountability of lower-level NHS agencies, the government set up a chain of administrative command that linked the Department of Health (DOH) to the national, regional, district, and unit (e.g., hospital) levels. To promote efficiency and cost containment, managers at all levels were instructed to rationalize decision processes (Packwood et al., 1991) and were held accountable for performance, which was to be assessed through reviews of measurable outputs. Full-time managers replaced the interdisciplinary teams that had previously run hospitals through 'consensus management'.

A growing number of hospitals also reorganized their departments as clinical directorates, which were to provide the crucial link between the hospital's top managers and its clinicians (Harrison and Pollitt, 1994; Packwood et al., 1991; Fitzgerald and Dufour, 1997). Directorates are responsible for managing the budget and non-clinical activities within a specialty or division, as well as overseeing clinical work. The directorate is run by a chief physician, a head nurse, and a business manager. They report directly to the hospital management or participate in hospital boards.

Hospital productivity rose dramatically during the 1980s, but these productivity improvements appear to have owed more to the simple fact that hospital staffs had to provide more services with fewer resources than to adoption of new, rational decision techniques. In fact, the General Management reforms did not lead to fundamental change in the prevailing occupational and organizational cultures of the hospitals. Managers continued to make decisions opportunistically and concentrated on balancing budgets. Hospital clinicians accepted the growing budgetary constraints, but the physicians carefully guarded their autonomy and continued to put traditional medical priorities before managerial ones (Harrison et al., 1992; Flynn, 1992).

32

Growth in the number of non-medical managers and in managerial influence were among the most significant changes introduced by General Management. This shift was accompanied by diffusion of concepts of operational efficiency and financial accountability from the world of business (Loveridge, 1992). Moreover, the government gradually ended its traditional pattern of 'policy-making by consent' (Godt, 1987), in which it consulted closely with physicians' organizations and other major stakeholders before initiating changes in health policy (Dohler, 1991; Ham, 1992).

The General Management reforms thus led to important structural, political, and interpretive changes within the NHS and laid the foundations for the formulation and implementation of the more radical, market reforms a few years later. Yet the short-run attainments of the reforms were few: Neither General Management, nor the government's broader drive for efficiency and cost-containment in the health system, helped bridge the growing gap between public demand for NHS services and the funds available to provide services. Furthermore, the cuts in hospital budgets seemed to hurt the quality of their services. Thus the reforms failed to diffuse growing criticism of the government's handling of NHS funding. By the late 1980s, the NHS faced a crisis of funding and public confidence, which weakened electoral support for the government.

In response, Prime Minister Thatcher and her senior ministers considered, but ultimately rejected, options for financial reorganization of the NHS. The government's decision reflected the wide popularity of the existing NHS among voters, opposition to financial or organizational change by the British Medical Association (BMA), and the higher costs of alternative systems of health-care finance (Butler, J. 1994; Klein, 1989).

LAUNCHING THE INTERNAL MARKET REFORMS

Instead of financial reorganization, the government proposed yet another structural reform, while also promising to boost NHS funding. The guiding thesis of the new reforms was that competition among NHS hospitals and among primary-care providers would unleash powerful incentives to use resources efficiently and improve the quality of care. This idea, which fit with the views of the New Public Management movement, was championed by neo-liberal economists, including three pro-market policy institutes (see Giamo and Manow, 1997) and Professor Alan Enthoven (1985) from the United States. Thus the 1989 White Paper, *Working for Patients*, announced the creation of an 'internal market' for health care. Besides boosting efficiency and quality, the reform was expected to insure greater representation and empowerment of patients within the organizations responsible for using public funds to purchase, or commission, care.

The reform proposals met with intense opposition by the BMA, the Labour opposition, and some portions of the general public. Nonetheless, Parliament quickly enacted the reforms into law. The 1990 NHS and Community Care Act took effect in 1991 for the hospital sector and in 1993 covered social care within the community – for example ambulatory care for chronically ill, retarded, and mentally ill patients. A new contract for general practitioners (GPs), who are self-employed, took effect in 1990.

The reform program contained four core elements: (1) separation of public pur-chasers and providers of hospital services; (2) reorganization of hospitals, ambu-lance services, and providers of community social care as semi-autonomous trusts; (3) strengthening the role of the GP in health-care delivery and creating an arrange-ment whereby GPs could become fundholders, acting as knowledgeable purchasers of health services for their patients; and (4) integrating health service sectors.

Despite the prevailing terminology, the 1990 NHS and Community Care Act provided for competition between public providers, which were state-owned or controlled, and private ones, as well as creating an 'internal market' among public providers. Under this act, public providers would continue to provide most medical care, and relations between purchasers and providers would be highly regulated by the DOH. In consequence, the reforms could best be characterized as creating a 'quasi-market' (Le Grand and Bartlett, 1993) for hospital care, and some other health services, rather than an open and highly competitive market.

To create market-like conditions within the NHS, the 1990 law relieved District Health Authorities of their responsibilities for direct administration of local hospitals, and made the new Health Authorities (HAs) responsible for assessing the health needs of their residents, setting priorities, and contracting for the best available services from hospitals and other public and private providers. In a similar fashion, the 1990 Act instructed local municipal authorities to contract for community-based services and residential care for the aged, retarded, and men-tally ill (Muijen and Ford, 1996; Wistow, 1997). The government steered district hospitals, ambulance services, and social care agencies toward reorganization as trusts. While owned by the government, trusts were allowed to make local agree-ments about pay and working conditions with their employees, including physi-cians. The trusts were expected to balance their expenses against revenues from care contracts and were made financially and operationally accountable to the government through the newly created NHS Management Executive Outposts.

Unlike the purchaser-provider split, the fundholding experiment encouraged GPs to become active purchasers of hospital care while continuing to provide most primary care – much as health maintenance organizations do in the United States. GPs who registered as fundholders thus received budgetary and adminis-trative responsibility for portions of their patients' ambulatory and elective hospital care. By choosing care providers and negotiating contracts with them, GP fundholders were expected to represent their patients' interests in the health-care market and form a countervailing force to the hospitals. Although fund-holders were not paid directly for managing the patients' care budgets, they were allowed to transfer savings between budget headings and use these savings to extend the range of services offered to patients within primary care clinics. The new GP contract aimed at further strengthening the role of health promotion within primary care by providing incentives for GPs to carry out specific forms of preventive care and minor surgery (Farmer, 1993; Silcock and Ratcliffe, 1996).

   To enhance integration among care sectors, in 1993 the DOH gave GP fund-holders budgets to pay for community health services, including nursing and health visitors, mental health care, and dietetics, but excluding midwifery and terminal care (Glennerster et al., 1994). To further enhance sectoral integration, in 1996 the government put the agency responsible for financing and supervising GPs under the Regional Health Authorities, which also supervised the HAs. The government also instructed the HAs to consult with GPs to find out which hospital and community services the GPs – and presumably their patients – preferred.

To improve resource use, provide a realistic basis for contracting and competition, and enhance the quality of care, the reformers envisioned providing all hospitals with new capacities and technologies for monitoring and controlling costs, procedures, and outcomes. Furthermore, contracts with hospital physicians were to contain clear job descriptions, and clinical audits were to render hospital consultants more accountable to local managers. To enhance and equalize the quality of hospital care, the government enacted a Patient's Charter in 1991. The Charter expounded a set of rights to which all patients were entitled – including detailed information about local health services and rights to have complaints investigated. The Charter also set performance standards for hospitals. The most closely monitored and widely publicized standard called for admission to hospital within two years of referral by a physician (McIver and Martin, 1996).

Between 1989 and the fall of the Conservative Party in 1997, much of the government's policy for the NHS followed the course originally charted by *Working for Patients*. Cabinet members and powerful figures within the DOH continued to celebrate the ability of the internal market reforms to enhance the efficiency and quality of NHS services. They prodded NHS staff to implement purchaser-provider contracting, extend and deepen GP fundholding, and strengthen service quality – with the main emphasis on reducing waiting times for surgery and achieving a few objectives in the Patient's Charters of 1991 and 1995. The national government also sought to enhance competition between public and private providers of community health services by requiring local social service departments to use 85% of a major national grant for community social services to purchase care from private or independent agencies.[3] In like manner, the government called on trusts to weigh the costs of purchasing services in the private market, instead of producing them ('The making ...', 1995). The Private Finance Initiative effectively precluded public financing of hospital construction. As a result, hospitals had to pay for the higher costs of private finance by reducing operating costs or selling off assets (Gaffney et al., 1999a, 1999b).

FURTHER POLICY INITIATIVES

As government policy for the NHS evolved, some new programs added administrative detail to the initial outlines for the internal market reforms. Other emerging policies led in new directions, some of which weakened the original drive to create a market for health services. These policy changes came in response to unanticipated developments during implementation – including actions by central government figures and other policy actors and explicit and implicit negotiations among policy actors. Particularly influential were physicians' responses to programs that they were supposed to implement, attacks by the Labour opposition, media coverage, electoral developments, and attitudes of the public at large. During the first half of the 1990s, opinion polls pointed to growing dissatisfaction with hospital inpatient services and the running of the NHS (Mulligan and Judge, 1997). Despite government efforts to please the electorate, popular opposition to the government's handling of the NHS contributed to the low levels of electoral support for Prime Minister John Major and his party during the mid-1990s (Labour's Health Policy, 1995).

The government's new policy initiatives led in five directions, which were only partially compatible with one another and with the initial pro-market policies. First, to assure success of the market reforms and relieve the funding crisis, the government greatly increased NHS budgets. During the first four fiscal years of the reform (1989–90 through 1992–93), the government boosted real spending on the NHS by 15.5% (Calculated from Appleby, 1999a, Table 2).[4] The NHS had not seen growth rates like these since the early 1970s. There was a freeze on expenditures in 1993–94. Then as municipal and national elections approached, the government again allowed substantial real growth in NHS total funding in 1994–96.

The torrent of additional funding during the formative years of the reform supported development of fundholding practices, rising managerial costs, and acquisition of management information systems by the NHS bureaucracy and trusts. The government also underwrote hiring of extra doctors by trusts and other trust expenditures that might quickly reduce waiting lists. Although spending grew, in 1996 total health expenditures still remained below the OECD average (see Figure 1.1 on page 4). Although the government was willing to spend more money on the NHS, it continued throughout the 1990s to press hard for efficiency savings in trusts and HAs. Hospital managers sometimes faced the ironic situation of receiving funds to pay for private doctors and extra operations, while they simultaneously cut hospital bed capacities and non-medical staffs (Ints.).

Second, top government policymakers shifted from initial enthusiasm about the benefits of a free market for health care towards a policy of 'managed competition' – which acknowledged that the government must actively regulate purchasers, providers, and negotiations among them. This drift toward regulation and intervention in the market reflected an effort to prevent discontinuities in health care and avoid or delay outcomes like hospital closures that would be unpopular with voters and physicians, labor unions, and other powerful interest groups. In accordance with these concerns, as will be seen below, the government intervened directly in the restructuring of London's hospital services. Elsewhere it moderated and cancelled plans for hospital closures and mergers (Ints.)[5] Thus the NHS Executive belatedly acknowledged that NHS hospitals provide important 'non-economic benefits' (Butler, P., 1994), like employment and public good, which need to be weighed before a hospital is allowed to fail like a private firm or is forced to reorganize.

Third, the government renewed and intensified its campaign from the 1980s for top-down control over health providers. These moves drew on a Tory tradition that valued centralized and hierarchical control and used these tools to curb the power of opposing policy actors (Giamo and Manow, 1997; Jenkins, 1995). Thus while proclaiming the virtues of the market, the government aimed at increasing the accountability of local NHS purchasers and providers to the DOH and the NHS Executive. This growing centralization of NHS operations clashed with the government's initial policy of devolving authority and budgets and allowing market forces to determine the distribution, quality, and costs of services. Steps toward centralization included placing GPs under HA supervision, controlling appointments to trust and HA boards, and merging 14 Regional Health Authorities into eight Regional Outposts. Rather than representing providers and patients, as Regional Health Authorities had done, the Outposts were staffed by civil servants. They reported directly to the DOH and followed DOH instructions (Stewart, 1996). The NHS Executive also developed close ties to the DOH, and government ministers used the Executive as a major channel for implementing their policies, sometimes bypassing the regions altogether. Thus the government began allocating funds directly to HAs and requiring HAs to transmit performance data directly to the NHS Executive (Dopson et al., 1999). With these data, the DOH and NHS Executive annually evaluated purchasers and providers on a narrow range of budgetary and performance outcomes (NHS Executive, 1996). Chief executives of trusts and HAs, and sometimes lower-level managers, then received performance-related pay. The main criteria in these reviews were the financial performance of HAs and trusts, improvements in hospital throughputs, and waiting-list reductions (Ints.) Throughout the reforms, the DOH and NHS Executives flooded local actors with directives. The government also took steps to strengthen regulatory control over the quality and content of primary care (Lunt et al., 1997).

Fourth, the government gradually intensified and extended its support for a 'primary-care led NHS', in which 'decisions about health care are taken as close to patients as possible, with a greater voice for patients and their carers in such decisions' (NHS Executive, 1996). Rapid expansion of GP fundholding was the most important expression of the policy of devolving authority toward primary care. The government also periodically extended the types of care which single fundholders could purchase. In addition, the government supported total fundholding experiments in which groups of GP fundholders came together to commission all health services for their patients (Mays and Dixon, 1996). Expansion of fundholding weakened the purchasing function of the HAs, leaving them with the strategic functions of defining the needs of the local population and specifying the most efficient and effective ways to deliver care and improve health. HAs sometimes sought to exercise their strategic role by shifting care from hospitals to the community, but their successes in these endeavors were quite limited (see Contracting by Health Authorities, below).

In the spirit of the primary-care led NHS, the government also gradually recognized and encouraged locality and GP commissioning experiments involving non-fundholding GPs and some fundholders. (Mays and Dixon, 1996). In these projects GPs advised HAs on purchasing decisions that affected the entire population within HA boundaries. Some of these groups of GPs also received delegated budgets for commissioning agreed-upon services. Through these programs GPs developed a wide range of linkages with their local HA, trusts, and municipal agencies and shared decisions with them about service configurations and contracts. This trend received official sanction in guidelines issued in 1995, that required HAs to contract with community-based providers for certain categories of community care that had previously been commissioned by municipal authorities. These guidelines sought an end to the increasingly unpopular tendency of HAs and hospital trusts to cut their services for geriatric, retarded, and mentally ill patients and shift the burden of care from the NHS onto means-tested social services, that were provided by the municipalities (Wistow, 1997).

37

Official endorsement of primary-care led commissioning and purchasing partly reflected the government's response to initiatives that were taking place within local health authorities (Dixon et al., 1998; Light, 1997a). Moreover, a broad consensus was emerging in support of a primary-care led NHS, as both the BMA and the Labour Opposition endorsed primary care commissioning (Butler, 1995 April 20; Chadda and Crail, 1996).

Devolution of authority to primary care led to important policy developments that were unanticipated by the original internal market policies. Chief among these was official sanction for levels and types of collaboration and integration among primary-care practices, health authorities, and social services that would have been regarded as anti-competitive just a few years earlier. Furthermore, locality and GP commissioning weakened the distinction between fundholding and non-fundholding practices. These new types of commissioning helped lay the ground for the subsequent elimination of fundholding by the Labour Government.

Finally, the government linked expansion of primary care to proposals that some GPs relinquish their self-employed status in favor of employment by primary care practices, community and hospital trusts, and even by private firms (Coulter and Mays, 1997; Groves, 1997). Employment of GPs would allow primary-care practices to save costs and expand the range of services they offered. Employment would also empower HAs to guide primary-care development by contributing to the pay of salaried GPs and reallocating primary-care funding as needed.

Fifth, during the 1990s the government placed additional stress on improving health outcomes, as well as boosting operating efficiency. The 1990 GP contract introduced financial incentives for immunization, health promotion, and cancer screening (Whynes and Baines, 1998). In 1992 the government launched its Health of the Nation strategy to promote a strategic approach to improving the population's overall health and shift energy from medical care to health promotion. The government set targets in key health areas including coronary disease, cancer, mental illness, sexual health (including AIDS) and accidents (Limb, 1996,

August 15). Furthermore, the government and publicly-funded agencies, like Oxford's Cochrane Centre, promoted evidence-based medicine as a way to increase the effectiveness of GP and HA commissioning (Harrison, 1998).

38

THE INTERNAL MARKET REFORMS IN PRACTICE

Let us now examine implementation of the government's reform policies within local districts and hospitals between 1991 and 1997. Our main focus will be on three crucial features of the quasi-market: new organizational structures, contracting by HAs and GPs, and management of acute hospital trusts. Although the structures of the purchaser-provider split were implemented quickly, the processes of market contracting and management emerged slowly. Moreover, these processes evolved in ways that were only partially compatible with the original vision of market reform.

Structural Foundations

The legal and structural foundations for the reorganization of primary and secondary care were rapidly put into place in England, while proceeding more slowly in the rest of Britain. By 1997 the administrative and structural distinctions among the UK countries were becoming less noticeable, although differences persisted in other areas, like funding (Dixon et al., 1999).[6]

The government had a strong mandate for reform proposals, since the Conservatives controlled Parliament in 1990 and were re-elected in 1992. This political constellation effectively undermined the plausibility and legitimacy of the shrill attack on the reforms by the BMA and other opponents. Hence by 1993 critics of the reforms felt the need to take more moderate positions (Chadda, 1993; Millar, 1994). As a senior BMA employee explained, 'We needed a different tactic – so we pointed to implementation problems, working with them to put it right'. In this spirit, after 1993, the BMA drew closer to the national organization representing trust directors and managers (Int.). Together these bodies opposed hospital closings (e.g., Butler, P. 1996, May 12). They also called for increased resource allocations to trusts, more constructive involvement of hospital consultants in hospital management ('In brief', 1995, Feb 9), and better deployment of managers – rather than reductions in their numbers (Limb and Chadda, 1996).

Overnight in 1991 former district managers (executives) – who had directly supervised the operations of district general hospitals – became HA managers.[7] These managers had responsibility for almost 90% of NHS purchasing. The procedures for appointing the top officers in trusts, HAs, and other NHS agencies greatly increased the influence of former businessmen over the HAs trusts and tightened governmental control over them. The government put managers in HA positions that had formerly gone to representatives from municipal authorities and professional groups. It directly appointed the chairs of HAs, regions, and trusts and the non-executive (i.e., non-managing) members of trusts (Int.; Ferlie et al., 1996). HA chairs and the HAs' non-executive boards were staffed mainly with white men from business backgrounds, who were loyal to the Tories and their programs (Ashburner and Cairncross, 1993). Many of the original HA chairs, who had strong pro-market approaches, left within a few years of their original appointments (Int.). Nonetheless, top managers in HAs continued to possess considerably stronger business skills and orientations than did the former general managers. After the 1996 reorganization, HA chairs from business backgrounds greatly outnumbered those coming from the NHS or other organizations in the public sector (Butler, 1996, January 4). The NHS reorganization also enhanced the roles of middle and lower-level managers and greatly expanded their numbers (Appleby, 1995).

Unlike the reorganization of the HAs, GP fundholding was implemented gradually. At first many officials within the DOH and the NHS were skeptical or critical of fundholding and unsure how much of a role to give it (Glennerster et al., 1994). Proposals for fundholding faced opposition by the BMA and the Labour party, hostility and skepticism among hospital administrators and consultants, and concern among GPs that fundholding might bring added fiscal and administrative burdens (Chadda, 1993; Glennerster et al., 1994). To promote fundholding the government offered generous start-up allowances to cover computer services and management costs (Farmer, 1993; Whitehead, 1994, p. 223). Gradually it extended financial benefits to fundholders. In addition, in a shift of its initial policy, the DOH gradually reduced the size requirements for fundholding practices and extended the range of services that could be purchased under the fundholding budgets.

In fact, GPs responded far more favorably to invitations to become fundholders than local or national administrators had anticipated. Besides strong financial incentives, the fundholding scheme provided the prospect that participating physicians would enjoy greater independence than their non-fundholding peers, along with greater freedom of referral and more control over treatment of their patients in hospital. In response to growing support for fundholding by its constituency, the BMA voted to recognize fundholding in 1993, and the new BMA chair adopted a more conciliatory stance toward the program's future development (Chadda, 1993).

Hence, fundholding spread rapidly among GPs. By April 1993 the third wave of fundholding extended the practice to GPs treating 25% of the population (Glennerster et al., 1994, p. 86). By mid-1996 around 50% of patients were enrolled in fundholding practices (Harrison and New, 1996).[8] Still GPs remained divided into fundholding and non-fundholding camps (Ints.; Whitfield, 1998).

The government planned to create provider trusts in a series of waves. Hospitals and other providers seeking trust status were told to submit business plans to the DOH demonstrating the financial viability of the proposed trust. The chairs of these new trusts came overwhelmingly from outside of the NHS (Ferlie et al., 1996, p. 128). Physicians led opposition among hospital staff to the transformation of district hospitals into trusts. But would-be trust managers overrode staff opposition, and the DOH rapidly and unselectively approved applications for trust status (Ints.; Ham, 1992, p. 56). Just two years after the reforms went into effect, hospital trusts were providing 55% of all NHS beds and accounted for 67% of NHS expenditures (Bartlett and Le Grand, 1994, p. 56). By the end of 1995, nearly all hospital, ambulance, and community social service providers were organized as trusts (Harrison and New, 1996).[9]

Considering the scope of the task and the initial opposition of the medical profession, the implementation of the new structures and reporting relations was quite rapid and extensive. There were, nonetheless, regional differences in rates of trust formation in England (Bartlett and Le Grand, 1994). Moreover, there were variations of practice and management among HAs, along with local differences in the content of services budgeted to fundholders, and the scope and mix of services provided by trusts (Harrison and New, 1996; 1997).

Contracting by Health Authorities

Despite the prevailing terminology, the contracts that HAs signed with hospitals and other providers were really service agreements, rather than legally binding contracts (Flynn and Williams, 1997; Savas et al., 1998). Most of these agreements took the form of block contracts for non-emergency care, which closely resembled the prospective budgets used before the reforms (Paton et al., 1997). In these contracts, HA purchasers arranged to pay for access to an agreed-upon range of facilities or services for a fixed fee and time period (usually a year), without specifying workload, procedure volumes, or the specific facilities to be used (Posnett, 1993). Much of the content of the service contracts reflected governmental instructions, rather than agreements between independent parties. NHS guidances and directives specified targets for HA performance and dictated crucial managerial and fiscal parameters for contracts – including time frames, pricing rules, dispute resolution procedures, and enforcement of the standards contained in the Patient's Charter, as well as adherence to other quality standards (Hughes et al., 1997; Walshe, Deakin, Smith, Spurgeon and Thomas, 1997).

Although many HA purchasers initially expressed interest in switching service providers, most HAs continued to sign contracts for the bulk of their services with the same district general hospitals that the HAs had directly managed before 1991 (Mulligan, 1998a). When HAs did contract for care with other public or private providers, these providers rarely operated under highly competitive conditions (Paton et al., 1997).

There are several explanations for the limited involvement of HAs in competitive commissioning. HA managers had long-standing ties to district general hospitals and generally preferred to work with hospital managers and physicians whom they knew and trusted, rather than purchasing new and unfamiliar services. In addition, HA managers were subject to local political pressures not to force hospitals in their area to compete with others hospitals or undergo painful cutbacks (Ints.).

Budgetary constraints also limited the ability of HAs to shop for services among competing providers. Despite increases in government spending, the dominant atmosphere throughout reforms was one of tight money for both HAs and trust. The government required HAs and trusts to make annual 'efficiency gains' by increasing production or cutting costs. Moreover, the government also refrained from compensating trusts for cost increases and imposed fiscal burdens, including charges for capital and requirements that trusts finance private capital construction by reducing expenditures in other categories (Pollock et al., 1999). The trusts responded to these burdens by increasing charges to HAs or reducing services.

Under these conditions, most HA managers struggled to maintain services in their local hospitals in the face of rising demand. A member of the executive team in a major urban HA contrasted the impact of these fiscal and political constraints with the rhetoric of pro-market reform:

Mr. G: This is not a market. Money doesn't follow the patient, because [purchasing] is cash limited.
MH: Could the local hospital trusts sell their services elsewhere?
Mr. G: Yes [in theory], but other HAs have no money [to purchase services outside of their district]. The HAs are too small and are wedded to their own patch. They spend their time trying to save their own hospitals.

When HAs did contract with hospitals other than their former district general hospital, they usually did so to reduce service costs, obtain services not available locally, or reduce waiting for elective surgery. As the following example suggests, these external purchases also helped them meet governmental expectations:

To conform to the Patients' Charter standard that waiting times for elective surgery not exceed one year, the manager in charge of commissioning special hospital services for a major HA contracted with providers outside of his area for several types of elective surgery. He described this move as 'politically useful', since it showed that the HA was engaging in a drive to 'expand the market', in keeping with the expectations of the NHS Executive. In the end, 13 of 16 patients who were to be sent 30 miles away for surgery refused to relocate and remained on their local hospital's waiting list.

London was an important exception to the prevailing pattern of relations between HAs and hospital trusts, because London had a bigger supply of beds than other parts of the country (Nicholls, 1997). Before the reforms, districts surrounding London had often obtained services from well-known hospitals in the city without forming strong ties to these institutions (Ints.). Under the market reforms, many HAs sought to shift some of this care to less expensive providers (Ints.: Mulligan, 1998a). In consequence, many of London's most prestigious hospitals encountered financial difficulties. Thus HA contracting heightened financial pressure on London's historic teaching hospitals and once again focused attention on their high capacities and costs.

Ironically, the emergence of market pressures on London's hospitals led to governmental intervention, rather than to a market shake-out, as market theorists might have expected. Bed reductions and proposals to close and merge

42

famous hospitals provoked storms of protests and heated debate. The government dealt with the controversy by setting up a high-level advisory commission, a bureaucratic implementation body, and a series of advisory reviews by hospital consultants of six of the city's major areas of medical specialization (James, 1995). The government also diverted extra funds to London's ailing hospitals and rescheduled closures of wards and hospitals. Still controversy over proposed reconfigurations raged in and around the trusts, often compromising the original proposals and delaying implementation of change for years (e.g., Chadda, 1998; Warden, 1998c) In this crucial test of the market, provider competition and purchaser choice worked primarily to surface and intensify long-standing debates about the viability of London's hospitals. But HA contracting per se produced little change. Instead top-down, governmental intervention, tempered by interest-group politics, formed the driving forces for trust consolidations and other structural changes.

Across Britain, HAs faced serious barriers to assessing the costs, nature, and quality of the services provided by trusts. Management information systems in HAs were unsophisticated and poorly integrated. As a result HA purchasers had no knowledge of large variations among providers in service charges. Nor could HA managers readily compile elementary data on their own purchase volumes and costs (Robins et al., 1996; Limb, 1997). Hence, purchasers had no valid and agreed-upon basis for costing hospital services or comparing prices and performance among trusts (Ints.: Goodwin, Neil, 2000; Hughes et al., 1997). A government-sponsored program to create a system-wide basis for recording clinical information into a database produced disappointing preliminary results (National Audit Office, 1996; Mitchell, 1998). The system was attacked by information specialists and ultimately became mired in charges of wastage and conflict of interest (Cross, 1998; Mitchell, 1998). The NHS also failed to implement systems for gathering and analyzing case-mix data – which are crucial to valid assessments of the efficiency and effectiveness of hospital units and entire hospitals. The NHS did not develop and mandate the use of case-mix codes until 1994 (Buckland, 1994). During the next few years, HA purchasers, trust managers, and clinical directors made very limited use of case-mix data (Ints.; Goodwin, Neil, 2000, May 15).

HA managers faced comparable difficulties in assessing the benefits of new programs and technology acquisitions. The managers usually relied on hospital clinicians to evaluate and justify the clinical value of the proposed innovations. Meanwhile HA and trust managers concentrated on the likely effects of such proposals on the financial and management performance of the trust (Ints.).

During the mid-1990s, in response to growing concern about clinical quality, HA managers tried to introduce contractual requirements that providers engage in quality assurance (Pugner and Glennerster, 1998). Some HAs also sent public health physicians into hospitals to conduct quality reviews of treatments of specific types of cancer or other targeted areas (Ints.). However, HAs typically did not gather systematic data on the clinical quality of services in particular hospitals and rarely used available data to shed light on the effectiveness and efficiency of care. Nor did NHS officials provide purchasers with quality data (Mulligan,

1998a). Instead, HA managers depended on providers for information on the quality of care and services and relied on voluntary cooperation in quality assurance. (Walshe et al., 1997).

The following summary of comments by a HA manager in charge of commissioning hospital services illustrates the difficulties HAs faced in their efforts to enhance clinical quality:

43

> Clinical audits conducted in hospitals are too 'long-winded' to help HA commissioners assess hospital quality. Moreover, the HA lacks the needed information system, including case-mix data, and does not have sufficient resources to conduct systematic assessments of the clinical quality of hospital services. The volume and complexity of services under contract are overwhelming, and the HA is 'unsystematic about requiring [quality] data and using it'. The HA does require hospitals to report whether they gave timely care that responded to patient needs, as specified by the Patient's Charter. But, neither these data, nor comparisons of length of stay by provider, influenced how the HA or the trust behaved.

The many technical, political, and financial constraints experienced by HAs made it very difficulty for them to develop a strategic approach to commissioning, as they were supposed to do (Drummond et al., 1997; Walshe and Ham, 1997). Strategic purchasing was supposed to be based on systematic assessments of the needs of residents; setting priorities for spending; and rational judgments about the most cost-effective mix of prevention, diagnosis, and intervention. By assigning high priority to public health, primary care, and evidence-based medicine, NHS officials hoped to lead to dramatic changes in HA purchasing patterns. In fact, change in the new direction was very limited and incremental (Ham, 1996; Klein et al., 1996). One manager succinctly summed up the dilemma confronting HAs: 'Our major budgetary commitments are fixed and hospital-based, so our ability to shift the configuration of services is limited'.

Even when they had the opportunities to shift resources, HA managers usually lacked the data and knowledge needed to chose alternative care configurations rationally. The much-heralded field of evidence-based medicine (EBM) failed to yield simple, unambiguous, and uncontroversial criteria for systematically evaluating the cost-effectiveness of alternative medical practices and procedures (Drummond et al., 1997). As an illustration of the hurdles to using EBM, consider the following comments by a public health physician serving on a HA management team. Dr. T was trying to explain how EBM justified her HA's decision to prefer home care to extended hospitalization:

> **Dr. T:** EBM can release funds. For example, if home care for stroke is as good as hospital care, [the HA] can save money [by commissioning home care].
>
> **MH:** Is it [as good]?
>
> **Dr. T:** I don't know. The patients perceive it to be better. They feel more looked after *if* the home is good, *if* there is a multi-disciplinary team *and* the [home] care continues longer [than would hospital care]. [*Emphases in original*]

Lacking hard data on care quality, Dr. T took refuge in patient perceptions. Moreover, she based her argument on a set of conditions for home care that could not be assured by the decision to shift the location of care.

In practice, HA managers rarely found evidence that was strong enough to convince clinicians and hospital managers to change treatments, reduce hospitalization periods, or shift care to the community. Moreover, most HA commissioners lacked the professional knowledge and influence needed to overcome resistance by hospital consultants to service cuts or reconfigurations. The following episode illustrates just how powerful such resistance could be:

> To speed identification and referral to treatment of urgent orthopedic cases, HA managers, in consultation with GPs and clinical directors of the local hospital, sought to move triage from the hospital's outpatient clinics to the primary care setting. Initial diagnosis in primary care clinics would come under the direction of physiotherapists. The Royal College of Orthopedic Surgeons rejected this initiative, arguing that waiting times could best be reduced by adding more orthopedic surgeons to hospital staffs.

HA commissioners thus had to be very cautious and selective in their attempts to ration or reconfigure care. HA managers risked legal actions if they imposed their views on the medical profession without sufficient evidence (Ints.). In consequence, HAs generally allowed physicians discretion in applying rationing decisions to individual cases (Locock, 2000; see also Klein et al., 1996).

Lack of public involvement created yet another barrier to strategic commissioning. The NHS Executive envisioned orderly public participation in defining local needs and setting health care priorities. In keeping with these expectations, HAs made some efforts to survey residents about their health care priorities and involve them in public discussions about purchasing priorities (Obermann and Tolley, 1997). However, these activities do not appear to have influenced HA decision making very much (see Chapter 3).

Lacking formal influence over HAs, the public often joined NHS staff, local government, and other interest groups in vigorously protesting HA decisions to reduce hospital services or reconfigure them (Ints.).[10] These protests usually delayed closings but did not halt them. HA managers sometimes avoided such vocal opposition by moderating plans for structural change or simply delaying them until after elections (Ints.). Managers usually paid even closer attention to the concerns of GPs and hospital consultants, who sometimes led public resistance to reconfigurations ('Public softens ...' 1996). Open conflict over reconfigurations gradually declined in the mid 1990s, as the public began to accept the inevitability of these changes. The tacit alliance between physicians and the public at large also seems to have grown weaker, as medical elites adopted the view that the quality of specialty services would improve if they were concentrated in a limited number of major medical centers (Department of Health, 1995; 'BMA favors ...' 1997; Chadda, 1998 July 2).

Although they worked under intense constraints, HAs did engage in limited and highly focused initiatives towards improving health services in their area. These frequently took the form of demonstration projects for enhancing coordination or quality of care for a specific ailment or category of patients. Other projects, which were part of the experiments in locality commissioning, sought to enhance cooperation between primary care givers and other service providers.

45

Generalizations about trends in HA contracting fail to do justice to substantial variations that emerged among HAs (e.g., Walshe et al., 1997). The profiles that follow summarize dramatic differences in orientations toward the market in two major metropolitan HAs. It is particularly noteworthy that these differences persisted six years after passage of the NHS and Community Care Act.

Top managers in Mellstock HA displayed pessimism about the prospects for market reform (Ints):

> Members of the executive team in Mellstock HA were skeptical about the ability of the purchaser-provider split to produce significant change. Instead, they described their HA as deeply committed to Mellstock's local hospitals, which had run up substantial deficits. Fiscal limitations, political pressures, and resistance by powerful hospital clinicians made it hard for Mellstock's managers to introduce changes in services. The HA was experimenting with collaboration with non-fundholding GPs. There were more than 40 major fundholding practices in the area, and area hospitals handled hundreds of separate contracts with fundholders. Nonetheless, HA executives doubted the ability of fundholders to generate major improvements in health services. Some saw fundholding as favoring the middle classes and providing unjustified financial benefits to participating GPs.

In contrast, Mr. R, the CEO of Sandbourne HA, and several members of his staff expressed enthusiasm about the ability of GP purchasing to generate competition among providers:

> Mr. R and his colleagues explained that local politics forced HAs to place most of their contracts with local trusts. Therefore, HAs could never really develop market relations with provider trusts. Only GP fundholders had sufficient freedom and discretion to act as purchasers in a market. For this reason, Sandbourne HA was rapidly delegating substantial portions of its budget to GP fundholders and was supporting an experiment in which fundholding and non-fundholding GPs cooperated in commissioning. Through both types of GP commissioning, Mr. R had found a way around the political constraints facing HAs. Explaining fundholding's ability to unleash market forces, Mr. R remarked gleefully 'We've torn up the constraints on the market! Price will no longer simply equal [provider] cost. That was Christmas for the providers!'

These very different orientations toward the purchaser-provider split and fundholding flowed in part from the divergent backgrounds of powerful actors in the two HAs. In Mellstock, as in most of the reorganized HAs (Ferlie et al., 1996), several members of the executive team had worked in the health system or in local government prior to the reorganization. They felt at home in the consultative atmosphere that had prevailed prior to the reforms. In contrast, Sandbourne's CEO (Mr. R), like other managers and non-executives who came directly from the private sector, held strong pro-market values. Moreover he was proud of his tough, confrontational style – one that was rather rare in the NHS prior to the market reforms, but is far more common in the world of business.

46   In conclusion, despite local variations, most HAs failed to contract for care among vigorously competing public and private providers. Instead, HAs remained dependent on local hospitals for the vast majority of their emergency and elective care. Nor could the HAs pursue distinctive community-based commissioning strategies without challenging the preferences of vocal patient groups or confronting the authority and expertise of hospital physicians. Thus, even in pro-market HAs, like Sandbourne, relations between purchasers and hospitals in the mid 1990s did not 'feel very different from what we did before [the reforms]'. (Int.) Cash constraints and governmental mandates severely limited the options open to HA managers. Moreover, most HA managers had neither the technical capacity, nor the political will and power to pursue market opportunities vigorously or implement distinctive care strategies. For similar reasons, HA activities on behalf of quality assurance in hospitals mainly pursued narrowly focused improvements in service quality, such as reductions in waiting times.

GP Fundholding

During the first few years of GP fundholding, participating physicians made more vigorous use of provider competition than did HA purchasers and thereby gained a reputation as the cutting edge of the internal market (e.g., Glennerster et al., 1994). Rather than relying on block contracts, as did HA purchasers, fundholders often signed contracts that specified prices for specific procedures (cost-per-case-contracts) or prices for procedures that were in excess of an agreed-upon workload (cost and volume contracts) (Glennerster et al., 1994; Posnett, 1993). The early fundholders showed less loyalty to particular hospitals than did HA managers. Unlike HAs, fundholders could renegotiate their small contracts without destabilizing hospitals or risking political repercussions for their actions. Thus early fundholders gained leverage over hospitals by threatening to shift contracts for elective hospital care and sometimes actively shopping for better or less expensive services in and out of hospitals. The GPs then used their influence over hospitals to win service gains for their patients. These included shorter waiting times, faster turnaround of lab results, better communication with GPs about patients referred to hospitals, and guarantees that consultants, rather than junior doctors, would see patients during an agreed-upon proportion of outpatient visits (Glennerster et al., 1994; Harrison and Choudrhy, 1996). The fundholders also negotiated reduced hospital charges, thereby saving part of their patient budgets (Audit Commission, 1996b; Goodwin, 1998).

Even when individual fundholders accounted for small proportions of a hospital's total budget, their impact on hospital managers and physicians could be quite substantial. Fundholding's impacts were well described by the finance director of a major metropolitan hospital, here called Greenham Hospital:

Mr. W: We have a problem with the GP fundholders. Together they account for around 12 to 14% of our budget. They take a very short-term approach. Each GP is interested first in the price of care and [second] in the length of the waiting list for his patients. They're particularly concerned about outpatient and discharge services. They threaten to move their contracts.

MH: Does this actually happen?

Mr. W: One big practice shifted its eye business. We argued [unsuccessfully] that Greenham's quality of care was higher. The fundholders have a potentially destabilizing effect. One group contracts for four to five million pounds of care per annum through a single negotiating office... We charge what the market will bear – not 'price equals cost' [as required by an NHS prohibition on cross-subsidization between services]. As the fundholders swing on price [expectations], you shift prices accordingly.

Besides seeking lower costs, many fundholders tried to improve the quality of care their patients received in hospital. Most often the GPs put quality standards into contracts. Sometimes fundholders directly pressed hospitals to improve services to the GPs' patients. In these ways fundholders were indeed able to reduce their patients' waiting times and improve the quality of information provided to GPs on hospital treatments (Dowling, 1997; Goodwin et al., 1998).

Despite these gains, fundholding did not significantly alter the character of clinical care in hospitals. Unlike the first few waves of fundholders, many of the physicians who joined the program later made less aggressive use of the market (Ints). Dr. U, a GP fundholder, who also served as an advisor on HA commissioning, explained the background to this more conservative approach to contracting:

According to Dr. U, a lot of the quality of care depends on relations between the GP and the hospital consultant, for instance when GPs follow up on hospitalized patients. Dr. U explained, 'If I know that the physician is both good technically and good at [delivering] bad news, I will feel better than if I buy a cheaper service [from a physician I don't know.]'

Fundholders, like HA managers, ultimately depended on consultants to assess and assure the clinical quality and appropriateness of care. Contracts between fundholders and hospital trusts contained no provisions for systematic evaluation or sanctioning of the trust's conformity to contract standards. Hospital clinicians, in turn, showed little concern for meeting quality and performance standards contained in fundholding contracts (Baeza and Calnan, 1997). Despite their medical training, fundholders were ill equipped to assess the cost effectiveness of hospital and community care, so as to insure that their contracts provided the best 'value for money' spent. Nor were most GPs disposed toward the research-based logic of evidence-based medicine (Harrison, S., 1998), on which assessments of cost-benefit rest. Flooded with conflicting and often ambiguous guidelines (Hibble et al., 1998; Cumbers and Donald, 1999; Woolf et al., 1999), fundholders and non-fundholders in total purchasing schemes continued to make decisions about clinical care much as they had prior to joining these schemes. They usually relied on their own clinical experience and inclinations and those of their immediate colleagues, rather than referring to empirical data on patients' needs, treatment effectiveness, or the cost-effectiveness of service alternatives (Audit Commission, 1996b; Mays and Mulligan, 1998).

In summary, GP fundholders were more willing and able than HA purchasers to take advantage of competition among hospitals. The GPs had fewer loyalties and ties to the hospitals than did HA purchasers, were less subject to political pressure to support hospitals, and were more sensitive to the needs and concerns of individual patients. Fundholders translated their newly gained leverage over hospitals into improvements in patient services and reduced hospital charges. Gradually fundholders – along with many non-fundholding GPs – forged more cooperative relations with HAs and providers of local social services. Besides encouraging GPs to use provider competition to reduce costs and enhance the quality of hospital care, fundholding was also expected to lead GPs to manage their patients' primary care more effectively (see Chapter 3). Despite its successes, fundholding divided the medical profession and was attacked by Labour and non-fundholding GPs as wasteful, divisive, and as creating a 'two-tiered NHS'. (Audit Commission, 1996b; Limb, 1996, March 14). These criticisms provided the impetus for the elimination of fundholding and creation of new forms of primary-care commissioning after Labour's election.

Managing Hospital Trusts

Acute hospital trusts formed the single largest source of NHS expenditures and provided most of the services contracted by HAs and GP fundholders. Trust activities and management therefore decisively shaped implementation of the internal market reforms and other non-market programs, like the government's drives for efficiency gains and quality assurance. As explained in Chapter 1, to understand how trusts responded to the reforms, it is particularly important to examine ways that hospital physicians influenced program implementation.

As noted, hospital trusts did not actively compete for most HA contracts. Nor did most trust managers actively seek to purchase vital clinical or administrative services from external providers, as the government urged them to do ('The making...' 1995; Decker, 1995). Instead, trust managers devoted most of their efforts to meeting targets imposed by NHS and DOH authorities for increasing service production while cutting costs.

For many trusts the internal market reorganization failed to create strong incentives and opportunities for market activity. In less densely settled areas, and even in some urban areas, former district general hospitals enjoyed effective monopolies over elective care (Appleby et al., 1994). Moreover, some urban hospitals provided clinical services that were unavailable nearby or were far more sophisticated than those provided by neighboring hospitals (Ints.). Even when HAs were able to refer patients elsewhere, patients often preferred to endure long waits for care in their local hospitals (Mahon et al., 1994). The block contracts used by most HAs further discouraged trust competition over quality or costs. These contracts failed to compensate providers for additional or improved services during the contract period (Bartlett and Le Grand, 1994; Ranade and Haywood, 1991). In the end annual variations in contracted expenditures depended more on governmental funding decisions than on the trust's performance during the prior year.

In contrast to their relations to HAs, acute hospitals competed directly for GP contracts. The experience of many trusts were typified by those of Nileston, a university-affiliated hospital, in Mellstock (see Contracting by HAs on page 45). As Nileston's CEO put it:

> The GP fundholders make their decisions on the basis of cost and patient access [e.g., waiting times]. We have had GPs switch on this basis. The HAs don't switch providers.

In response to competition for fundholders' contracts, trust managers made clear to their clinicians that it was important to satisfy fundholding physicians and their patients. The best way to do so was by reducing charges, minimizing waiting times, and improving responsiveness to patients' needs. Some trusts vigorously marketed hospital services to fundholders (e.g., McNulty et al., 1994). One marketing strategy involved devolving budgetary authority to clinical directorates and rewarding clinical directors formally and informally for success in gaining contracts (e.g., Propper and Bartlett, 1997).

The following summary of activities at Greenham Hospital (see pages 46–47), illustrates the range of tactics used by managers and physicians to attract and retain fundholding contracts:

> Physicians at Greenham reported that consultants and managers examined referral patterns to determine why GPs referred patients to their hospital or preferred other ones. Dr. B, a particularly entrepreneurial clinical director, actively solicited GP referrals by running GP training sessions on clinical developments in his specialty. Dr. B also maintained a 'GP hotline' to enhance communication with referring physicians. Physicians in the outpatient clinic of another department at Greenham took steps to 'deliver to purchasers'. They made sure that GPs quickly got the results of their patients' diagnostic tests. Departing from the tradition of keeping GPs at arms length, department members met periodically with GPs and solicited their comments on clinical practices and suggestions for improvement. According to a junior physician in the department, this initiative sought to 'make a good impression' on the GPs, rather than seeking to produce fundamental changes in clinical decisionmaking.

Although some hospitals actively marketed their services, most trust managers faced many internal constraints on marketing and entrepreneurial ventures. These powerful constraints also posed barriers to the implementation of other managerial programs that were not primarily oriented toward market competition – such as cost containment, rationalization of resource usage, and quality assurance. As noted, trusts and HAs faced opposition from staff unions and local politicians whenever they sought to reconfigure services or alter working conditions.

Trust managers also found it hard to gain their physicians' support for efficiency drives and other organizational changes. The managers depended directly on clinicians to improve existing services, develop new ones, acquire new medical technologies (Rosen and Mays, 1998), and market services to purchasers (Ints.). But hospital consultants typically showed more interest in advancing their own medical specialties and careers than in cooperating with managerial efforts to enhance hospital revenues and market share.[11]

Hospital physicians begrudgingly coped with the fiscal constraints and stepped-up work loads initiated by management, even as national physicians' organizations protested these developments. Here is a junior doctor's description of the effects of managerial pressures in an outpatient clinic:

> When I see a manager get up and tell me [what to do], it irritates me. [I say to myself,] 'You don't have a clue as to what I do'. It irritates a lot of us. The numbers impinge on outpatient treatments. The numbers and the time allocations are important [for the managers]. They don't allow enough time [per patient]. So you cut corners, or you run late, and then everyone gets annoyed.

Hospital physicians often did not comply with proposed organizational changes that directly threatened their livelihood, power, and clinical autonomy. Both junior and senior physicians frequently failed to sign government-mandated work contracts and did not conform to limitations on private practice (Audit Commission, 1995, 1996a). In like manner, hospital physicians resisted managerial steps, like the imposition of drug lists and budgets, that the physicians viewed as infringing on clinical autonomy (Ints.; Sibbald et al., 1992).

When trust managers sought to make personnel changes or reorganize services, they sometimes faced bitter opposition by their clinicians: in six well-publicized instances (e.g., 'Top doctor ...', 1994; Crail, 1997), conflicts over proposals to fire physicians or reorganize hospitals ended in the resignation of trust chairs, CEOs, or medical directors. Trust CEOs quickly learned that to survive and succeed, they had to avoid confrontations with physicians, other staff groups, and local politicians. As the CEO of Milford Hospital, a major urban specialty hospital, put it when describing the challenges he faced, 'These are burn out jobs. You have to be careful how you approach it. One mistake is one too many'.

Institutional constraints also undercut the capacity of trust managers to reward and sanction compliance with managerial programs. Local pay, which had been a fundamental feature of the original reform plan, was successfully resisted by the physicians and other NHS staff groups (Crail, 1995; Mailly, 1997). Hence, national bargaining frameworks and agreements remained in place after 1991. However, trusts were given authority for deciding on small annual pay increments for all staff, except physicians. In the mid-1990s a new procedure was adopted for assigning merit pay to physicians ('C' payments), which allowed for some local influence. However, consultants, rather than managers, retained most of the control over merit raises (Ints.). Other reward contingencies, like career advancement and opportunities for private practice, depended on professional and market forces that lay beyond managerial control. Moreover, tight hospital budgets and high demand left few opportunities for management to reward staff by improving working conditions.

Ironically, the central government contributed to external constraints on the ability of trust heads to act like independent business managers. Instead of treating trusts like the semi-autonomous corporate actors described in *Working for Patients*, the DOH severely restricted trusts' ability to borrow money in the private capital markets, acquire assets, and manage revenues and surpluses (Bartlett and Le Grand, 1994). The government's Private Finance Initiative (PFI) required private financing for new capital projects and imposed heavy borrowing costs on the hospitals (Gaffney et al., 1999a, b, c). Managers and clinicians in trusts worried about these costs and about losing control to private investors of new facilities financed under the PFI (Ints.). As a result, few trusts introduced new construction projects within the PFI framework.

Poor management information systems also made it hard for trust managers to engage in systematic assessment, planning, and control of trust operations. In most cases trust managers lacked accurate data on the costs, activities, and outcomes of specific hospital services and units (Ints.). Without such data, managers could not rationally price and market services or adequately carry out internal control functions.

While limited in their capacity to engage the market, trust managers were subject to powerful pressure to meet performance targets imposed by central government (Hamblin, 1998). The DOH set these targets and then passed them down from the NHS Executive, to the regions, the HAs, and on to the trusts. The government and the NHS Executive concentrated mainly on costs, other financial measures, and hospital throughputs. Their quality drive aimed most directly at reducing waiting lists and promoting other standards reflecting rapid movement of patients through general hospitals. Other rights and values articulated in the Charter received far less attention in practice (Cole, 1995; Dyke, 1998). The government annually evaluated each hospital's financial performance and its success in meeting other targets. Trust heads who failed to attain fiscal and production objectives risked losing their appointments, while managers at high-performing hospitals received bonuses. The publication of league tables, which ranked hospital performance, further intensified pressure for fiscal and operational improvements.

Rather than developing bold market strategies, most hospital managers responded conservatively and defensively to the operating conditions imposed by central government and lower-level agencies. As they labored to meet government expectations, hospital managers simultaneously tried to cope with demand for services that rose much faster than available resources. Annual winter hospitalization crises were one of the most visible signs of this situation. To enhance throughput and make required efficiency gains, trust managers drew up lists of recommended drugs, encouraged day surgery, and reviewed data on length of stay with clinicians (Ints.; Lyall, 1995; Stewart, 1994). Some hospitals deployed bed managers to oversee the stays of geriatric patients and urge medical staff to release them as quickly as possible (Ints.).

While significant, operating improvements like these often proved insufficient to attain fiscal targets. So trusts across Britain closed wards, cut bed capacities and staff, and reduced hospital stays. Trust managers also reduced skill mix in wards by employing lower-ranking nurses or health-care assistants and gradually shifted nurses and other staff members from full-time to part-time contracts, which carried fewer benefits. Unfortunately, agreed-upon quantitative data on these staffing changes are very scarce.[12] According to the analysis of one member of the Labour opposition, the number of nurses fell in almost all regions during 1992–93, while the number of managers rose, in some areas dramatically ('Management growth...', 1994). When the Tories left office in 1996, there were 43,000 fewer nurses (in full-time equivalents) than in 1989 at the start of the market reforms – a decline of 11.6% (OECD, 2001).[13] Declines in hospital capacities were equally dramatic: Nine percent of hospitals with Accident and Emergency Units closed them between 1991 and 1994 (In brief, 1995 February 16). Between the start of 1990 and the end of 1996, more than one out of every four hospital beds (25.8%) in Britain were eliminated, with the heaviest cuts falling on psychiatric, geriatric, and maternity beds (OECD, 2001). For the most part, these reductions in hospital capacity followed the path of least political resistance, rather than responding to local demand, as reflected in contracts or analyses by health services planners.

While emphasizing fiscal and performance targets, governmental officials also urged the hospitals to enhance managerial control over clinical quality. The hospitals' most important efforts in this direction turned on improving information on clinical practices, implementing clinical audits, and devolving management responsibilities to clinical directorates.

Hospital physicians often viewed these developments as threats to their professional autonomy. Without openly opposing them, the physicians succeeded in stalling, encapsulating, or undermining most moves that might have further intensified managerial control over the medical profession. Thus hospital physicians joined the chorus of critics of league tables, which ranked hospital performance and costs without reference to case mix or care quality (e.g., Parry et al., 1998). Clinicians also raised apparently legitimate doubts about the validity of proposed NHS activity and case-mix measures (Ints.).

In like manner, hospital physicians were quick to pick up on limitations of locally designed information systems (Ints.):

The Clinical Director of Oncology in Milford Hospital reported that his colleagues reacted angrily to coding categories that made it look as if their department had produced no outputs in two months: 'They said this was nonsense, and that it was a waste of time to investigate [this finding]. So distrust [of the system] just grew further'.

The history of clinical directorate structures shows dramatically how hospital physicians diverted reform programs from their original trajectory. From the

1980s, the government had envisioned the directorates as a means of integrating disparate clinical and non-clinical activities and enhancing managerial control over health professionals (see pp. 31–32). In the early 1990s it seemed that directorates could make costs and outputs of clinical units more visible to external purchasers, as well as to trust managers. **53**

Although directorate structures had diffused widely by the mid 1990s, relations among top managers, clinical directors, and physicians in their directorate usually undermined the structure's main managerial functions. For the most part neither trust managers nor external purchasers could rely on clinical directors to help monitor or reshape medical practice within trusts. Instead, most directorates operated mainly as administrative frameworks for distributing centrally controlled budgets, rather than as autonomous budget units (Audit Commission, 1995, p. 64). This situation developed in part because top managers feared they would lose control over costs if they delegated budgetary authority to the directorates. In addition the BMA rejected governmental proposals to give clinical directors disciplinary authority over their colleagues (Int.; Orchard, 1993), and hospital physicians resisted managerial control by clinical directors (Ints.). Hence, medical directors or other members of top management, rather than clinical directors, became responsible for reviewing consultants' contracts and their work practices (Int.). A further blow to the power and authority of clinical directors came from retention of parallel supervisory hierarchies among nurses, paramedical professionals, and non-professional employees (Audit Commission, 1995).

In practice, both physicians and managers recognized that power and influence among hospital physicians still flowed more from clinical expertise and professional prestige than from formal administrative authority. Within the trusts, powerful consultants maintained direct access to top hospital managers and their boards, thereby bypassing clinical directors (Audit Commission, 1995; Ints.). To satisfy their clinicians, hospital managers retained structures that divided services into traditional, quasi-autonomous specialties. In most cases, these traditional structural divisions thwarted the development of market or patient-centered groupings capable of integrating services within hospitals and bridging gaps between hospital and community-based services (Laing and Galbraith, 1996).

Consultants, rather than clinical directors, kept control over the scheduling of both NHS and privately-funded operations within NHS hospitals. In this fashion, consultants influenced the length of cues for elective surgery. Throughout the reforms, consultants with private practices continued to benefit from long waiting lists for NHS–funded operations (Yates, 1995; Light, 1997b).

Under these conditions, clinical directors felt caught between the peer-oriented culture of medicine and the financial and operating constraints imposed by management (Ints.). Most clinical directors were prominent senior physicians, who were elected to their positions by their peers or appointed by management after consultation with the medical staff. Hence, clinical directors depended on their colleagues for legitimacy and professional support. At the same time, most clinical directors relied heavily on non-medical managers for logistical assistance and information (Ints.). Having little or no management training and limited expertise in management, clinical directors sometimes found themselves at a disadvantage in their negotiations with trained managers (Ints.).

The conflicting pressures to which the directors were subject made them understandably reluctant to try to exercise their authority over their colleagues. One clinical director (as reported by a colleague) nicely summed up his loyalties: 'I'm not a manager. I represent my colleagues!'. Dr. J, the Clinical Director who headed the medical division at Nileston Hospital, also made clear how hard it is for him to manage clinicians:

> There's a common understanding by clinicians and management. The common approach is not to impose imperatives [on clinicians]. [Dr. J then describes the difficulties of getting good data on medical activities within the division and convincing staff members to deal with statistical evidence of practice variations:] There's marked variation among my colleagues. Some have no interest outside their own patch. They say if variations in practices or outcomes were a major issue, we'd already know it [without the data] ... My colleagues are happy for me to run the show. They don't need to dabble in it.

Clinical audits were yet another means whereby the government sought to enhance managerial knowledge of clinical practice and control over it. This program encountered many of the same forces that affected implementation of clinical directorates and followed a similar path. Despite governmental efforts (Dent, 1995; Harrison et al., 1992), throughout the 1980s quality assurance in hospitals remained the nearly exclusive terrain of hospital clinicians. The internal market reforms envisioned a fundamental change in this situation (Packwood et al., 1994). Audits of clinical practice, in which all hospital physicians and GPs were required to take part, would assure that quality of care would be subject to managerial and public scrutiny. Trust managers would obtain control over clinical quality, since clinical directors would report on audit outcomes to managers and would cooperate in enforcing medical quality standards.

Contrary to initial expectations, compromises between the DOH and the physicians prevented audits from supplying systematic information about clinical practices to trust and NHS managers and rendering these practices subject to managerial control. The DOH quickly bent to pressure from the BMA and redefined audit as a confidential peer-review process, controlled and directed by physicians. To avoid conflicts between management and physicians, no sanctions were specified for non-participation in the audit process (Harrison and Pollitt, 1994; Macpherson and Mann, 1992). These compromises between the DOH and the BMA effectively encapsulated audit as a form of professional education. The DOH distributed the funds for audit to local and regional audit committees composed solely of physicians. The results of these policies were that most audits were local, criteria-based efforts to evaluate a single clinical technique (Kerrison et al., 1994). Hospital and HA managers had little input into the audit process and limited access to the results (Ints.). The impact of medical audits was further limited by disagreements among participants over the criteria used to assess clinical procedures, difficulties in using computerized databases, and confusion about what should be done with audit findings. Managers and clinicians seemed to feel that audit was something they had to do to satisfy purchasers, but that it was not really an integral part of their work (Ints.).

A description of audit procedures provided by the Medical Director of Milford Hospital captured well (and probably unintentionally) the very specialized focus of audit investigations. The Director's comments make it clear that his hospital had failed to integrate audit processes and findings into decision processes within clinical directorates or higher levels of management:

> All consultants have it in their contract that they have to participate in audits. Cardiologists don't understand Neurology and so on, so we devolve the responsibility for audit to the specialty level. The Clinical Director, [who oversees several specialties,] is [only] responsible to make sure that something goes on. If there's a problem in the specialty, the specialists would go and speak to the head of that specialty.

As it became clear that clinical audits would not yield tangible care improvements for entire hospitals, HA managers began to press hospitals to take additional steps toward monitoring quality and providing quality data. These efforts concentrated mainly on assessing the trusts' conformity to Patient's Charter standards (Ints.). Sometimes, HAs also required trusts to audit practices in specific medical areas, such as colon and breast cancer. Besides making hospital-wide efforts to meet Patient Charter standards, many hospitals also engaged in audits of nursing practices (Ints.) and total quality management projects. Due to their lack of popularity with physicians, projects in total quality management did not typically deal with purely clinical practices (Harrison and Pollitt, 1994, p. 97) and usually did not actively involve physicians (Ovretveit, 1994).

At the national level, specialty associations and national agencies, like the Cochrane Centre, responded to concern over clinical quality by developing protocols that specified best practices for specific ailments and treatments. During the market reforms, these protocols and guidelines informed the clinical practices of individual physicians and even of entire specialty groups, but they did not lead to managerially-led programs for reducing practice variations and enhancing the quality of hospital care. Under pressure from public opinion and the government to enhance medical accountability for hospital quality, the head of the General Medical Council affirmed the value of external review of practices based on national professional standards (e.g., Irvine, 1997b).[14] The emerging protocols and practice recommendations are filled with ambiguities and complexities, which clinicians quickly identify (Lawton and Parker, 1999). Thus clinicians continued to champion their autonomy to deviate from protocols and guidelines and expressed concern that managers might try to force conformity to such standards (Ints.). In some cases, managers resisted implementation of guidelines that called for use of costly drugs or equipment, while clinicians applauded the recommendations (Ints.). In light of all these implementation hurdles, protocols seem unlikely in the near future to provide trust or HA managers with unassailable criteria for assessing and controlling clinical practice.

In summary, except for efforts to attract contracts from GP fundholders, trust managers had limited opportunities and incentives to engage in market competition. Throughout the period of the internal market reforms, hospital managers devoted most of their energy to maintaining adequate hospital services with increasingly tight resources. At the same time they struggled to attain efficiency gains and waiting list reductions imposed by central government. The trust managers faced severe limitations in their capacity to rationalize services, improve their quality, and market them to purchasers. Chief among these constraints were government intervention and regulation, limited information-management capacities, and opposition to change by physicians and other stakeholders. During the internal market reforms, hospital physicians' successfully resisted most efforts by trust managers, HAs, and the central government to rationalize hospital care and gain control of quality management.

CONCLUSION

This chapter showed how the government's tight fiscal and managerial controls over NHS hospitals and public purchasing agencies (health authorities) often hampered its own policies of generating competition among NHS providers. Moreover, the chapter examined how political, organizational, and technical barriers restricted choice of providers by public purchasers and limited the effectiveness of purchasing contracts. In contrast, GP fundholders were more able to switch providers and attain service improvements and price concessions from them. Hospital managers faced severe funding constraints and many additional limitations to their capacity to rationalize and market services.

NOTES

1 This background sketch is too brief to portray the complex process of negotiations among health-policy actors that led to formulation and implementation of the General Management programs and the Internal Market reforms (see Klein, 1995; Wistow and Harrison, 1998).

2 The Community Care reform (Wistow and Harrison, 1998), which shifted responsibilities to local government, was an important exception to the trend toward centralization of governmental control.

3 This grant covered about one third of local Social Service Department expenditures, while national grants together accounted for around 85% of municipal expenditures (Wistow, 1997).

4 That is, spending in 1992–93 was 115% of spending in 1989–90. See Chapter 1, footnote 4 on reporting of changes over time.

5 In 1997 additional reports on decisions to moderate reconfiguration plans appeared in the *Health Service Journal* and *Lancet*.

6 This chapter concentrates on data from England. For data on Wales see Warner (1993). For Scotland see Kendrick (1995).

7 The newly reorganized HAs originally followed the geographic lines of the former districts. However, there were many subsequent mergers and boundary changes (Harrison and New, 1996). A further reorganization in 1996 eliminated the former Regions and District HAs, while preserving the HA form.

8 In Scotland GP fundholding was running at only about half the level of England and Wales (Kendrick, 1995).

9 In Scotland as well, most hospitals had become trusts by 1995 (Kendrick, 1995).

10 Reports of protests often appeared in the *Health Service Journal* and the daily press.

11 See pp. 70–72 in Chapter 3.

12 The trend in deployment of nurses was reported in my interviews and is often mentioned in articles on cost-saving in hospitals.

13 There was a steady rise in nurses throughout the 1980s, a small drop in 1990, an increase for 1991 and 1992, and then a steady decline through to 1997.

14 The General Medical Council is a body charged by law with assuring the competence and professional behavior of physicians. Financed by the medical profession, its membership and policies are dominated by physicians (Smith, 2001).

3

Outcomes of Market Reform in the United Kingdom and Labour's New Health Policies

This chapter examines outcomes triggered by the Conservatives' internal market programs in terms of the four implementation frames developed in Chapter 1. It then shows how Prime Minister Blair and his colleagues abandoned pursuit of reform through competitive forces, while retaining many other features of the health policies of previous governments.

OUTCOMES

It is hard to distinguish effects of the nascent quasi-market on NHS purchasers and providers from the more direct and powerful effects of government-imposed incentives and controls. Throughout the reforms, the central government enforced strict fiscal and performance targets for HAs. While reigning in spending for many HA and trust operations, the government simultaneously boosted allocations for fundholding, new managerial positions, information processing, and reduction of waiting lists. A further challenge to evaluating the reforms comes from the concurrent impact on the health system of unrelated social and technological changes, such as diffusion of minimally invasive forms of diagnosis and surgery (Ints., see Chapter 1). In addition, by the mid-1990s increased training requirements for junior doctors (Paice et al., 2000), made it harder for hospitals to employ juniors as an 'extra pair of hands' and led to the closure of hospital units that could not provide adequate specialty training (Ints.).

Lack of solid data and systematic evaluation studies further hinders assessment of market reform in the UK (Le Grand et al., 1998), as in other countries (see

Chapter 1 and Kalo, 2000/2001). Furthermore, the official NHS measure of hospital activity in terms of Finished Consultant Episodes (FCEs), adopted on the eve of the reforms, seriously overstates service production and the treatment of individual patients (Ints. Seng et al., 1993; Radical Statistics Health Group, 1995; Hamblin, 1998). Each time a patient is transferred to another specialist or unit within the hospital, the FCE measure the movement as a completed episode. FCEs and other official NHS measures, such as occupancy levels, day surgery rates, length of stay, and waiting times for hospital admission have been repeatedly attacked as invalid, non-comprehensive, and vulnerable to manipulation by managers anxious to demonstrate improvements in performance (Clarke et al., 1993; Pettiger, 1997; Morgan et al., 1999).[1] A further assessment difficulty is that improvements on hospital-wide measures can mask enduring inefficiencies in crucial fields like orthopedic surgery – which contribute substantially to waiting lists and lead patients to turn to private practitioners (Millar, 1996; Yates et al., 2000).

The outcomes of the reforms appear very mixed when viewed through the *administrative frame* – which focuses on top-down implementation and attainment of declared policy objectives. The central government did succeed in rapidly enacting and diffusing the main structural changes needed to launch a market for publicly-funded health care. The government also succeeded in its efforts to privatize some NHS operations – including capital construction and social care for geriatric patients – while encouraging gradual privatization in other areas, like dentistry. The trend toward privatization is partly reflected in a rise in out-of-pocket payments as a proportion of total health expenditures – from 10.6% in 1990 (the first year for which data are available) to 11.1% in 1996. However, figures on the proportion of total health expenditure coming from the private sector in the early 1990s do not show an impact of privatization.[2]

More importantly, however, there was only partial implementation of the market-like *processes* that were supposed to help purchasers obtain value for money. Governmental interventions and controls prevented the development of the market-like exchanges that were expected to lead providers to become more efficient and improve service quality. By tightening its chain of command, the central government forced HAs and trusts to devote much of their energy to meeting just a few fiscal and performance targets. Moreover, the DOH and NHS Executive upstaged the market by controlling HA budgets and steering decisions by HAs and regions about service reductions and reconfigurations.

In the end, the reforms failed to create two critical conditions under which neo-liberal theories expect market forces to create incentives for provider efficiency and quality: vigorous provider competition and rational choice of services by commissioners (purchasers). Competition among hospital trusts was largely restricted to attempts to attract contracts from fundholders, rather than HAs. HA managers typically remained loyal to former district general hospitals. When they did contemplate contracting for services elsewhere, they encountered reluctance among patients and local political opposition.

Contracting between the trusts and HA commissioners more closely resembled budgeting processes like those used before the market reforms, than systematic, rational choice of value in the market. Neither HA managers nor GP fundholders developed the needed capacity to assess the quality and costs of provider services or judge the cost-effectiveness of services. Thus HAs and fundholders could not really reward efficient and high-quality providers, and HAs could hardly engage in strategic purchasing. Trust managers, in turn, usually lacked the power, autonomy, information systems, and managerial controls needed to run the hospitals as competitive, not-for-profit firms. Carefully guarding their clinical autonomy and power, hospital physicians blocked or delayed many efforts by hospital managers to introduce business practices that would tighten managerial control over their work or reduce hospital services. In contrast, many specialists did cooperate in marketing services to GP fundholders.

When judged in terms of the reforms' declared objectives, the record of the internal market reforms is not impressive. Where limited provider competition did emerge, it did not typically yield the many positive effects that were anticipated by its advocates. On the positive side of the market reforms' balance sheet, official statistics show greater increases in hospital activity during the period than in earlier periods (Mulligan, 1998a). There were also reductions in waiting lists and further declines in length of stay between 1991 and 1996 (Le Grand et al., 1998). Average length of stay in acute settings, which had plummeted by over 30% during the 1980s, dropped 14% between 1989 and 1996 (from 5.8 to 5.0 days) (OECD, 2001).[3] Furthermore, according to official figures, real costs rose more slowly than hospital activity, so that efficiency increased during the reforms (Le Grand, 1999). As noted, market competition was not the primary driving force for these changes. Moreover, gains in productivity (activity divided by cost) only constitute efficiency improvements if quality remains constant or improves. As will be seen below, along some dimensions hospital quality may actually have declined during the reforms.

The gains in hospital activity just discussed were accompanied by substantial growth in managerial costs for both purchasers and providers. These expenditures reflected the proliferation of contracts, data management, monitoring, and decision activities associated with the market reforms, along with the intensification of governmental controls over HAs and trusts (Le Grand et al., 1998). Besides adding managers, during the 1990s, NHS trusts assigned extra managerial tasks and responsibilities to many nurses, physicians, and other health professionals (Ints.). Management costs were particularly heavy in fundholding practices (Goodwin, 1998) and, contrary to expectations, turned out to be even higher for the larger, total purchasing pilots, than for the smaller fundholders (Killoran et al., 1998). It is difficult to estimate precisely the increased managerial costs or their impact on service production.[4] Nor is it clear how much of the increased transaction costs resulted directly from the internal market, as opposed to gradual expansion in the NHS managerial infrastructure, which had begun in the 1980s (Appleby, 1995).

Even if the productivity improvements reported by the NHS are genuine, they cannot be attributed mainly to the introduction of the quasi-market. There is no convincing evidence that greater exposure to competition produced more substantial improvements in trust production and efficiency (i.e., productivity)

(Hamblin, 1998), as anticipated by neo-liberal economists, advocates of the New Public Management, and government spokespersons.[5] A further reason not to attribute productivity changes to market forces is that improvements on key indicators of throughput, such as length of stay and outpatient treatment, began long *before* the market reforms. These improvements responded to powerful non-market forces, including new medical technologies and top-down governmental pressure for cost-containment. Rather than reflecting market forces, most genuine productivity improvements during the early 1990s probably simply reflected dramatic improvements in cash flows from the government (Appleby et al., 1994; Maynard, 1993).

Research on GP fundholding also yielded very mixed evidence on the impacts of competitive contracting on trust and system efficiency. Advocates of fundholding expected the scheme to enhance hospital efficiency and effectiveness by creating incentives for fundholder savings similar to those found in American health maintenance organizations. To bring down costs, fundholders would trim unnecessary referrals to hospitals, reduce their patients' hospital stays, and substitute services within primary care clinics for hospital services. The fundholders would then reinvest their budget savings in improvements in primary and community care. In practice, fundholders in the early waves mainly reduced costs by negotiating lower hospital charges. Early fundholders gained faster treatment for their patients but were no more successful than non-fundholders in reducing their patients' length of stay (Goodwin, 1998). On the other hand, fundholders in total purchasing schemes, who received delegated budgets from HAs and directly purchased hospital care, did attain shorter hospital stays (Goodwin et al., 1998). Since reduced hospital charges to fundholders raised HA costs (Le Grand et al.,1998), the savings obtained by the fundholders did not contribute to savings or efficiency for whole NHS areas or the entire NHS.

Except for fundholding's impact on hospital services, its documented attainments fell short of its advocates' expectations. Longitudinal and comparative research uncovered no consistent evidence that fundholding led to changes in referral practices or produced significant substitution of community services for those previously provided by hospitals (Godsen and Torgersen, 1997; Goodwin, 1998). More fundholders than non-fundholders expanded their primary care practices into areas like physiotherapy, ophthalmology, and care of the chronically ill. However, other forces had a greater influence than fundholding on practice expansion and related steps towards more effective primary care. These forces included the GP contract and a wide range of individual, organizational, managerial, and contextual factors. (Goodwin, 1998; Mays and Dixon, 1996; Mays and Mulligan, 1998; Mulligan, 1998b). Fundholders were somewhat more successful than non-fundholding GPs at holding down growth in drug costs (Godsen and Torgersen, 1997). However, the cost advantages of fundholders compared to non-fundholders were most dramatic during the first year of fundholding and disappeared after the third year (Harris and Scrivener, 1996).[6]

There is considerable debate as to whether fundholders spent their savings in ways that provided good 'value for money' for patients and the health system as a whole (Audit Commission, 1996b, p. 72) or mainly translated governmental subsidies and budget savings into personal gain. Fundholders spent most of their budgetary savings on improvements in their primary care premises and equipment, while investing much smaller amounts in extra hospital and community care. Despite very high management costs, most GP fundholders failed to develop important contracting, monitoring, and budgeting processes, which could have directly contributed to the efficiency and effectiveness of contracting for care (Audit Commission, 1996b).

The modest gains for patients created by fundholding have to be weighed against its high costs, which stemmed from generous government support to fundholding practices and high management costs. In addition, the fundholding program deepened inequality among NHS patients (Glennerster et al., 1994; Goodwin, 1998). The available evidence shows that fundholding led to preferential hospital treatment for patients of fundholders (Goodwin, 1998; Hamblin, 1998; Ints.). What is more, fundholding was considerably less common in inner cities and other areas of social and economic deprivation than in the better-off areas (Audit Commission, 1966b, p. 10). Hence, the scheme further aggravated prior socio-economic differences in access to hospital services.

In summary, the reform outcomes reviewed so far raise serious doubts about the feasibility of using market forces to boost provider and health system efficiency in the UK. So long as the politicians responsible for overseeing the health system remain publicly committed to providing comprehensive health care that is universal, equitable, and affordable, there are limited prospects for market-driven change.[7]

Another set of outcomes that warrant close examination through the administrative frame relate to the quality of NHS care. Waiting times for elective admissions are a form of service quality that is closely linked to hospital efficiency. The declines that occurred in waiting times during the reforms cannot be attributed mainly to market processes, since waiting time became the target of top-down programs and earmarked funding in 1987, several years before implementation of the market reforms. Moreover, between 1991 and 1993 hospitals that had reorganized as trusts reported smaller improvements in waiting times than hospitals that continued under the direct management of the HAs (Hamblin, 1998). Measurement of time to admission for elective patients masked other features of service, like time to treatment for patients visiting Accident and Emergency departments, which did not improve and even worsened as the reforms moved into full swing (Gould, 1998). Moreover, hospitals diverted energy to meeting measured standards, at the expense of other dimensions of service. For instance, the national Audit Commission found that hospitals with the shortest waiting times between emergency admission and assessment – a measure of conformity to a Patient's Charter standard – had the longest times for treatment and discharge – processes that were not assessed under the Patient's Charter (Butler, 1995 December 7).

The improvements in waiting times and other trust services that GP fundholders attained for their patients did not produce system-wide benefits. Thus, for the NHS as a whole, fundholding failed to push hospital and community providers toward higher quality, more effective, and less costly care (Audit Commission, 1996b).

On the whole, the internal market reforms had no direct positive effects on clinical quality in trusts (Hamblin, 1998). Nor is there any evidence that clinical audit programs, which were to help providers meet purchaser demand for higher quality, actually improved clinical quality in either hospitals or community settings (Cervi, 1996).

In fact, introduction of the internal market seems to have harmed certain aspects of clinical quality, while weakening the continuity and coordination of care across organizational and sectoral boundaries. According to GPs and other primary caregivers, there was a growing tendency during the reforms for hospital trusts to 'dump' patients onto primary care, by releasing them earlier than was advisable (Ints.; Francome and Marks, 1996, p. 69; Scott; and Wordsworth, 1999).[8] A report by the Health Advisory Service attributed the hospitals' overemphasis on rapid throughput of elderly people in acute wards to perverse incentives built into the productivity measures used in hospital contracts (Millar, 1997). The government's requirement that hospitals attain annual efficiency gains probably also contributed to premature release of patients. Statistical analysis of data on the first four years of the reform in Scottish hospitals also points to mixed results on clinical quality, as measured by post-hospital mortality (Maniadakis et al., 1999).[9]

Another indication of declining hospital quality came in emergency care crises that recurred each winter (Chadda, 1997). Rather than directly resulting from the internal market reforms, these crises reflected loss of spare capacity by hospitals, as a result of bed cuts that had gone on since the 1980s.[10] The admissions' crises also indicated that reorganization of directly managed hospitals as trusts did not substantially enhance their flexibility in resource allocation. Moreover, the crises pointed to the failure of HA contracts to anticipate predictable seasonal fluctuations in demand and shift elective work from winter to summer (Jones, 1997).

Disturbing episodes of clinical and organizational ineffectiveness in hospitals also came to light during the reforms ('An unhealthy...', 1997; Dyer, 1995). There was no direct connection between these episodes and governmental programs. Moreover, the underlying quality problems predated the reforms and were characteristic of other advanced nations (e.g., Rosenthal, 1995; Committee on Quality of Health Care in America, 2001). Nonetheless, the quality scandals made clear that the reforms of the 1980s and early 1990s had not prevented failures of both managerial supervision and professional self-regulation (Smith, 1998). Exposure of these failures triggered efforts by the Blair Government and the medical profession to tighten regulation of professional work.

While polls showed continuing confidence in the NHS, dissatisfaction with the quality of the services grew during the reforms (Mulligan and Judge, 1997). In like manner, complaints against doctors increased rapidly during the reforms (Irvine, 1999), and malpractice awards continued to rise (Harrison and New, 1997). Politicians also expressed increasing concern about NHS quality. These trends probably reflect critical media coverage of NHS quality, changing attitudes, and legal developments, more than changes in objective conditions.

Coordination among caregivers and continuity of care, which are crucial to quality, suffered under the reforms. The purchaser-provider split and fundholding deepened existing structural and financial divisions within and between primary care, hospitals, and social-care and heightened the potential for rivalry and conflict among care sectors and providers (Millar, B. 1997; Muijen and Ford, 1996; Wistow, 1995). The mentally ill especially suffered from lack of coordination among care sectors, as the closure of long-term care beds made them ever more dependent on community care ('From Bedlam to bedsit' 1995). Toward the end of the market reform period, governmental policy makers, local commissioners, and providers acknowledged the serious problem of care discontinuity and began to seek solutions to it (Ints., Hamblin, 1998; Mc Cormick, 1998; Wistow, 1997)

Enhancing patient choice and empowerment were yet additional system-wide goals for the reforms, as declared in *Working for Patients* and later policy statements. The reforms did give patients more flexibility in their choice of GPs, and the Patient's Charter promoted specific service improvements that were important to much of the public. Moreover, GP fundholders acted as advocates for patients within the hospital system. However, other practices associated with the reforms actually reduced the unmediated influence of patients and public representatives within the NHS. Patients could no longer ask their GPs to refer them to the specialist or hospital of their choice. Instead, the contracts that HAs and GP fundholders signed with hospitals determined referrals. Patients and local interest groups also lost political power under the reforms. Representation of local politicians on HA boards was eliminated, and these boards became directly accountable only to the Secretary of State for Health (Ferlie et al., 1996). In response to government pressure, HAs attempted to solicit the views of patients and involve them in decisions about purchasing and planning decisions. These activities were mostly short-term, superficial exercises, that focused on narrowly-selected groups (Milewa et al., 1998; Mulligan, 1998a). The dissemination of information to the public was also very limited. In the end, the reforms failed to make decisionmaking in either the trusts or the HAs more transparent to the public at large (Le Grand et al., 1998).

Neither the introduction of the internal market nor the subsequent massive increase in funds set the NHS on sound financial ground, as the government promised would be the case. Instead, funding levels continued to lag far behind demand and fell short of spending levels in most other advanced industrial nations (see Figure 1.1 on page 4). Many trusts experienced intense cost pressures during the reforms (Dixon, 1997), and the number of HAs operating in the red tripled between the fiscal years of 1994–95 and 1995–96 ('Three quarters...', 1997). These funding pressures resulted from macro-level trends like population demographics, local factors, and unintended outcomes of incentives to cut waiting lists and increase throughputs in many trusts (Dixon et al., 1996).

According to official pronouncements, the reforms aimed to preserve and even enhance the capacity of the NHS to provide health care to the public on the basis of clinical need, regardless of ability to pay – a traditional NHS goal, that was rearticulated in the Patient's Charters of 1991 and 1995. When the reforms are evaluated in terms of such broad NHS goals, fundamental failures become evident. Instead of extending publicly-funded health care, the internal market reforms continued a trend that prevailed throughout the 1980s of curtailing NHS services and shifting them to the private sector. During the market reforms the government introduced ever-stricter limits and higher co-payments for NHS dental care, increased co-payments for ophthalmology and privatized much of this field, and withdrew NHS-funded nursing care for the elderly. (Harrison and New, 1996; Paton, 2000). There were also increases in co-payments for pharmaceuticals (Heath, 1994). By placing heavy stress on the financial accountability of each purchaser and provider, the government also encouraged local NHS decisionmakers to curtail services or attempt to shift them out of their budgets.[11]

In the final analysis, the market reforms further reduced the capacity of the NHS to pursue its most fundamental mandate of improving the health of the population. Attainment of this goal required sustaining specialized, hospital care while strengthening patient education and preventive medicine in the community, adapting local services to the needs of special groups, enhancing links between community care and hospitals, and coordinating social and health services. Instead of promoting wellness and a strategic approach to health care, as proposed by the Health of the Nation policies (Secretary of State for Health, 1992), the government directed attention toward formal structural change and narrow fiscal and performance targets for hospital (Ints., Mulligan, 1998a). As a result, none of the key actors in the NHS and in local authorities invested much time or resources in activities that could have contributed to meeting the targets set by the Health of the Nation strategy (Department of Health, 1998)

The *bargaining frame* calls attention to a very different set of outcomes than those just reviewed. From this perspective, the most dramatic *national-level* development was further centralization of governmental power over health politics and health system operations (Klein, 1998c). This process of centralization was not directly related to purchaser competition, but it did make use of the business accounting and reporting procedures that were a central feature of the internal market reorganization. Rather than curtailing heavy-handed governmental control over the health system, as advocated by neo-classical economic theorists and the Conservative Party, between 1989 and 1996 the governments of Margaret Thatcher and John Major continued to tighten their chain of control over NHS organizations and practitioners. These Governments also directly intervened in the workings of the market in places like London, so as to minimize disruption of services that were popular with voters and powerful stakeholder groups.

Governmental policies and actions also gradually curtailed the national strategic influence of the medical profession and made some inroads into physicians' clinical autonomy. Most notably, the government excluded the physicians' national representatives from traditional policymaking channels, thereby bypassing opposition to its programs. The GP Contract of 1990 constrained the GPs' economic and operational control over their work by specifying health promotion tasks which were to be reported in detail and were subject to performance-based pay (Calnan and Williams, 1995). Later, the government developed provisions that would shift some GPs from their traditional status as independent contractors to that of salaried employees within practices. The government also tried, without much success, to enforce hospital consultants' contracts in ways that would tie pay more closely to performance and reduce opportunities for private practice.

The empowerment of GPs as fundholders appears to be the most notable exception to this governmental drive for control over the medical professions. Yet fundholding weakened the medical profession's *national* influence by creating two divergent camps among primary care physicians and deepening long-standing divisions between GPs and hospital clinicians. Hence fundholding made it harder for the BMA or the GPs to adopt a united stance on national reforms and other health policies. In contrast, as will be seen below, fundholding policies enhanced the GPs' *district-level* influence on HAs and hospital physicians.

Despite these inroads into the physicians' national strategic influence, governmental pressures for medical accountability had the unexpected effect of strengthening the operational control of national professional bodies over their members (Allsop, 1998). Faced with growing public demand for restrictions on problematic doctors and assurance of the quality of medical practice (Stacey, 1992), the General Medical Council, and the Royal Colleges (which represent medical specialties), accepted increasing responsibility for supervision of practitioners, development and application of quality standards, and promotion of evidence-based medicine (Irvine, 1997a, 1997b). These moves were supported by the cabinet and Parliament.

At the *district and organization* levels, the reforms expanded the ranks and influence of managers, and particularly of finance managers, within trusts and HAs (Ferlie et al., 1996). Evaluation of hospital managers on the basis of the trust's financial performance often drove a wedge between cost-conscious managers and health professionals, who generally sought to preserve and even expand existing services. Tension rose between managers and health professionals, as managerial influence over physicians and nurses grew. Hospital physicians faced increasingly tight resources, stress on financial accountability and performance improvements, and pressure to give preference to patients who had waited longest for elective surgery (Ints.; Moore, 1995) or had been referred by fundholders. The burden of extra clinical and administrative work that resulted from these organizational changes fell even more heavily on nurses than physicians (Harrison and Pollit, 1994; Robinson, 1993).

Physicians in former district general hospitals felt greater pressures from service cutbacks and provider competition than physicians in specialty hospitals. The specialty hospitals were less vulnerable, because they often provided unique services for an entire district or region (Ints.). But even in specialty hospitals, tight cash constraints provided consultants with less opportunities to initiate changes that would gradually influence hospital strategy. When physicians did propose technology acquisition and new services, non-medical managers judged the proposals more in terms of cost than potential clinical benefits (Ints.).

Notwithstanding such tensions, informal coalitions between managers and consultants periodically developed. In some hospitals, trust managers rewarded consultants who attracted contracts from fundholders or generated other additional sources of revenues. As the Medical Director of Greenham Hospital bluntly put it, 'In the end, if patients are paid for, they bring power'. Managers in both trusts and HAs also made common cause with their professional employees and with local politicians in efforts to avoid closures of hospital facilities or funding cuts.

Although hospital consultants lost some strategic and managerial control within trusts, these senior clinicians continued to be very influential and to enjoy substantial clinical and economic autonomy. Highly prestigious and influential consultants were especially able to resist control by non-medical managers and clinical directors (Ints.). The power of these elite consultants stemmed from the fact that both clinical directors and non-medical managers ultimately depended on the consultants for medical expertise (Ints., Rosen and Mays, 1998), cooperation in attaining performance targets, implementing change, and mobilizing informal political support among the medical staff (Ints.). In consequence, non-medical managers and clinical directors usually avoided direct confrontations with senior physicians over issues of medical practice. Moreover, hospital physicians retained control over clinical audits and remained highly autonomous in their clinical practices (Ints.). Consultants also continued to enjoy much flexibility in their allocations of their time – as they took advantage of spotty enforcement of job plans and contracts, which had changed little since the pre-reform period (Int., Moore, 1999; Yates, 1995; Audit Commission, 1996a).

Unlike hospital physicians, many primary care physicians directly benefited from the reforms. Fundholding gave GPs more economic, managerial, and strategic control over their work by creating opportunities to deploy patient care budgets in keeping with their professional judgment and personal preferences. Nor did fundholders sacrifice operational autonomy in exchange for participation in the program. For the most part, fundholders do not appear to have altered their clinical behavior in areas like diagnosis and surgery in response to financial incentives contained within the fundholding scheme (Coulter, 1998). Moreover, there is no evidence that either fundholders or non-fundholding GPs ordinarily changed their clinical practices in response to clinical audits or exposure to clinical protocols. What is more, both types of GPs often bypassed potential constraints on their autonomy contained within the GP Contract. Instead of personally carrying out the health promotion tasks listed in the Contract, GPs assigned the tasks to their practice nurses. Then the physicians reported performing the tasks and received payment for them (Broadbent, 1998).

Total fundholding, locality commissioning, and GP commissioning programs all enhanced communication and cooperation among groups of GPs, gave the GPs more influence over the delivery of care within the community, and enhanced their influence over decisions made within HAs. Fundholding also strengthened the leverage that GPs could exercise over hospital consultants and managers. However, the power and influence of the new forms of primary care organization over HAs and trusts should not be exaggerated. In the final analysis, fundholding and the other GP commissioning experiments could not bridge the gap in status and professional expertise between GPs and hospital consultants (Ints.) and did not radically modify prevailing attitudes and patterns of interaction between the two groups (e.g., Somerset et al., 1999; Marshall, 1999).

Probably the most visible and dramatic *interpretive* outcome was the transformation of NHS rhetoric. This shift in discourse did more than rename existing NHS activities and provide labels for new ones. It implied new ways of valuing, justifying, and evaluating the activities of HAs, hospitals, GPs, and the NHS as a system. As implementation progressed, language from the realms of the marketplace and corporate management displaced much of the terminology of bureaucratic budgeting and control. Managerial memos and talk were filled with terms like purchasing (and later, commissioning), contracting, providing, attaining value for money, competition, marketing, pricing, costs, financial returns, and efficiency. In annual performance reviews of trusts, HAs, and their chief executives, staff from the NHS Executive concentrated on financial and operational performance standards 'where it can see immediate results'. These reviews left little room for assessment of the quality of hospital care (Ints.).

Top government and NHS officials led this sea change in NHS rhetoric. Mid-level officers in the NHS, executives in trusts and HAs quickly adopted the new terminology and symbolism (Bennett and Ferlie, 1996; Kitchener, 1998; Walshe et al., 1997). They did so either because they identified with the goals and means of the new programs or sought to conform to normative pressures to adopt the new discourse. As shown above, the behavior of the central government and of local purchasers and providers changed far less than their discourse.

Although trust and HA managers – and to a lesser degree health professionals – learned to use terms from the market and corporate accounting, they also continued to use discourse that predated the market reforms. Physicians, for example, continued to talk – and presumably to think – more in terms of their individual practices, advances in medical practice and technology, and their own career paths than in terms of competition, contracts, and prices (Ints.). Managers in HAs and trusts also continued to use terms and phrases that fit the pre-market regime and the everyday realities of bureaucratic control and health politics. Here, for example, is what a general hospital director said about the difficulty of reducing a serious, recurring operating deficit and also meeting the 3% efficiency target imposed by central government:

> The purchasers [HAs] are enforcing a national policy of efficiency gains, and this can be difficult ... I want to cut services [to meet the target] and want to know if they [i.e., HA and the regional managers] back the cuts. They said they weren't politically acceptable and preferred the deficit in a pre-election year.

As this quotation suggests, when interviewed under conditions of anonymity, managers did not describe contracting in the market place as a prime concern. Instead, they talked about their struggle to keep the system running and meet the conflicting expectations of central government and multiple stakeholders.

As the difficulties and political risks of implementing market-like competition among trusts became evident, officials in central government and at the top of the NHS hierarchy began to shift their rhetoric. Gradually their new catchwords and vocabularies diffused to HAs, trusts, and community clinics. Chief among these new waves of rhetoric was an emphasis on cooperation and coordination among NHS providers and purchasers. Talk of 'commissioning' and 'consultation', rather than purchasing and competition, signaled the shift. Official talk and activity also began to express the need for HAs to ration care and choose systematically among care through evidence-based medicine.

A related theme concerned strategic commissioning by HAs, which was to reflect the needs of the local population and the cost-effectiveness of alternative forms and settings for prevention, diagnosis, and treatment. At the same time that the government advocated sensitivity to local health care needs, the GP Contract, with its behavioristic approach to promoting preventive medicine and patient education, embodied a narrow and less flexible conception of health improvement. In like manner, the Health Improvement Strategy of 1992 set out a very narrow range of operational targets, even though its architects spoke of encouraging a strategic approach to health enhancement. In the end, these initiatives had very little effect on the ways that health purchasers and providers defined their missions and responsibilities (Crail, 1998; Department of Health, 1998).

Empowerment of patients as consumers was yet another theme sounded periodically by Government and NHS spokespersons. The HAs took up this theme at times, but they did not often rework their operating priorities to fit the new rhetoric (Jordan et al., 1998). Instead, according to one in-depth study (Harrison and Mort, 1998), local NHS managers selectively evoked user input in ways that supported the managers' own views and helped legitimate the HA's role in the community.

It was harder for managers in HAs and trusts and health professionals to implement the policies signalled by the many shifts in government rhetoric than for senior governmental and NHS officials to enunciate new policies or reaffirm old ones. Still, by adopting the new vocabularies of action and reporting on progress toward new policy objectives, local managers could sometimes satisfy senior health officials and politicians and improve their standing and legitimacy with their immediate supervisors and external stakeholders. As is often the case in professional organizations (Meyer and Rowan, 1977), adoption of new terms and symbols may actually have helped insulate NHS professionals and managers from pressure to make concrete changes in well-established practices.

Although adoption of fashionable rhetoric brought organizational benefits, rapid shifts in NHS terminology and program objectives made many local managers and professionals feel stressed, vulnerable to the whims of policy fashion, and skeptical about prospects for meaningful change. Dr. J, head of the medical division at Nileston, clearly expressed this sense of overload and skepticism as he listed the hospital's many quality programs and the new roles and units established to run the programs – including an audit department, clinical practice groups, and Patient's Charter units:

> We have half a dozen departments looking at parallel developments in quality of care. We ought to have a good wheel by now, since we have reinvented it a half a dozen times! But there is a lack of integration [among units and programs]. We

need a negotiated process of pooling resources [and involving people]. We have an inadequate information technology structure. The data to support clinical effectiveness programs are lacking.

70

Although the reforms led to a transformation of NHS discourse, it is not clear how deeply they changed managerial and professional culture. On the one hand, recruitment of many managers from industry and commerce, combined with short-term contracts, forged a cadre of managers who voiced few fundamental reservations about governmental policies. On the other hand, insiders suggested that managers held more divergent views than those they expressed in public. A former NHS researcher described the situation this way: 'The [Thatcher–Major] Government has been in power long enough, so that to work in NHS [as a manager] you either have to be right wing or keep your mouth shut'. In like manner, my interviews uncovered a wide variety of managerial orientations, ranging from enthusiastic embracement of the reforms to skepticism (see, for example, the profiles of Mellstock and Sandbourne HAs in Chapter 2). Some informants expressed hope that the coming elections would bring an end to the government's over-emphasis on short-term outcomes and market processes, while others took for granted that the reform process would continue and would be accompanied by further shifts in policies and programs.

In stark contrast to managerial culture, the occupational culture of hospital physicians changed more slowly during the reforms. Although specialists became more aware of budgetary and market considerations, few seem to have viewed these external forces as anything other than unavoidable constraints on sound medical practice (Ints.; Jones and Dewing, 1997; McNulty et al., 1995; Laing and Galbraith, 1996). For example, a specialist bitterly contrasted his hospital's lack of funds for new diagnostic instruments with the 'glossy-image of round-the-clock care' projected by hospital management.

Instead of acknowledging the centrality of budgets and marketing, most hospital physicians continued to treat specialized clinical expertise and individual clinical autonomy as unalterable foundations of modern medical practice. These underlying orientations came to the fore in the physicians' hostility to the imposition of non-clinical priorities on their work. For instance, physicians objected to pursuit of targets like reduction of waiting lists, because attention to these targets could force hospital staff to give preference to less clinically urgent patients (Ints.). In like manner, many physicians expressed distrust and skepticism about attempts by non-medical managers to measure and monitor the nature and outcomes of medical work. Many clinicians even doubted the value of physician-led programs of quality assessment and assurance, like clinical audit. 'We do it because the purchasers want it', was the laconic evaluation of audit offered by one clinical director (Int.).

Even though they might acknowledge the research benefits of developing case mix and hospital activity codes, many hospital physicians seem to have agreed with the physician who described the actual coding processes as 'rubbish and laughable' (Int.). Some hospital physicians also resented pressures to pay more attention to the preferences of fundholders and patients (Ints.). GPs, like patients, traditionally exercised little influence on hospital practice, and many hospital specialists continued to view them as lacking in both medical knowledge and prestige.

The consultants' traditional orientations toward clinical autonomy and expertise also came to light in their resistance to managerial control or guidance by clinical directors. In consequence, clinical directors were loath to challenge consultants on non-clinical grounds, even when the directors did not fully accept their colleagues' norms and assumptions (Ints.). This hesitation is evident in the comments of Dr. P, Clinical Director of Oncology at Milford:

Dr. P: There are places that the clinical director has responsibility for supervising clinical practice, but not here.

MH: Why?

Dr. P: We have consultants with national and international reputations. You can't challenge their clinical practice as you could in a District General Hospital's general surgery [ward]. The issue is fundamental: The right of the doctor to do what he sees is right is enshrined in many documents, but it clashes with resource considerations.

MH: One way might be to get doctors to agree to protocols.

Dr. P: I've tried this in the area of drug budgets for oncology. Finance says [the costs are] spiraling. Most of our patients are taking part in clinical trials involving new drugs. These are hot spots – very expensive drugs. I am close to having to say 'We can't afford the expensive drug'. The clinicians are not sympathetic to management doing this. They say we have crossed the divide. You run the risk of adverse publicity [from] colleagues. You have to do it [restrict costs] on the basis of evidence. You have got to be seen as clinically committed and lacking in [professional] defects.

Although the majority of hospital specialists failed to identify with the principles of marketing and corporate management, a small group did begin to adopt these business orientations. Sometimes they blended the market approach with fierce loyalty to their specialty. In hospitals that delegated budgets to directorates, consultants in marketable specialties could reap benefits for their unit and themselves by aggressively generating revenues while controlling costs. Consider, for example, the views of Dr. B, the entrepreneurially-oriented clinical director in Greenham Hospital, whose outreach work with GPs was described in Chapter 2:

Dr. B made it clear that he expected the finance department to reward his unit for bringing in revenues from GP contracts and outpatient services provided for other hospitals. He took a dim view of colleagues who objected to management's policy of linking departmental budgets to the generation of extra revenues. As he explained, 'There is no reason why my team should subsidize other teams that underperform due to idleness, mismanagement, or poor expertise. If you don't take my approach, you might as well go back to the old system where budget allocations depended on how much you wept or shouted. The whole principle of the NHS is that money should follow the patient'.

In his uncompromising endorsement of the new rules for departmental budgeting, Dr. B treats the hospital as a set of autonomous and competing specialties. He completely ignores objective differences within and among specialties in the marketability of services.

Fundholders – and particularly those in the first waves of fundholding (see Glennerster et al., 1994) – more often embraced the principles of the internal market than did other types of physicians. However, there were substantial variations in the fundholders' degree of conviction about market principles (Francome and Marks, 1996, p. 70, Table 4.2; Calnan and Williams, 1995). Many physicians who joined the earliest waves of fundholding (e.g., Maddox, 1999) saw the program as providing opportunities for enhancing the care they could provide their patients. The contrast between support for the reforms among these GPs and the hostility to the early market reforms shown by many hospital clinicians reflects fundamental organizational and institutional divergences between the two sectors. The internal market policies presaged a much less radical break with past practices for GPs than was the case for hospital physicians. Since 1948, GPs had operated as independent entrepreneurs under contract with the NHS. Under the 1990 GP contract, 60% of the GP's income came from capitation payments (Farmer, 1993). In contrast, until the market reforms, hospital clinicians received salaries that were unrelated to their productivity in the hospital or to their contributions to hospital revenue flows. Consultants who wanted to act as independent practitioners established lucrative private practices outside the hospital, while still enjoying the facilities, prestige, and security of hospital employment.

Despite the GPs' initial support for fundholding, only a small proportion of all fundholders implemented care and planning practices that reflected strong identification with the fundholding program's objectives (Audit Commission, 1996b). Moreover, GPs in and out of fundholding worried about the program's impact on equality and patient care (Calnan and Williams, 1995) and saw purchasing as a threat to long-term cooperative relations with providers of community services (Williams et al., 1997). Many GPs – including participants in the Primary Care Groups established after the elections – regarded practice management as a burden that would detract from clinical work. The head of one large non-fundholding practice put this view clearly when commenting on total purchasing arrangements, which were favored by Labour on the eve of the general elections:

> I don't think GPs want to get that involved in non-clinical activities. I don't. Purchasing is a managerial skill. I don't want to spend hours getting fluffed up [i.e., hot and bothered] if I'm 10,000 pounds overspent. I want to spend time seeing patients.

In summary, the reforms did not radically alter the physicians' occupational subcultures or span gaps between rank and file physicians and non-medical managers. Fundholders, who were more active in the emerging market than other groups of physicians, used fundholding to build up their own practices.

Only a small proportion of GPs showed interest in the broader goals of the reforms, such as coordinating community services and directing purchasing toward a primary-led NHS. Long-standing barriers of status, power, and medical orientations continued to separate GPs and hospital clinicians. Hospital physicians continued striving to give care without regard to cost, keep up-to-date with technical and clinical advances in their specialties, and enhance their income and career prospects. Sometimes clinicians found ways to make the new market rules work to their personal benefit and that of their specialty. Otherwise, they showed little enthusiasm for the market. Furthermore, because clinicians viewed medicine from the perspective of their own specialty, they were slow to warm to appeals by management to place the good of the hospital before partisan interests. As one trust director put it, seven years after the launch of the internal market, hospital managers and clinicians still formed 'two different and some-times hostile groups of people' (Int.).

The institutional frame directs attention to four ways in which the internal market reforms created important precedents for future health policies and restructured basic institutional arrangements for bargaining and interaction among health policy actors. First, the reforms contributed to an ongoing trend toward centralization of governmental control over health system actors. NHS managers came under tighter fiscal and operational control from the DOH and the NHS executive, while managerial constraints on hospital physicians also intensified. Patients and public representatives lost direct access to NHS decision channels, but fundholding and the Patient's Charter made hospitals more sensitive to some of the patients' needs.

Second, the creation of markets for health and social care – with their processes of costing, contracting, and competition among market players – made the health system even more differentiated than it had been and more subject to market-like negotiation among health-related organizations. The trend toward differentiation gave NHS managers and health practitioners opportunities to work with a wider range of actors than in the past, for example, by contracting for services from external sources. Moreover, differentiation created conditions under which the activities of both purchasers and providers might become more transparent – at least when their activities could be reasonably measured. However, market arrangements like contracting and the new stress within NHS agencies on business management and marketing, pitted provider agencies – and sometimes even units within agencies – against one another in a struggle for scarce resources. As a result of these developments, care delivery became ever more fragmented than it had been prior to the reforms. As contractual relations proliferated, HAs and other agencies faced increasing difficulties in planning and guiding health service development for entire geographical areas or population groups. Furthermore, the market reforms, in tandem with the government's passion for assessing and publicizing short-term results, created incentives for self-interested, calculative behavior, which clashed with norms of reciprocity, cooperation, and trust (Harrison and Lachmann, 1996). One result was gaming the system to meet performance and financial targets (Light, 1990).

Third, the reforms gave rise to growing public, managerial, and governmental pressures for more efficient and higher-quality medical care. Hospital physicians and nurses faced managerial drives to meet government performance targets and use ever-tighter resources to handle increasing patient demand. Moreover, managers increasingly expected doctors and nurses to account for their activities in terms of costs and performance. Evoking the principle of self-regulation, the medical profession succeeded in warding off most efforts at direct managerial or political supervision of clinical work. However, if hospital trusts devolve budgets more fully to clinical directorships, physicians will gradually become more fully exposed to market forces and managerial controls.

Fourth, the reforms helped shift power and resources away from hospitals toward primary care. The trend toward curtailment of hospital facilities and reduction in the proportion of the health budget devoted to hospitals was actually stronger in the 1980s than during the market reforms (OECD, 2001). Nonetheless, the market reforms created organizational structures that enhanced the power and strategic influence of primary care. These structural changes began with fundholding, extended into total purchasing and GP commissioning, and continued in the creation of Primary Care Groups and Primary Care Trusts after the formation of the Labour Government in 1997. Some advocates of the primary-care led NHS envisioned a more radical shift from *medical* care, which revolves around hospitals, to promotion of *health and wellbeing* through community-based services. This radical budgetary and cultural transformation did not take place.

These institutional developments created important precedents for the policies developed by Tony Blair and his Labour Party while they were in opposition and after their election by an overwhelming majority in May, 1997. Chief among these policy precedents were the shift toward primary-care commissioning and the attendant reduction in the centrality of acute hospitals. More broadly, the Blair reform proposals took as their starting point market institutions like the purchaser-provider split, contracting, and the organization of providers as semi-autonomous trusts. Labour also gradually adopted the Conservative's tendency to use private providers to construct NHS facilities and supply portions of publicly-funded medical and social services. Finally, Labour's reforms, like those of previous governments, continued to rely heavily on centralized control over NHS purchasers and providers.

A NEW NHS?

Shortly after the elections, the Blair Government announced its vision for 'A New NHS'. (Secretary of State for Health, 1997) and for major revisions in social services (Secretary of State for Health, 1998). These bold policy statements and the programs that were subsequently implemented (Dobson, 1999; Dixon and Dewar, 2000) promised to chart a 'third way' between centralized control and market regulation of the NHS.[12] In practice, during its first few years, the new government pursued policies that led in contradictory directions: It sought devolution of authority for commissioning and delivery of NHS services yet continued to centralize control over NHS funding, strategies, and clinical practice standards (Klein, 1998a).

In keeping with the policy of a primary-care led NHS, the government planned to devolve budgets and responsibility for primary care, other health services, and some social services to groups of GPs (Goodwin, Nick, 2000). In England and Wales around 500 Primary Care Groups (PCGs) – about three or four per HA – received prescribing budgets and capitated funds in exchange for provision of primary care services to around 100,000 patients. These agencies gradually received additional commissioning budgets and were urged to reorganize as Primary Care Trusts (PCTs). These semi-autonomous bodies, which cover twice the population served by PCGs, receive capitated budgets for commissioning all of their patients' hospital and social care, as well as delivering or commissioning primary care and community health services care. PCTs pay GPs and deliver or commission services that were previously delivered by separate community trusts – including services that involve some forms of means-tested social care (Pollock, 2000). It is planned that PCTs will eventually handle 75% of the entire NHS budget and will integrate commissioning and provision of services formerly covered by separate health and social care budgets (White, 2002). As commissioning devolves to the PCTS, the 99 HAs will lose their purchasing functions and be merged into just 30 Strategic Health Authorities. These new bodies will be responsible for strategic planning, health improvement programs, and monitoring the performance of PCTs (Wise, 2001).

The new government established a National Institute for Clinical Excellence (NICE), with a mandate to develop NHS standards and guidelines for effective practice derived from evidence-based medicine. NICE evaluates the desirability of introducing new drugs and technologies. The task of diffusing NICE guidelines and overseeing their implementation fell to yet another new central agency, known as the Commission for Health Improvement (CHI, or CHIMP, as some call it.) CHI was also made responsible for assessing the operations of NHS trusts and making sure that provider trusts meet new statutory obligations for quality assurance through Clinical Governance programs (Halligan and Donaldson, 2001). These programs include compulsory audits of all specialists (Warden, 1998a). CHI and other government agencies are to assess trust performance using new standards of clinical quality, efficiency, and accessibility. Through these initiatives, the NHS Executive and DOH expect that 'best practice will be identified and spread' while 'poor performance will be rooted out' (NHS Executive, 1998). The government also declared its intention to improve the nation's health by setting new health improvement targets, promoting integration of social and health services, and reducing health and social inequalities (Dean, 1997; Marmot, 1999; Secretary of State for Health, 1999).

In pursuit of its diverse goals for reform and in order to provide tangible evidence of improvements in NHS performance, the government subsequently announced a wide range of modernization programs, many of which are centrally funded and directed (Appleby, 1999b). These aim at improving scheduling and access to primary and outpatient specialty care, reducing use of

Accident and Emergency wards, and boosting hospital capacities. Among the widely publicized programs are walk-in clinics in commercial areas and a 24-hour NHS telephone help line, both staffed by nurses (Beecham, 1999a). In addition the NHS announced new hospital construction programs and plans for modernization of Accident and Emergency departments (Dixon and Dewar, 2000).

The funds for these new programs came from unprecedented increases in health budgets for the four years beginning in April 2000. With real increases averaging 6.1% per year, the government aims to bring the UK close to average European levels. The government anticipates that the funding increases will put an end to what the public and many analysts viewed as long-term underfunding of the NHS (Warden, 1998b).The additional funds will support dramatic growth in the numbers of hospital physicians, nurses, and GPs, medical equipment, information technology, and expansion of bed capacity – including a new network of intermediary-care beds outside of acute hospitals (Pollock, 2000). The government plans to retain tight control over these new cash outlays. In 2000, for example, the government made it clear that modernization funds would be awarded to providers who performed well on national quality standards, while other providers would be subject to scrutiny by CHI and related agencies (Dixon and Dewar, 2000).

At first glance, the Labour Government's reforms seemed to break radically with the pro-market policies that had prevailed under a succession of Tory governments. When Prime Minister Blair committed himself to financing NHS expansion through new taxes and set up a host of new supervisory agencies, he implicitly acknowledged the difficulties of relying on market forces to promote provider efficiency and quality. In like manner, the New NHS policies suggested that private finance would be insufficient to support national health needs. Furthermore, the new government abolished GP fundholding – the institution that came closest to realizing the ideal of the internal market. The PCTs, which replaced fundholding, are much larger and will grow even bigger through mergers. PCTs will sign three-year contracts, and require HA approval for contracts. Hence PCTs will be less able than fundholders to influence trusts by threatening to shift contracts (Boyce and Lamont, 1998; Light, 1999). In addition, the New NHS reforms urged cooperation, rather than competition, among providers and commissioners of care.[13] To help break down the 'Berlin Wall' separating social and health care, the government called for pooling budgets for social care and the NHS (Secretary of State for Health, 1998), joint priority setting for local services, and the creation of Health Improvement Zones and Health Improvement Projects that would build on cooperation among service providers from both sectors.[14] In the hospital sector, as well, the government abandoned or weakened market mechanisms. Mergers among hospitals were encouraged (Garside, 1999; Harrison, A.,1998), while local pay and compulsory market testing for trust purchases were dropped (Crail, 1994; Butler, 1997).

Although the proposals and programs for the New NHS departed from previous market policies and practices, they nonetheless exhibit remarkably strong continuities with underlying assumptions, policies, and institutional arrangements that emerged during the 1980s and 1990s. First, the main institutions of contracting and some features of the former purchaser-provider split were retained. Second, by locating responsibility for most commissioning in PCGs and PCTS, the New NHS program continued and even deepened the former government's commitment to a primary-care led NHS. Thus, as PCGs and PCTs begin to develop new forms of managed care, they will draw directly on experience gained during GP fundholding and GP commissioning. The new government's enthusiastic commitment to a primary-care-led NHS is particularly noteworthy, because there is so little evidence that this type of restructuring will indeed quickly deliver sought-for improvements in care quality and health outcomes.

Third, like previous Tory governments, the Labour Government sought private-sector financing for health-related care and sometimes preferred private providers to public ones. Thus the government continued to require means testing for social care for the aged and declined to restore free NHS coverage for geriatric care. It also continued the Private Finance Initiative for hospital construction, despite objections by trust managers and physicians (Fisher, 1999; Ward, 2002). In addition the government encouraged expansion of private financing of primary care facilities and movement of private firms into provision of ambulatory care (Pollock, 2001a). Investment in more sophisticated ambulatory facilities, including creation of intermediate beds to supplement the dwindling supply of hospital beds, are creating incentives for PCTs to shift care to private providers and engage in risk selection (Pollock, 2000; Pollock, 2001b).

Fourth, the architects of the New NHS programs continued efforts by prior Conservative governments to rationalize medical care and replace professional autonomy and self-regulation with governmental and managerial controls. New Labour, like the Conservatives before them, operated on the untested and debatable assumption that restructuring and top-down control can ultimately lead to complex behavioral changes among local NHS managers and professionals (Harrison, 1999). In this case the government's aim was that quality would become 'the focus of decisionmaking at every level of services' and a new spirit of cooperation and teamwork would prevail among divergent occupations and organizations. In adopting this stance, the government failed to recognize that cultural change in complex systems requires decentralization and encouragement of local initiatives, as well as strong leadership. With little attention to local sources of variation, the Labour Government, like its predecessors, strove to eliminate 'unacceptable variations' in services. To this end the government sought to require providers to implement national best practice guidelines under the supervision of CHI, regional watchdogs, and the HAs.

Fifth, the DOH and NHS Executive continued to use a centralistic and bureaucratic implementation style which closely resembled that of their predecessors. These agencies issued many directives, received little input from local health managers and professionals, imposed tight timetables on them, provided few resources to facilitate the implementation process, and made limited allowance for local conditions and problems (Goodwin, Neil, 2000; Yamey, 1999).

Some important trends in the implementation of the New NHS reforms are already evident, even though it is too soon for their systematic evaluation. From the administrative and bargaining perspectives, this latest drive for NHS reforms has proceeded rapidly and remained remarkably on course. On the other hand, rapid and demonstrable progress toward desired outcomes has proved more illusive. As anticipated, expenditures for the NHS rose substantially, as did their share in total national expenditures. After four years without growth, total health expenditures rose by 4.4% in 1999 and gained another 2.8% in 2000 at which point, health expenditures accounted for 7.3% of GDP (OECD, 2002).[15] What is more, in 2002, the government committed itself to massive spending increases for the NHS, which will amount to a 7.4% increase in real terms for each year between 2003–4 and 2007–8.

Nonetheless, doubts remain about the feasibility of implementing the modernization program (Appleby and Coote, 2002; Robinson, 2002; Ferriman, 2000). It remains unclear whether the government can sustain such an ambitious level of spending, while also spending more for education and other deserving services. In addition, the government faces an uphill struggle to overcome serious shortages of staff and beds and keep British expenditures apace with growth in other countries. Further concerns are that most of the new funds are earmarked for hospital care, despite the government's commitment to strengthen primary care (King's Fund, 2001). In addition, there are questions as to whether the spending will be directed where it is most needed and can be most effective.

The structures required by the reforms have been quickly established. As the government moved the enabling legislation through Parliament, the NHS executive instructed NHS staff to get ready for the transition to PCGs. Health Authorities and primary care physicians prepared hastily to begin operating under the new rules (e.g., Proctor and Campbell, 1999). The 481 PCGs went live in April of 1999. While still struggling to get organized, the PCGs received instructions to prepare for the transition to PCTs. In April 2002 the first 302 English PCTs began operation.[16] In like manner English HAs have merged into strategic health authorities, as planned.

Negotiations between the physicians and the government at both the national and community levels directly shaped the character of the new PCGs and PCTs. During preparations for the PCGs, the GPs lobbied vigorously for control over decisionmaking in PCGs and sought to preserve their status as independent practitioners (Beecham, 1998a, 1998b; Oldham and Rutter, 1999; Wise, 1998). In the end, GPs and nurses gained strong representation in PCG management, and the physicians' interests were preserved (Gilley, 1999; Wilkin et al., 2000). However, PCTs may develop in ways that lead to salaried employment of GPs or otherwise curtail their autonomy and influence. Thus the NHS Executive will subject the PCTs to strict budgetary constraints. Although GPs form the majority of PCT executives, who run daily operations, laypersons control PCT boards. These boards supervise trust executives and bear responsibility for the PCT's financial performance (Beecham, 1999c). In their first few years of operation, PCGs and pilot PCTs did not successfully involve members of the local community and voluntary groups in decisionmaking (Wilkin et al., 2001).

The new PCGs struggled to meet difficult managerial and developmental challenges but received limited assistance in these areas from the central government or the HAs (Boyce and Lamont, 1998). In particular, the PCGs suffered from serious limits on their information and management and capacities (Majeed, 1999; Wilkin, 2000). The PCGs also faced the challenges of developing effective forms of inter-professional team work and coping with pressing local issues (Goodwin, Neil, 2000).

Changes in commissioning occurred gradually, since many PCGs took over agreements that had been previously negotiated by HAs. PCGs extended primary care services and improved their accessibility, provided integrated nursing services, and began to develop partnerships with municipalities and other providers of social care and community services, including housing and education. The PCGs and PCTs also took steps toward promoting clinical quality and health improvement, particularly for coronary heart disease (Wilkin et al., 2001; Regen et al., 2001).

NICE began its operations in 1999 and quickly made several controversial decisions concerning NHS funding for new drugs. The debates over these decisions made it clear once again that rationing of NHS resources is unavoidable (Smith, 1999b) and can never be an entirely rational process. Nor can decisions about priorities satisfy all NHS stakeholders (Klein, 1998b; see Thomson, 1998 for a critical view of the prospects for CHI).

At both the national and local levels there was progress toward implementation of the government's policies for strengthening quality through clinical governance. However, it is far from certain that the new formal governance programs will ultimately transform deeply entrenched forms of professional practice and thought – a goal that clinical audit and other previous quality programs had failed to attain. During its first year of operation, CHI published four reviews of hospitals and launched 40 others, with over 500 to be conducted by 2004 (Commission for Health Improvement, 2001a, 2001b). The CHI reports, which rated hospitals and targeted problem areas, helped precipitate decisions by the government to remove senior managers in several hospitals that were performing poorly. The trust managers will be replaced by managers from other trusts, who will be appointed for a three-year period (Hawkes, 2002). In 2002 the government further strengthened CHI's supervisory and assessment functions by announcing plans for a new Commission for Healthcare Audit and Inspection (CHAI), which will encompass CHI, the Audit Commission's work on the NHS, and private health inspection (Moore, 2002).

PCGs and PCTs also began to set up structures and targets for clinical governance, but they have just begun to translate these formal arrangements into quality improvement processes (Wilkin et al., 2001; Wilkin et al., 2000; Dowswell et al., 2002). Hospital trusts also started putting formal clinical governance mechanisms in place, with most changes occurring at the trust directorate level, rather than within departments. Governance practices rested on existing quality assurance activities, which were fragmented and suffered from weaknesses in information systems and the overall knowledge base (Walshe, 2000; Freeman et al., 1999; Latham et al., 1999).

To avoid costly confrontations with the medical profession, the government sought the profession's cooperation in implementing national quality standards and clinical governance (Klein, 1998c). Beleaguered by scandals involving professional incompetence and misconduct, the physicians' organizations adopted a generally favorable view of the government's quality initiatives, while seeking to maintain the principle of professional self-regulation.[17] In an attempt to restore public confidence in the profession, the General Medical Council announced new procedures for revalidating physicians. These procedures would rely on peer review and build on the Council's existing structures and practices. In contrast, England's chief medical officer called for compulsory appraisal of all doctors using external assessment centers (Beecham, 1999b). Most members of the medical profession opposed compulsory assessment, but the General Medical Council eventually endorsed the controversial procedure (Smith, 2001; Burke, 2001). Thereafter, the Minister of Health outlined plans for revalidation reviews that would cover all doctors by 2005 (Eaton, 2002). During this period, members of the Royal Colleges (specialty bodies), along with the General Medical Council, declared their willingness to cooperate with NICE and other agencies in the development of binding clinical standards and protocols (Salter, 1999). A dramatic break-through toward government-enforced review of physician behavior came with the announcement that beginning in 2004 the government will publish data on post-operative mortality for heart surgery centers and individual surgeons (Vass, 2002). The Society of Cardiothoracic Surgeons reluctantly agreed to cooperate with this initiative, which they viewed as inevitable. Similar steps are likely for other specialties, even though physicians worry that publication of such data may be misinterpreted and will lead surgeons to avoid high-risk cases.

Progress toward other reform objectives was slow. Integration of health and social services required cooperation among groups long divided by structures, budgets, occupation, and training (Robinson and Poxton, 1998). The government called on HAs to develop programs for reducing inequality and integrating services and launched demonstration programs in deprived areas ('Health action...', 1999). Nonetheless, the government proved reluctant to take more controversial and expensive political steps that could promote health gains for the aged and the poor and reduce socio-economic inequalities underlying many differences in health status. For example, concerns about revenue losses and pressure from lobbyists led the government to abandon its opposition to tobacco advertising, in spite of its declared objectives of reducing cancer and heart disease ('Pains, strains...', 1998).

During their first four years, the New NHS reforms produced very few discernable improvements in service production and quality. So far, an all-too-familiar litany of problems continues to make headlines and worry politicians and policy analysts: incompetent physicians, poor quality, insufficient quality assurance, overcrowding, delays in access to hospital care, unsatisfactory outcomes, inadequate information systems, and failure to use available performance data (Warden, 1998d; 'Public inquiry...', 2000; Feachem et al., 2002; Smith, 2002). With time, the benefits of modernization and funding increases should produce improvements in NHS service production and may enhance quality and health outcomes. Moreover, PCTs could become an effective instrument for delivering managed care if the government supports quality care, local learning, and initiative – rather than focusing mainly on cost containment and standardization of practice (Klein and Dixon, 2000; Smith, 1999a).

When viewed from the bargaining and interpretive perspectives, the potential long-term impacts of the new policies outweigh their effects thus far. Although official discourse abandoned much of the language of the market place, the stress on business management techniques continues. Moreover, there is growing use of evidenced-based standards as a basis for evaluating and controlling the performance of hospitals and community care (Harrison, Moran, and Wood, 2002). Neither hospital physicians nor general practitioners are openly resisting this drift toward increased managerial and governmental supervision and standardization of their work (Dowswell, Harrison, and Wright, 2002). In fact, general practitioners and their nurses appear to accept control over their work by the new primary care organizations and are trying to comply with NHS clinical guidelines (Harrison and Dowswell, 2002; Harrison, Dowswell and Wright, 2002).

Despite these trends, many features of the old NHS culture remain. Perhaps the most damaging assessment of the culture of NHS hospitals – and by extension of recent attempts to reform the NHS as a whole – came from a government-commissioned inquiry into the circumstances surrounding the high mortality rates of children who underwent cardiac surgery in the Bristol Royal Infirmary between 1984 and 1995 (Dyer, 2001). The report on that hospital described a 'club culture', in which a small number of senior consultants held inordinate power (Secretary of State for Health, 2001). Cooperation between these physicians and trust managers 'makes it difficult to bring about change'. According to the report, the hospital was 'awash in data', and there was enough information from the late 1980s onward to point to poor mortality outcomes at Bristol and elsewhere. Still, few people in or out of the hospital showed much concern about the mortality rates. The commission did not view these and other features of the NHS culture as unique to the offending hospital:

> The NHS is still failing to learn from the things that go wrong and has no system to put this right. This must change. Even today, it is not possible to say, categorically, that events similar to those which happened at Bristol could not happen again in the UK, indeed, are not happening at this moment.

In contrast to this grim assessment, the New NHS reforms are leading to two institutional developments that could fundamentally alter the culture of NHS hospitals, as characterized by the Bristol inquiry and detailed earlier in this chapter. First, the government's drive for increased accountability and transparency in the health services runs broad and deep. This drive focuses on clinical quality, hospital organization, and a wide range of performance indicators in the hospital and ambulatory sectors. These indicators cover many important features of hospital operations that were not measured by the narrow band of financial and service indicators used by previous governments. The government is investing unprecedented amounts of energy and resources to sustain its drive to improve care quality. Furthermore, the medical profession is displaying a new willingness to cooperate with the public call for quality standards and quality control. Second, the government's steps toward creating a primary-care-led NHS may ultimately lead to a fundamental redirection of NHS activities – from emphasis on sophisticated, hospital-led interventions toward stress on prevention of illness and promotion of wellness.

If the government sustains its efforts on behalf of these transformations and successfully mobilizes the medical profession in support of its goals, the New NHS reforms could attain much of the unrealized potential of earlier reform programs. Moreover, this new wave of reforms could produce these dramatic transformations without buffeting the NHS with the shocks of market forces. On the other hand, the New NHS reforms are unlikely to produce such fundamental institutional and cultural changes if the government continues to launch wave upon wave of new policies and directives. Instead, the government must give NHS managers and health professionals the guidance, time, resources, and authority to implement fundamental change.

Unfortunately, significant reform of a system as complex as the NHS apparently requires more money, greater local experimentation, better data and information management, mobilization of health professionals on behalf of reform objectives, and a longer time frame than are tolerated by the realities of health politics in the United Kingdom and most other nations. Political pressures and public expectations encourage dramatic announcements of new funding and new programs. Thus neither the continuity of the New NHS policies, nor their outcomes are assured.

CONCLUSION

During the first half of the 1990s the Thatcher and Major governments restructured the NHS as a market containing public purchasers and providers. The government also fostered private finance and provision of health care. While espousing the benefits of market forces, the government strengthened its already tight grip over NHS purchasers and providers. NHS and DOH elites placed managers in HAs and hospitals under intense pressure to attain efficiency gains and cut waiting lists. Only GP fundholders retained sufficient freedom and flexibility to take advantage of the contracting process.

Judged from an administrative perspective, the attainments of the market reforms were few. Fundholders did use the market to bargain for better prices and services for their patients, but they made little progress toward shifting care out of hospitals and developing a genuinely primary-care-led NHS. Purchasing by GPs and HAs made little use of evidence-based medicine or other guides to rational decisions. Hospital productivity rose, but this development resulted more from a combination of tight global budgets and targeted funding increments than from market forces. The clinical quality of care showed little improvement overall and seems to have declined in some specialties and settings. Opposition by hospital physicians slowed progress toward assessment and assurance of clinical quality. Patients gained neither freedom of choice nor influence over NHS purchasing agencies. The internal market did not produce aggregate cost reductions and further fragmented relations among the many health agencies and sectors.

Nonetheless, the reforms produced lasting legacies, which can best be viewed through the bargaining, interpretive, and institutional frames: business concepts and practices diffused throughout NHS management. The reforms increased governmental and managerial control over physicians and intensified pressure for assessment of clinical behavior and outcomes. The reforms also began to shift power from the hospitals toward the primary care sector.

The Blair government modified or abandoned many of the NHS' market mechanisms, including fundholding, and favored an ethos of cooperation instead of competition. To overcome chronic shortages of beds and staff, massive new investments were planned, which would be funded by new taxes. Despite this move away from reliance on the market and the private sector, the Blair government retained the contracting process and private finance of hospital construction. In addition, the New NHS reforms made substantial progress toward a primary-care-led NHS. The new government also strongly supported the ongoing drive for greater accountability and transparency among provider agencies and clinicians. Reeling from scandalous revelations of the failure of professional self-regulation, the physicians reluctantly accepted these moves. The government's new programs and its more generous funding for health care hold promise for major improvements in the NHS. It is too early to judge whether they will prove sufficient to revitalize the system as a whole.

NOTES

1 For these reasons the OECD (2001) data on acute bed turnover in the United Kingdom, which rely on the FCE measure, are not reported here.

2 This proportion rose dramatically during the 1980s from 10.6% to 16% but declined somewhat from 1992 through 1995; it reached 16.3% in both 1996 and 1997 and rose to 16.7% in 1998 and 1999 (OECD, 2001).

3 See Chapter 1, footnote 4 on reporting of changes over time.

4 Söderlund, et al. (1999, Table 2) calculate total hospital administrative costs at 8.73% of total expenditures in 1993/94 – in contrast to 8.07% for 1991/92. According to their analysis, for the first three years of the reforms, increased spending for management had moderate *negative* effects on hospital productivity.

5 One sophisticated statistical analysis did turn up evidence that trusts achieved lower costs per patient than directly managed hospitals during the first three years of the reforms (Söderland et al., 1997). These findings have been challenged on the grounds that managers of hospitals that were about to become trusts may have intentionally reduced productivity before assuming trust status so as to look good after the reform (Hamblin, 1998). Moreover, in their multiple regression analysis, Söderland and his colleagues did not find any independent impact on efficiency of the competitiveness of the markets to which hospitals were exposed. On the contrary, hospitals facing less competition (i.e., higher proportions of their patients coming from the local HA) attained significantly *higher* efficiency levels than hospitals facing more competitive markets.

6 This finding may reflect the fact that the Family Health Service Authorities, which funded GPs until 1996, created disincentives for continuing savings among fundholders

by reducing the annual drug budgets of fundholders who saved money on drug costs during the previous year (Goodwin 1998).

7 Other health policy researchers who reached similar conclusions about Britain's reforms include Walshe et al., 1997; Hamblin, 1998; and Hunter, 1999.

8 In their study of GPs in England, Francome and Marks (1996) found a jump of 270% between 1992 and 1994 in the proportion of physicians reporting that they had sent people back to hospital after premature discharge. Trust competition effectively began in 1992, after a year during which the government held the internal market in a 'steady state' (Bartlett and Le Grand, 1994).

9 For the period 1991/92–1995/96, 27 hospitals showed progress on mortality, 21 had no change, and 27 regressed.

10 In fact, the annual rate of bed reduction was considerably higher in the 1980s than between 1990–91 and 1993–94 (Hensher and Edwards, 1999).

11 Surprisingly, there was little growth in the proportion of people carrying private health insurance between 1989 and 2000 (Association of British Insurers, 2000, Table 2). In 2002 just 9% of British households held any kind of private medical insurance (Association of British Insurers, 2002, Table 2).

12 Unless noted otherwise, the phrases in quotation marks in this section appear in the White Paper, *The New NHS* (Secretary of State for Health, 1997).

13 In an apparent reversal of this direction late in 2002, the government announced its plan to designate hospitals as foundation trusts. This model, which will eventually be widely applied, gives hospitals substantial financial and managerial autonomy and requires them to compete for both patients and funds – much like the trusts in the original plan for an internal market (Wintour, 2002; Watt, 2002).

14 Interest in fostering cooperation between social and health care began when John Major was Prime Minister but became more central to the policies of the newly elected Labour Government.

15 Per capita health expenditures in dollars, based on purchasing power parities (PPPs), grew by 9.1% in 1999 and 5.8% in 2000. On PPPs see Chapter 1, note 24.

16 In Scotland, commissioning was eliminated, and primary care was immediately organized into PCTS, which cooperate with health boards in strategic planning (Hopton and Heany, 1999).

17 See the many public statements and position papers, beginning with Irvine (1997a, 1997b), that appear in or are reported by the *British Medical Journal* and the *Health Service Journal* from 1997 through 1999.

4

Market Experimentation within Swedish Health System Reform

At the end of the 1980s and the start of the 1990s, some of Sweden's county councils (CCs), which fund and manage most health care, experimented with creating quasi-markets for care. These CCs funded independent and competing family physicians, granted greater autonomy to publicly owned hospitals, and separated hospital providers from public purchasing bodies. Patients were allowed to choose hospitals, which would be reimbursed for patient visits. Public purchasers were to allocate CC funds to hospitals through contracts. The national government supported the drive toward competition among health care providers by allowing patients free choice of hospitals and providing public funding for self-employed family doctors, as well as physicians employed by the traditional community clinics. Although several of the Swedish market programs resembled those implemented in Britain, Sweden's market activities were more decentralized, aimed more directly at satisfying patients, and were more self-consciously experimental and evolutionary than were Britain's reforms.

Besides introducing market forces, Sweden's national and county governments also took more bureaucratic, top-down steps toward restructuring the financing and delivery of medical and geriatric care. Both the market and the top-down reforms aimed at a broad spectrum of objectives – including containing health costs, making the health system more efficient, reducing waiting for elective surgery, giving patients greater choice of providers, strengthening primary care, and integrating care sectors.

After providing background on Sweden's health system policies during the 1980s, the first part of this chapter uses the bargaining frame to analyze the emergence of extensive experimentation with market reform by CCs and the national government between 1989 and 1993, the reorientation of these market reforms beginning in 1994, and the rise of competing policy agendas. This analysis also periodically adopts an institutional perspective, which illuminates the ways in which historic political arrangements led to different paths of reform implementation in Sweden and Britain. The second part of the chapter examines in detail the implementation of national health system reforms. Some of these programs used national authority to foster quasi-markets for health services, whereas others mandated top-down reorganizations and fiscal controls over CCs and health care providers. The third part of the chapter analyzes implementation of three of the more prominent market experiments that took place within counties. This analysis highlights similarities and differences in the purchasing processes of Stockholm, Dalarna (formerly Koppaberg), Bohus, and other counties, along with responses to county programs within hospitals. The account of policy implementation in the second and third parts of the chapter blends administrative, bargaining, and interpretive perspectives. Using all four implementation frames, Chapter 5 examines outcomes of Sweden's market and non-market reforms and recent movement toward a more complex mix of public and private health care.

MARKET REFORMS

Background

Sweden's national politicians and civil servants share responsibility with their counterparts in the CCs for setting policies for the nation's public health and welfare systems. The national government typically uses fiscal controls and regulations to steer health policies, while devolving responsibility for the financing, ownership, and running of medical and social care facilities to the CCs and municipalities. The trend toward devolution began in the 1960s and 1970s and has continued to the present day (Heidenheimer and Elvander, 1980; Twaddle, 1999).

To hold down health expenditures Sweden's central government imposed constraints on national and county health budgets throughout the 1980s and 1990s. The government relied mainly on ceilings on CC expenditures and restrictions on CC taxation (Calltorp, 1995). The central government also sought to influence national pay agreements between the Federation of Swedish County Councils (Federation of CCs) and health care employees so as to contain costs and moderate government spending. In 1991, as it faced the deepest recession in 50 years, the central government imposed constraints on fees for ambulatory services and restricted growth in the CC's total expenditures. It also froze CC tax levels, thus effectively blocking revenue flows to the health system. This 'tax stop' was renewed each year through 1994. In response to these constraints and the growing burden of unemployment benefits, the CCs placed strict budgetary caps on health expenditures. Largely as a result of these moves by the central and county governments, health expenditures as a proportion of GDP declined in real terms during the 1980s and remained stable during the early 1990s, with some decline after 1993 (see Figure 1.1 on page 4). Although the budget ceilings succeeded in reigning in total expenditures, they did not provide solutions for officials in CCs and elsewhere who were responsible for providing health services. Moreover, the budget cuts did not address, and even intensified, other problems facing the health system (Diderichsen, 1993).

County managers, political parties, unions, the manufacturer's associations, and other policy actors developed very divergent definitions of the problems facing the system and appropriate solutions to these problems.[1] At the end of the 1980s the most pressing problem for CC politicians and managers was how to cope with rising health care costs and growing demand for health care in the face of falling tax revenues, rising unemployment, and growing welfare outlays. Business groups, along with many politicians in the CCs and the national government, feared that high taxes and public budgets were undermining Sweden's ability to compete in world markets and blocking the country's ability to reduce its budget deficit in accordance with requirements for entry into the European Community. Members of the Moderate (Conservative) opposition party were among the most vocal advocates of this view, but it was also held by many Social Democrats.

Equally important for the Social Democrats was the need to reduce waiting times for elective surgery and make the system more responsive to the needs and preferences of patients. This concern was shared by journalists, policy analysts from both the left and the right, and much of the electorate. A related concern was lack of direct representation of citizens in decisionmaking about health policy and services. As these criticisms mounted during the second half of the 1980s, they threatened to undermine the legitimacy of the health system.

To enhance the responsiveness of the health system, many advocates of patients' interests championed permitting patients to choose hospitals and care-givers, rather than assigning them on the basis of residence or bureaucratic considerations. In keeping with this proposal, the Liberal Party, which controlled the Ministry of Health from 1991 through 1994, proposed allowing patients to choose as their family physicians either physicians in CC clinics or private physicians, who are self-employed and reimbursed by the public insurance system.[2] The Family Doctor system would have replaced the arrangement whereby clinic doctors and nurses saw patients on a rotating basis. Assignment of patients to family physicians was intended to create more personalized and higher quality care than that given in the clinics. Referrals to hospital by the GP would be recommended, but self-referrals, which would incur higher co-payments, would be permitted (Anell and Jendteg, 1993, p.3). The Family Doctor program would have led gradually to reorganization of the health system around a primary-care based model (Expert Group, 1994) involving a new type of primary-care provider, who was reimbursed through capitation, and acted as a gatekeeper to specialists and hospitals. Some versions of this proposal envisioned family doctors holding budgets for portions of their patients' care, as GP fundholders did in Britain (Bergman, 1997). The Swedish Medical Association (SMA) strongly backed the Family Doctor reform, which allowed salaried primary-care physicians to become independent practitioners.[3] In addition, the program would increase the demand for community-based physicians and improve their earning prospects. In contrast, the Social Democrats and the unions representing nurses and other health employees opposed the plan, which threatened to undermine employment in the polyclinics. Many politicians, health planners, and managers also favored preserving and even strengthening the clinic system. These champions of the clinic system cited its contribution to preventive medicine and its potential for reducing reliance on expensive hospital services. This emphasis on community care fit recommendations by the World Health Association, that had been endorsed by the Swedish government in 1985.

Gradually some grounds for agreement and joint action emerged out of this welter of conflicting diagnoses of the ills facing the system and the best ways to cure them. Thus there was agreement among the politicians in power, many opposition politicians, and most of the public, that Sweden's system of high quality health care should be preserved, along with its principles of universal and equal access to publicly funded, government-managed services. This position reflected the legitimacy that citizens and their representatives granted to the country's cradle-to-grave welfare system. To preserve the health system, most actors agreed that it was necessary to improve the productivity and efficiency of health care and make it more responsive to the people's needs (Saltman, 1992; Swedish Institute, 1993). Hence, by the late 1980s the major political parties, the SMA, and representatives of business, all expressed interest in further deregulating the system (Riska, 1993). Among the most widely supported changes were programs that guaranteed patients rapid access to elective surgery and free choice of hospitals.

Rise of Competitive Reforms, 1989–1993

Over a period of several years, a broad and informal coalition emerged that favored addressing the health system's problems by experimenting with market mechanisms in health finance and delivery. Politicians and policy analysts who advocated market reform for Sweden cited Britain's drive toward creating an internal market within the National Health Service as worthy of emulation (Whitehead, Gustafsson and Diderichsen, 1997). These advocates of reform recommended separating purchasers and providers so as to relieve hospitals of direct CC management and turn them into semi-autonomous public firms (Culyer et al., 1991; Saltman and von Otter, 1992; Blomqvist, 1992). As in Britain, these recommendations often reflected local applications of neo-liberal economic views,[4] along with growing international interest in the New Public Management.

The advocates of market reform expected that separating hospitals from purchasing boards would promote hospital competition over the accessibility and quality of their services. The new contracting system was also expected to create incentives for efficiency since hospitals could not turn away patients, continued to be reimbursed for services on the basis of fees set by the CCs, and were subject to strict budgetary limits. CCs that had multiple purchasers also laid the ground for purchasing boards to compete with one another in terms of their ability to obtain value for money.

CCs under the leadership of the Social Democrats introduced the earliest reforms employing purchaser-provider splits. By 1991 the parties in the Federation of CCs had agreed to support provider competition, purchaser-provider splits, and freedom of choice for hospital patients. The elections of 1991 ended decades of nearly uninterrupted dominance by the Social Democrats and swept center and right-wing parties into the governing coalitions of the national government and most CCs. From 1992 through 1994 these coalitions gave strong backing to market reforms at both the county and national levels.

Political caution, coalition politics, and CC autonomy resulted in much slower diffusion of purchaser-provider splits in Sweden than in Britain. In Britain, a single ruling party initiated the market reforms and implemented them with the aid of institutions that gave central government much power over regional and local bodies. Although many CCs experimented with new purchasing arrangements, by 1993 only six (out of 26) had implemented formal 'models' – programs and major structural reorganizations – featuring purchaser-provider splits. Other counties created purchasing units within their central administration. At least in theory, these units could purchase services from providers outside of the county. Despite these developments, in 1994 most CCs still relied on the traditional budget process for allocating resources to health care.[5]

Although neo-conservative views on markets influenced Swedish politicians and policy analysts, their approach to change was eclectic, pragmatic, and experimental. For example, even at the height of Sweden's market experiments, when center-right coalitions were in power, most politicians and health-system actors did not question the wisdom of central government intervention into health finance and structure. Hence, the central government continued to set annual limits on direct payments by patients during the 1990s, rather than allowing CCs to experiment with varying fee levels and formulae. To take another example, the advocates of market reform sought provider autonomy for hospitals. But these reformers did not change the legal status of hospitals, as had been done in Britain. Nor did they press the central government and the health-employee unions to dismantle well-established mechanisms for negotiating national wage agreements. In contrast, the British planners of the internal market, who were more hostile to organized labor, planned to substitute local pay for national negotiations with health employee unions.

Reorientation of Market Policies and New Policy Agendas, 1994–1999

By the mid-1990s most of the Swedish counties that had pioneered British-type internal markets had recentralized their purchasing functions, while other CCs established contracting functions that were centralized and had limited auto-nomy. Contracting between CC agencies and hospitals thus developed a broader, longer-term, and more cooperative style than that envisioned by the original competitive reforms. In like manner, the national government and many coun-ties stopped assigning additional patients to independent general practitioners, as mandated by the Family Doctor program.

This scaling back of market programs gained momentum after the elections of 1994, when the conservative parties lost power in the national government and in all but a few CCs. However, movement away from market policies had begun in the early 1990s, while center-right coalitions still prevailed in the national government and most CCs. Moreover, many of the same politicians, managers, and experts who had originally favored market experimentation supported modification of the original market policies and programs. As will be seen in the next two parts of the chapter, much of this policy shift flowed from encounters with complexities and unintended consequences of implementing purchaser-provider splits.

The reorientation and decline of some of the early market policies also stemmed from the emergence of competing policy agendas within the CCs and at national and regional levels of government. Among the most important developments were revival of regional government during the 1990s and growing cooperation among CCs in planning, budgeting, and delivering health care. The trend toward regionalization built on regional parliaments, agencies, and agreements that had existed since the 1980s.[6] Four CCs in Western Sweden and several in the South developed joint plans for tertiary hospital care and plans to coordinate or merge hospitals across CC boundaries. Plans were also made for the merger of five CCs in Western Sweden and three in Southern Sweden.[7] As they moved toward merger, the CCs began substituting regional purchasing and administration of hospital care for purchasing within separate CCs. These steps toward regionalization spelled the end of the purchaser-provider split as originally envisioned, although contracting with hospitals continued.

The trend toward regionalization strengthened an ongoing wave of hospital mergers. Many CC politicians and some policy analysts advocated partial or total mergers of hospitals as a means of attaining cost savings (Calltorp, 1999b). By early 1997 ten mergers of hospitals were in various stages of execution across the nation, and by 1999, 13 mergers had been completed (Bergman, 1999).

By the early 1990s, a new set of policy issues reduced excitement about market reform and directed the attention of politicians and analysts to problems that did not seem amenable to market solutions and could even be aggravated by too much stress on competitive incentives. One of the most critical new issues centered on setting priorities for funding and delivering care under tight budgets (Honigsbaum et al., 1995). Two other areas of concern were assurance of quality of clinical care in hospitals (e.g., Garpenby and Carlsson, 1994; Garpenby, 1995), and coordination of care and services across care sectors – for example, between hospitals, community clinics, and municipal services, like housing and geriatric care. To understand why Sweden's market reforms were so short lived, let us now look more closely at the implementation of these reforms and more traditional, top-down programs for cost containment.

IMPLEMENTATION OF NATIONAL PROGRAMS

Rather than flowing from a coherent national initiative, as occurred in Britain, Sweden's national market reforms responded to county-level experiments. These

CC experiments promoted a very diverse, and even contradictory, set of goals. Unlike the one-party Tory governments in Britain, Sweden's coalition governments had neither the will nor the power to impose a comprehensive restructuring of the health system on many powerful health-system stakeholders. Hence, significant inconsistencies and contradictions emerged among national policies and programs, as well as within specific programs. Diversity in policy implementation in Sweden also reflected its decentralization of health finance and provision. Reform policies varied among the CCs, as did the ways in which CCs implemented national programs.

Tension prevailed throughout the 1990s between national programs favoring decentralized, market-like forms of finance and delivery and programs through which the national government intervened directly in the financing and structure of health services. Before examining national market programs in greater depth, let us consider how the national government used non-market, hierarchical controls to contain costs and 'steer' county and municipal actors toward other national objectives.

Steering from the Top

During the early 1990s, the national government imposed ever-tighter ceilings on health expenditures, taxes, and payments by CCs. In response, CC politicians continued to seek cost reductions in hospitals, since inpatient care still accounted for over half of total public expenditures, despite substantial reductions during the 1980s (OECD, 2001). In response to the national limits on expenditures and tax revenues, the CCs capped hospital budgets and sought to close or merge small hospitals or convert them from acute to geriatric status (Ints.). As the recession deepened and professionals replaced politicians on hospital boards in some areas, it became easier for CCs to overcome local opposition to closing or restructuring local facilities (Ints.). However, the greatest impact of the fiscal restraints was on bed capacities, which continued to decline in the 1990s after substantial reductions during the 1980s. From early 1990 to the end of 1994, 22% of the country's acute care beds were eliminated (OECD 2001).[8]

Two other national government programs contributed to hospital change and cost containment during the 1990s. The Clinical Chief reform and the introduction of diagnosis related groups (DRGs) did not use competitive mechanisms, but they nonetheless facilitated adoption of market-like thinking and practices. Introduction of both programs facilitated supervision of expenditures by hospital managers, made hospital operations more transparent to CC managers and politicians, and introduced payment and budgetary arrangements that could be used to contain costs. The Clinical Chief reform restructured the management of hospital departments. The Health and Medical Services Act (effective 7/91) created a clinical directorate structure, much like the one introduced a few years earlier in Britain. A single functionary, known as the Clinical Chief, was given responsibility within hospital clinics for both medical care and administration, including the budget. The chief must be a physician in clinical departments and in many medical service departments (e.g., diagnostic radiology). The reorganization was accomplished quickly, and by 1993 some 2000 clinical chiefs headed the nation's hospital departments (Calltorp, 1993). In addition, some large hospitals introduced divisional-level directorates (Ints.).

The SMA endorsed the Clinical Chief reform, because it eliminated management of clinical departments by non-medical administrators and practitioners from para-medical fields, as had sometimes occurred in the past (Int.). This reform, also eliminated sectoral hierarchies within the hospitals, under which nurses reported to a chief nurse and physicians to a chief physician. At the same time, the reform removed managerial responsibilities from around 8000 hospital consultants (senior level specialists) and district physicians, who were not heads of clinics. By assigning accountability for clinical management to one person, the clinical chief structure made it easier for managers in the hospitals and, to some extent in the CCs, to focus on issues of resource allocation and case-mix management (Ints.; Paulson, 1993)

Despite formalization of reporting relations under the clinical chief reform, interactions between clinical chiefs and their staffs continued to be more consultative than hierarchical. Clinical chiefs had to persuade or pressure their colleagues to cooperate with budgetary constraints, rather than instructing them to do so (Ints). The tensions between the hierarchical and collegial modes of interaction were well captured in the comments of Dr. B, a senior physician in a small (200 bed), suburban hospital, referred to here as Brookside:[9]

> **MH:** Has the job of the clinical chief changed during your 12 years in the department? Does the chief have more or less power than in the past?
>
> **Dr. B:** As a senior physician you work for yourself and try to make progress in your area. The chief is a coach for a team... Our CC wants to have a chief-centered system, and I don't like it.
>
> **MH:** Why not?
>
> **Dr. B:** It's a bit like an industrial or military system. You can't do that. Our profession is to carry out diagnoses and treatments.
>
> **MH:** [encourages further comments].
>
> **Dr. B:** We have a biological system, not a mechanical one... You don't have a chief who has knowledge of what's happening in different areas [within the department]. He'd have to be God himself to be chief over so many areas. The CC is saying you should have chiefs who people [follow], but that's impossible. [As a physician] you're dependent on colleagues and nurses. There has been an attempt to make chiefs more like officers, but you cannot do that.

Introduction of DRGs took place gradually during the 1980s and early 1990s. In 1980, after several years of research supported by the national government and the Federation of CCs, the government began supporting CCs which used DRGs to enhance the productivity of the health services (Paulson, 1993). By 1992 ten CCs were using per-case payments based on DRGs for at least some hospital procedures (Forsberg and Calltorp, 1993). At that time, almost half of the CCs planned to introduce payment per performance in all care units by 1995, and almost all the other CCs planned to do so after 1995.

Hospital managers adapted to tighter budgets and new payment systems by working with clinical chiefs to cut staff and bed capacities and encourage staff members to reduce patient stays and expenditures, without sacrificing quality of care (Ints.). The hospital directors set budgetary targets for the departments and sometimes provided informal incentives for departments that obtained the sought-for savings (Ints.; Saltman, 1990). Drug committees recommended drugs to hospital physicians (Ljungkvist, et al., 1997). In planning these cutbacks and other cost-saving measures, the hospital managers avoided arousing the ire of their local physicians or threatening physicians with unemployment (Ints.).

The physicians largely opposed the cutbacks of the 1980s and early 1990s and worried about their impact. For instance, physicians surveyed in late 1992 reported that patients were being released prematurely (Forsberg and Calltorp, 1993). In like manner doctors and nurses whom I interviewed expressed some concern that financial considerations might compromise care. Nonetheless, the SMA and the hospital employees' unions did not actively fight the cutbacks in hospital facilities. Moreover, physicians and nurses within hospital departments largely accepted and cooperated with budgetary constraints.

Why was there so little organized resistance to hospital retrenchment among health professionals? One explanation is that physicians and nurses, along with most members of the public at large, recognized that the economic downturn posed a serious threat to the country and its welfare institutions. Hence, the health professionals were in a weak bargaining position (Ints.). Second, within the medical sector, as elsewhere (Rehn and Viklund, 1990), there were strong norms that restrained action by organized labor in exchange for job security and generous social welfare benefits (Ints.). The government's austerity moves tested this 'Swedish model' of the welfare state but did not break it. In keeping with this institution, the counties protected veteran health professionals from the impact of staff reductions. The CCs mainly cut temporary and part-time employees and occupants of the lowest nursing grade (Ints.). Third, even if the SMA had chosen to challenge the government, it lacked the power to do so. The SMA's capacity for confrontation was reduced by a growing surplus of physicians, limited organization at the hospital and CC level, and limited influence over the critical early stages of national policy formation (Ints.: Duffy, 1989, Immergut, 1989, 1992). The SMA and the hospital employee unions may also have been chastened by the knowledge that a nurses' strike in 1986 had failed to produce substantial wage gains (Int.).

Besides using budgets, the national government launched the Ädel reform, which sought to contain acute hospital costs, while improving geriatric care (Styrborn and Thorslund, 1993; Andersson and Karlberg, 2000). This program aimed at reducing acute hospital stays among chronically ill 'bedblockers', while at the same time enhancing coordination of geriatric services, and providing the elderly with freedom of choice of social and medical services. Before the Ädel reform the CCs were responsible for all medical and nursing care for the elderly, while the municipalities were only responsible for social services, including home care. As of January 1992, the responsibility for geriatric nursing services – including nursing homes, shelters and old age homes – was transferred from CCs to the municipalities. The reform also gave municipalities financial incentives for quickly accepting responsibility for any elderly patients who were ready for release from acute hospitals. Nurses and physicians in general hospitals viewed the program as a positive step toward relieving the problem of bed blockers and acted to expedite the transfer of those geriatric patients who did not require acute hospital care (Ints.).

The government's budgetary ceilings, the Ädel reform, and the Clinical Chief reform affected all counties and most providers within them. In hospitals throughout the country these programs created an atmosphere of constraint among hospital professionals and increased awareness of the cost implications of medical practice. This atmosphere, in turn, probably made hospital managers and health professionals more responsive to the market experiments that were introduced in many locales. There were, of course, local variations in the timing and depth of response to the national cost containment programs. For example, one CC, which had a long history of budget surpluses, was less vulnerable to the effects of the tax stop than others. But it too eventually had to introduce a program of retrenchment and reconfiguration of hospital services (Ints.).

Market Reforms

In contrast to the top-down governmental interventions into health finance and structure just examined, the government's Patient Choice, Care Guarantee, and Family Doctor programs sought to create market mechanisms that would generate incentives for providers to contain costs, boost efficiency, and become more responsive to patient preferences. These three programs all contributed toward decentralization of national governmental control over providers and strengthened competition among them.

Patient Choice and the Care Guarantee were the most enduring and most widely implemented national programs that promoted market conditions within the public health services (Ints.; Hanning, 1996). These programs aimed at providing patients with prompt elective care for procedures such as hip replacements, cataract removal, and coronary bypass, which had long waiting lines. The programs also introduced choice of hospitals and thereby fostered competition among hospital providers. The competition centered on access to care and to a lesser degree on perceived quality, but not on price.

The Care Guarantee began in 1989, when the national government earmarked extra funds for procedures with long waiting lists. Stockholm CC introduced patient choice of hospitals in 1989, and the program spread rapidly among other CCs. In 1991 the Federation of CCs endorsed the principle of hospital choice. A year later the national government granted patients who did not receive care within three months the right to seek treatment elsewhere. Instead of assigning patients to hospitals on the basis of residence, the counties now gave patients their choice of where to obtain elective care. In most counties, money was to follow the patient, rather than being budgeted in advance to the hospital. In other words, the local hospital or CC was to pay for care that patients received outside of their local area. Some CCs translated the program into a direct productivity incentive for hospitals: only hospitals that treated patients within three months would receive the funds that the national government had earmarked for reducing waiting lists.

The logic behind Patient Choice and the Care Guarantee was simple: by allowing money to follow the patient, the reform would generate strong incentives for hospital managers and professionals to increase hospital productivity and efficiency. By treating patients quickly, hospitals could avoid losing patients from their catchment area and could attract patients from surrounding areas. The allocation of funds in response to patient choice would thus remove the 'perverse incentive' for managers and physicians to allow long waiting lines to develop so as to justify additional funding.

Patient Choice had a significant impact on urban and suburban hospitals in metropolitan areas, where patients could readily reach hospitals outside of their residential area. For example, suburban hospitals in Western Sweden found themselves losing patients to prestigious hospitals in the city centers, which were accessible to patients who worked there or could easily travel to the cities. For some smaller hospitals these losses contributed to other forces threatening their viability as independent institutions (Ints.). In response to patient flows, urban and suburban hospitals began to compete with one another to provide prompt access to elective surgery. Some hospitals strengthened their surgical departments and publicized elective services, so as to attract patients or reduce the risk of losing them.

However, as the comments of Mr. T, the Associate Director of Brookside hospital suggest, small hospitals could not generate much revenue though proactive marketing:

Mr. T indicated that Brookside has supported expansion of its orthopedic services, which could generate income under Patient Choice and the Care Guarantee and that they do 'some marketing', by including an article on the skills of their orthopedic surgeons in a hospital flyer that is periodically distributed to all households in the vicinity. Mr. T added that they are trying to improve the reputation of the department, 'which was not good [in the recent past]'. Brookside's efforts in this area aim more at warding off threatened reductions or even elimination of the hospitals' surgical and internal medicine departments than at generating substantial additional income. 95% of general medicine patients and 70% of surgery patients present themselves through the emergency room, rather than seeking elective procedures covered under Patient Choice.

In contrast, in Stockholm, where half of the referrals came through private specialists working in the community, hospital managers and physicians had strong incentives to market services to these specialists (Int.).[10]

Patient Choice was implemented throughout the country and quickly became very popular with citizens and CC politicians (Ints.; Anell et al., 1997). Because of its popularity, many CC politicians continued to support the program even when they realized that it complicated health budgeting and sometimes hurt the CC financially. The program's impact was uneven, since hospitals in rural areas were far apart, and patients were reluctant to travel long distances for elective care (Ints.). Altogether the program affected around five percent of all patient visits between 1991 and 1993 (Ramström and Dahlström, 1995) and led to reallocation of two to five percent of total health care resources during the early 1990s (Rehnberg, 1995).

The Family Doctor reform created competition for patients among independent physicians and between independent physicians and their salaried colleagues in local clinics. This competition turned mainly on the accessibility of the physicians and the perceived quality of their care. Steps toward implementation of a Family Doctor system began in the late 1980s in Stockholm and other counties, when private GPs and ambulatory specialists were encouraged to provide services on a fee-for-service basis, outside of the clinics. In 1993 the national government passed a bill requiring patients to choose a private physician or a member of their community polyclinic staff as their Family Doctor. After January 1994 the national government required CCs to reimburse private physicians and physiotherapists on a fee-for-service basis and increased the levels of these fees (Whitehead, et al., 1997). By September of 1994, over three-quarters of the population had chosen a Family Doctor (Wilhelmsson et al., 1998). As a result of the reform, the number of GPs per capita was more than 20% higher in 1991 than it had been in 1986 (Federation of CCs, 1993).

After the elections of 1994, the Social Democrats, who favored organizing primary care around community clinics, moved quickly to weaken the Family Doctor system. New legislation allowed CCs to continue the Family Doctor arrangement, but few left it unaltered. The Social Democratic majorities in most CCs did allow patients to chose Family Doctors and permitted physicians who had entered private practice prior to mid-1995 to retain that status. However, the CCs subjected the private physicians to tighter regulation and control. By 2001 nearly half of the CCs had implemented some form of capitation payments to Family Doctors (Bergman, 2002).

Although the SMA had enthusiastically backed the Family Doctor reform, neither the doctors nor any other group actively opposed these moves to curtail the reform. In contrast to Britain, Sweden lacked a strong institutional basis for restructuring health care around GPs. While appealing to the desires of many citizens for more freedom in choosing their primary care physician, the reform had assigned priority to physicians whom most citizens viewed as less expert and lower in prestige than hospital specialists (Ints.). Moreover, unlike the British, Swedish patients were not used to relying on the judgment of primary-care physicians (Ints.). Hence, the program flew in the face of a longstanding tradition of direct patient access to specialists and hospitals.

MARKET EXPERIMENTS IN THE COUNTIES

Experiments by CCs with purchaser-provider splits generated the most dramatic and widely publicized market reforms in Sweden. The reforms in Stockholm, Dalarna, and Bohus counties illustrate the main types of health purchasing arrangements created by CCs and the divergent ways that CCs implemented provider competition. After examining variations among these counties, we will note important continuities in public purchasing experiments across Sweden. These continuities reflected behavior that was very different from that anticipated by neoliberal models of market competition.[11] This section closes with an analysis of the values, beliefs and political actions that contributed to disillusion with market reform in health care and undermined support for the reforms within the CCs.

Stockholm

In the late 1980s and early 1990s, the county council that delivers health care for around 1.7 million residents in Stockholm's metropolitan area pioneered patient choice and family physician programs which became prototypes for the national programs. At the same time Stockholm CC developed a distinctive model for public purchasing of hospital care. By 1994, just two years after the formal launch of Stockholm's 'buy-sell' model, conflicts between market programs and the CC's tight-money policies had produced substantial disaffection with market reforms in Stockholm and throughout the country.

Like other CCs, Stockholm enforced tight budgets during most of the 1980s, and its hospital managers responded by cutting beds, reducing staff, and restructuring units. When the Conservatives gained control of the CC after the 1992 elections, they intensified support for markets in ambulatory and hospital care. At the same time the new CC government introduced even deeper budget cuts than those required by the national tax stop.

Provider competition in Stockholm began in 1989 with a program granting patients choice of primary health care center. Then the CC encouraged medical specialists and general practitioners to become independent, self-employed practitioners. In early 1994 the CC assigned patients to independent family physicians, who were paid on a capitation basis. After the national government rescinded the Family Doctor reform, Stockholm continued to allow patients to chose private family doctors. As a result, the number of independent physicians in the community grew. These physicians were not given incentives to reduce referrals to hospital, and no substantial relocation of care took place. Furthermore, the vast majority of Stockholm's patients continued to go directly to hospitals without referral or obtained referrals from independent specialists.

In 1991 Stockholm began introducing a purchaser-provider split much like the one being implemented in Britain at that time. Beginning in 1992, Stockholm was divided into area boards, each representing between 200,000 and 300,000 people. These boards had responsibility for purchasing health services with funds allocated by the CC. Purchasing board members, who were chosen by election and remunerated by the CCs, had little direct contact with the citizens they were to represent. Instead the boards were to assess the needs of the population through surveys and epidemiological studies.

The public hospitals in these areas remained under CC ownership but attained the status of semi-autonomous organizations. As such, they were responsible for balancing their revenues and expenditures and no longer had to serve the population of a specific geographic area. The hospitals were governed by supervisory boards composed of professionals and business people. These boards replaced supervisory boards made up of politicians, who had often served as intermediaries between hospitals and the CC and as advocates of their hospital's particular needs and interests. Under the reform, hospitals directors could deal directly with purchasers and were empowered to develop and implement broad administrative goals and strategies for their institutions.

'Buyers' (area boards) and 'sellers' (hospitals) were to negotiate prices for hospital services, with central Stockholm boards setting price ceilings and overseeing quality. Originally, contracts were based on per-diem payments. Prospective budgeting based on DRGs was introduced for surgery in 1992, internal medicine in 1993, and all other areas in 1994. To hold down hospital expenditures, DRG rates were to decrease if activity exceeded target levels (Ints.). The CC allowed hospitals to keep budget surpluses and made each hospital responsible for its deficits. In response to these reforms, several hospitals gave their departments budgetary autonomy and experimented with internal pricing (Forsberg and Calltorp, 1993).

In practice, the contracts that area boards negotiated with hospitals were really purchase agreements, which lacked the status of legal contracts and contained no provisions for enforcement. Gradually purchasers required hospitals to commit themselves in the contracts to implementing quality assurance programs and to cooperate with quality initiatives run by the various medical specialties. The medical specialties concentrated on gathering regional data on practices and their outcomes and developed consensus documents on best practices. Toward the mid-1990s, purchasers also began to require hospitals to develop plans for 'chains of care', which integrate hospital and community care in areas like geriatrics.

Stockholm's purchasing boards also made efforts to convince hospitals to shift care to the community. In practice, purchasers met with resistance and were often unable to negotiate meaningful changes. Hence they tried to use budgetary allocations to achieve their goal. The tensions that emerged between purchasers and hospitals were evident in comments by a physician with managerial responsibility in one of Stockholm's main hospitals:

> Dr. R described how the purchasers were developing community-based services that overlapped with internal medicine services already provided by the hospital. As investment in primary care grew, the hospital was forced to cut outpatient services 'that we think are fine', in areas like cardiology and skin care. 'Primary care is [now] supposed to take care of [these areas], but we know they can't...' A committee made up of physicians from the hospital and primary care, along with purchasing administrators, concluded that only five percent of hospital cases might readily be transferred to community care. Unfortunately, 'the purchasers don't believe in our conclusions'.

Despite these conflicts, department heads and physicians in the hospitals sought closer links with primary care centers and referring physicians in the communities. The providers also made efforts to assure that community physicians and their patients were satisfied with hospital care. Besides enhancing hospital revenues, these links to the community helped promote continuity and co-ordination of care across sectors – a goal which became increasingly important to both practitioners and politicians.

Many of Stockholm's physicians and nurses expressed concerns that cost con-siderations might harm the quality of their work and their clinical autonomy (Forsberg and Calltorp, 1993, p. 9; Ints.). But health professionals had little influ-ence over the design of the 'buy-sell' system. There was little or no negotiation with them during the planning of the reforms, nor were hospital staffs trained to implement them. Instead, the CC and its boards simply announced the various stages of the reforms and expected conformity and cooperation. As one administrator in Stockholm's CC explained:

> We just decided to start [the program], and [the providers] reacted to the eco-nomic incentives. The doctors had a lot of reservations but acted as we wanted.

When the CC planned to introduce DRGs, it consulted with department heads in the hospitals about DRG weights, but overrode their recommendations just before implementation. Thereafter, recurring negotiations between practitioners and CC administrators over DRG prices and frequent changes in DRG criteria created many financial uncertainties for hospital managers and physicians.

The prospect of productivity-based revenues created incentives for hospitals to boost their activity levels. The hospitals also experienced pressure to increase productivity, because patient demand was rising faster than hospital budgets. In some cases, clinic chiefs took anticipatory steps toward increasing savings and production in their units before the DRG payments became operative. One clinic head was reported to want to prove that he could introduce efficiencies before being forced to do so. Some clinical chiefs saw their ability to introduce effi-ciencies as improving their ability to bargain with hospital directors. While con-tinuing to cut staff and beds, hospital managers and clinical chiefs introduced more flexible work arrangements and encouraged staff to work longer hours. When DRG reimbursements declined, hospital staff sought to preserve their department's revenues by redoubling efforts to cut hospital stays and hasten patient throughput. There were also reports that hospital physicians sometimes favored procedures with better reimbursement rates, reclassified procedures under more favorable DRG categories, shifted patients to less costly treatment settings, and encouraged repeat hospitalizations, rather than completing treat-ment in a single stay (see also Charpentier and Samuelson, 1996).

By 1993 it was clear that Stockholm's purchaser-provider split and DRG-based remuneration system encouraged hospital production more than cost contain-ment. Moreover, costs for hospital care and private practitioners in primary care were rising while CC income from taxation and government transfers was falling. This situation contributed to a sense of loss of financial control within the Stockholm CC (Whitehead et al., 1997) and intensified pressure for cost con-straint. To combat rising budget overruns, CC politicians imposed the deficits on the hospitals and directly capped their budgets. These moves overruled the area boards' purchasing commitments and deprived hospitals and departments of control over revenues deriving from patient flows. In addition, CC politicians intervened more directly in hospital restructuring, rather than leaving decisions on how to cut costs up to hospital managers and their staffs.

Hospital physicians and managers reacted to this rapid policy shift with shock and frustration. Here is how the head of an internal medicine department described the turnabout:

> In 1993 we were happy. We said, 'now we'll work hard'. We looked at the DRG classifications to see what revenues we would get from them... When we got paid more for [a particular treatment],... we increased patient visits, especially in outpatient clinics. Then six months later, the CC said 'Stop!' The balloon burst.

The DRG system quickly lost its credibility among providers. Backed by their managers, hospital physicians ignored hospital deficits and cuts in DRG rates and maintained previous rates of service provision. In like manner, the physicians refused to implement an activity-based pricing system for outpatient care. At the same time, organized labor and neighborhood constituencies put pressure on local politicians to withdraw plans to close local hospitals. Aware that it was losing ground in the polls, members of the CC's governing coalition sought to avoid further confrontations with providers and the public. They put off plans to cut beds by another 15% and concentrated on reconfiguring services within and between hospitals, rather than closing hospitals altogether.

By 1995 the CC had abandoned the original Stockholm model. Providers spoke of its 'disintegration' and 'collapse', CC members struggled to come up with a satisfactory successor that would preserve purchasing, while tightly capping expenditures. Researchers (e.g., Bergman, 1993; Håkansson, 1993) and health system actors outside of Stockholm (Ints.), who had carefully followed developments there, concluded that the new purchasing system was driving costs and volumes upward, rather than helping to control costs by enhancing system efficiency and effectiveness.

In 1996, in yet a further move toward tightening control over expenditures, the CC gave its central health board responsibility for coordinating purchasing of hospital services by the nine district boards (Bergman, 1997). It reassigned contracts to hospitals, rather than departments, and proposed changes in the prospective payment system. In 1996 and 1997, the Stockholm CC further restricted the autonomy of purchasers and hospitals. Now purchasing had to conform to plans for hospital services, which were drawn up by a new committee within the CC. Furthermore, the CC imposed cooperation on one pair of hospitals and cut services at Stockholm's smallest hospital.

Dalarna

In June 1990, Dalarna County launched the 'Dalamodel' for health system reform. The CC created 15 primary health districts, each with its own politically elected board.[12] Each board owned and operated a primary-care center and had responsibility for purchasing specialist and hospital care from a prospective budget. Local boards signed contracts with hospital departments and clinics. Patients could choose their primary-care centers annually.

By assigning purchasing functions to the boards, the CC intended to reduce hospital referrals and generate competitive incentives for hospital efficiency. To further enhance provider competition, the primary-care centers were allowed to purchase care from private providers and from public providers outside of Dalarna County (Bergman, 1993). The structure, location, and size of boards – the smallest of which covered less than 10,000 inhabitants – encouraged close contacts between purchasers, patients, and primary-care staff. Moreover, in an arrangement that anticipated the British fundholding model, the Dalamodel gave GPs direct inputs into decisions about contracts for hospital care.

Prices were to be set locally through direct negotiations between the district board and the provider. Remuneration was to be based on the services given – either in terms of fees per visit, per day, or some combination of the two. In some cases the CC sought to set prices centrally. The use of price ceilings and DRGs was debated for several years (Bergman, 1993), but DRGs were not implemented. Patients were free to choose their own hospitals and specialists, although extra charges were imposed for visits to specialists without referrals from the GP.

To enhance the hospital sector's efficiency, the county's four hospitals were to be merged into one, thus eliminating 150–200 positions. The hospital sector was then to be placed under the supervision of a single politically appointed board (Federation of CCs, 1990). Each hospital clinic (department) was to operate as a profit center, which would be financed with the income from selling services to the district boards (Paulson, 1993). Bonus payments to employees based on productivity were also planned (Saltman, 1990).

In practice, this bold experiment failed to meet the expectations of most of its planners and participants (Borgert, 1993). The small and non-professional purchasing boards were unable to exercise much influence over the hospitals. Limited opportunities emerged for provider competition, even though the hospitals did not merge, as planned. Distances between hospitals made it impractical for boards to move contracts from one hospital to another. In addition, there were not enough funds available in the system to attract additional providers. Hence, a group of physicians failed in their attempt to establish a privately operated hospital clinic, which would have competed for public funds.

Rather than attaining savings, the boards faced extra costs, as they devoted substantial resources to negotiating contracts and monitoring results. Thus they had less money available than previously for direct care. In theory, boards could shift care from hospitals to primary care, but in practice they were unable to do so. Rather than becoming more efficient, several hospital departments faced serious cost overruns. Costs of administering contracts in the hospitals were one source of rising costs per patient. Hospital physicians were reported to view the experiment as a 'nightmare', because of recurring negotiations over pricing and administrative arrangements.

Unable to obtain cost reductions through the market, the CC's Executive Committee intervened directly to reduce hospital budgets. Moreover, politicians and planners restructured their purchasing model once the high costs of running many local purchasing boards became evident. In 1993, in an effort to strengthen the power of primary care purchasing and reduce the costs and confusion generated by local purchasing boards, the CC reorganized primary care under the auspices of a single, integrated purchasing function. This team was also given responsibility for purchasing hospital care. These moves effectively eliminated possibilities for patient choice among primary care centers or competition among purchasers. Rather than merging the hospitals, the CC established a politically elected board and a single hospital management team to oversee them. The result, which further weakened the purchasers, was a cooperating network of autonomous provider units, which critics viewed as a 'cartel' (Borgert, 1994). Instead of creating a quasi-market for health care, these reorganizations generated a cooperative network of interdependent politicians, purchasers, and providers.

By the mid 1990s, Dalarna's politicians, like their colleagues in other counties, had redefined the objectives of the purchaser-provider split. Now the system was supposed to help coordinate care across caregivers, rather than contain costs or enhance patient choice. Here is how Dalarna CC's Chief Executive summarized this radical change in vision:

> If we stressed costs when starting the Dalamodel, now the stress is on cooperation... How to treat patients, where to treat them, [how to develop] a chain of care, how does the patient pass through the care system, how do CC [medical] caregivers cooperate with municipalities [which provide social care].

Bohusland

After earlier experiments in public purchasing, in the early 1990s Bohus County restructured its health care around 14 Primary Health Councils, each with around 20,000 citizens. These were run by a health board, to which members were elected. The board members served on a voluntary basis, with the support of one or two paid staff members. Boards sometimes shared staff and services. Each board was to gear its purchasing plans to the needs of its own population. After initial experiments with local purchasing, the CC grouped the boards into three geographic areas for purchasing purposes. Bohus' hospitals remained in public hands, but since 1989 had been governed by professional, non-political boards, which were responsible to the CC for the hospital performance.

Until 1992, the CC had assigned each purchasing board a weighted, capitated budget on the basis of which the board was to sign block contracts with community-based specialists and their local hospital, but not with other hospitals or individual hospital departments. After 1992, the Bohus model allowed for market-like behavior by public purchasers, but the purchasers rarely switched providers. DRGs were introduced as an accounting mechanism, but not as an incentive for productivity in inpatient care. The CC developed a separate system for pricing outpatient activities. Gradually purchasing contracts expanded to cover participation in national quality registers and patient care standards, including waiting times.

Comments by Mr. J, a manager responsible for contracts for one of Bohus' purchasing areas, provide a vivid illustration of the ways in which local politics limited the ability of purchasers to gain leverage over providers through market mechanisms:

> Mr. J explained that purchasing contracts spell out goals for increasing day surgery. Through negotiations with hospitals, the purchasers are moving 'step by step toward the goals of the boards. This type of change in medical care takes time. We can't do it in a few years'.
>
> MH: Take the example of surgery. You meet with the department chief and the hospital director. You say you want more outpatient treatments. What if he says it can't be done? Do you have outside advice [to rely on]?
> Mr. J: Yes, we live close to [a major hospital]. If there is a big difference [in use of outpatient surgery] between hospitals, we could buy from another hospital. We could say we want to go on the open market.
> MH: Have you done this?
> Mr. J: No, it's a theoretical possibility.
> MH: Has it happened elsewhere in Bohusland?
> Mr. J: Not on the hospital level [because of local] politicians in the [communes. Citizens] can go to them to get [their] needs met... If there's unemployment [because of hospital restructuring], they [the communes] must bear the responsibility.

Decisions by purchasers faced resistance by hospital managers and physicians, as well as local politicians, as the following episode shows:

> In keeping with its policy of encouraging transfer of care from the hospitals to the community, the Bohus CC initiated a professional assessment in its northern purchasing area of the feasibility of relocating care. The community physicians who took part in the assessment generally agreed with hospital specialists that 90 to 95% of the cases being treated in hospitals could best be handled there. Some forms of care were relocated after the assessment.

For the most part, such judgments by physicians and constraints on primary care budgets provided few opportunities for substantial substitution of community care for hospital services.

The volunteers who staffed Bohus' local boards had even less influence over hospitals than area purchasers. In most cases, local board members lacked the expertise, technical capacities, and political influence needed to evaluate hospital performance and enforce contract standards.

> When asked about quality and other contract standards, the head of a local purchasing board only cited requirements concerning professional certification, waiting times, and keeping appointments. She did not mention any clinical

process or outcome measures. She reported that information on compliance with contract standards comes in quarterly computer printouts from hospitals and periodic complaints from individual patients. But the board head seemed unsure as to what to do with the printouts. In addition, she had no means of enforcing conformity to contract standards. For example, when the hospital seemed likely to exceed its volume limits, she could only 'ask the hospital to hold more discussions with the board and [recognize that] it's better to reduce production earlier instead of later'.

Hospital physicians with managerial responsibility generally held a skeptical view of the competence and efficacy of the local and area boards and viewed quality assurance as a professional responsibility and prerogative. Here is how Dr. N, the head of a surgical department put it, when asked whether contracts included quality standards:

The purchasing board members don't have the competencies to follow up. These purchasers are politicians. You can't expect them to have insight into how we treat patients. These issues are a professional responsibility.

Despite his position, Dr. N admitted that his specialty's development of quality indicators for Western Sweden and their efforts to develop best practice standards reflected 'the wishes of the political system'. Still he saw these forces as weaker than the aspirations of surgeons throughout the region, who 'want to compete on quality' [while guaranteeing adherence to treatment standards].

Dissatisfaction with the purchasing system grew within Bohus CC, as patient demand outpaced budget allocations. Gradually the CC began to intervene actively in the purchasing process. At first the CC tried to cope with cost overruns by centralizing purchasing within three area boards. However, by transferring surpluses from boards that achieved savings to those running deficits, the CC effectively eliminated the boards' autonomy. By 1994, the CC had undermined local purchasing by centralizing hospital purchasing and planning mergers between hospitals within Bohusland and adjoining counties. These mergers partially reflected a belief that larger hospitals would deliver care more efficiently and effectively than smaller ones. Another force for regional cooperation came from planning uncertainties and operational difficulties stemming from the movement of hospital patients across county borders.

Common Features of County Experiments

Although there were many variations in the purchasing arrangements implemented by these and other CCs (Bergman and Dahlbäck, 1995), the key actors in the CC experiments behaved in remarkably similar ways. Their actions contrasted radically with those envisioned by neoliberal theories of quasi-market competition.

First, consider the actions of Sweden's health purchasers: they did not ordinarily foster competition among hospitals by 'shopping' for the most cost-effective services, switching contracts, or threatening to do so (Expert Group, 1994). In fact there was very little movement of funds among providers, and most of what did occur stemmed from patient choice programs, rather than decisions by purchasers. One reason that contracting did not increase fund movement was that CC purchasers typically signed block contracts, which committed them to obtaining entire packages of care from a single provider. Moreover, many CCs had few options for shifting contracts, because of geographical barriers and a lack of independent providers of specialty care outside of the largest cities. CC politicians also discouraged purchasers from switching contracts lest market pressures destabilize local hospitals. Politicians and purchasers that did plan reconfigurations often met resistance by local politicians and labor unions.

The purchasers also faced additional barriers to market behavior. In particular they lacked the knowledge, skills, and data that could support rational choices among services. Nor did purchasers go far toward developing their capacities to assess provider performance and compliance with contracts. Neither purchasers nor hospital managers obtained much valid data on the costs of specific hospital departments and services (e.g., Lindkvist, 1996). Moreover, purchasers had virtually no data on the clinical quality of care and limited information on service and other quality dimensions. Thus the purchasing experiments did little to reverse the asymmetric relations that had prevailed before the reforms: physicians continued to hold almost all the expertise and information needed to assess the medical needs of the public and the degree to which these needs were being met (Bergman and Dahlbäck, 1995).

Budgetary constraints imposed by the CCs led the purchasers to devote much of their energy to keeping hospitals within their budgets, rather than focusing on longer-term objectives. As these constraints grew, the purchasers found fewer and fewer opportunities to transfer care from hospitals to the community, enhance prevention and health education, follow-up on hospital quality initiatives, or encourage integration of hospital and community care.

Rather than relieving the budget problems as anticipated, the market experiments added to them. The CCs encountered unanticipated managerial costs. Patient movement among hospitals and across county borders added expenditures and fiscal uncertainties. Payments to independent family physicians added to the costs of community care.

Second, the behavior of hospital managers and specialists, who were the most important health care providers, did not conform to the scenarios of market reformers. Providers did compete for individual patients under the Patient Choice program, but they rarely competed for CC contracts. Instead, they responded mainly to budget constraints. Outside of Stockholm, hospital managers typically introduced changes in an incremental and reactive fashion, in response to pressure from the CC.[13] Even when managers had opportunities to market their services to more than one purchaser, they channelled more energy into coping with ever-more difficult operating conditions. Tighter budgets, frequent changes in reimbursement techniques and prices, resistance to job cuts by unions, and local political opposition to service reconfigurations limited the hospital managers' opportunities to seize the initiative. Hence, they concentrated on preserving or even improving existing levels of output, despite cuts in beds and staff.

When hospital managers did reconfigure services, they proceeded with caution, consulting with department heads as to how best to attain cost savings. The managers could obtain very limited guidance about these changes from existing information systems. With the exception of a few hospitals that introduced American management information systems for calculating the costs of inpatient care (for example, Brookside Hospital, which is described in Chapter 5), most hospital managers obtained very limited data on the costs of specific services and departments. For the most part the hospitals achieved their staff reductions through attrition in numbers of nurses aides, who had minimal training, and under-nurses, who lacked university degrees in nursing (Ints.; Federation of CCs, 2002, Table 1, p. 18). This tactic fit prevailing governmental policies that encouraged retention and upgrading of skilled nurses. Political and managerial wisdom argued against cutting positions for physicians.

Third, as cost pressures rose, politicians actively intervened in the nascent market. Their interventions were unanticipated by market theories, which largely relegated politicians to a secondary function of assuring fair competition and exchange among purchasers and providers. Unable to cut expenditures through purchasing and unwilling to halt popular programs like Patient Choice, CC politicians quickly reasserted their control over hospital budgets and patient flows. In Western Sweden, counties that were losing patients introduced marketing rules that curtailed patient choice (Anell, 1995). Moreover, many of the CCs that had experimented with purchaser-provider splits consolidated and centralized their decentralized purchasing schemes.

CCs that introduced purchasing later often favored centralized purchasing functions, which allowed less room for market behavior. The preference for centralized purchasing apparently reflected an attempt to capture some of the flavor of the purchasing process, while avoiding the old system of direct, top-down management of the hospitals by the CCs (Brommels, 1997). However, integrated purchasers did not enjoy freedom from fiscal and political intervention by the CC. Nor did they usually engage in market-like interactions with providers, like those envisioned in the original purchasing experiments in Dalarna County and Stockholm. Centralized purchasing grew in popularity, as the original buy-sell models lost their appeal. By early 1997, around half of the CCs had purchasing functions, and by 1999 the proportion had risen to two-thirds of CCs and covered a similar proportion of the population (Calltorp, 1999a).

Disillusion and Reorientation

As the trend toward centralized purchasing indicates, CC politicians gradually withdrew their support for vigorous market experiments. Drawing on the bargaining and interpretive frames, this discussion examines the changes in beliefs and political alliances that led to this pull back from market reform within the counties and contributed to a reorientation toward purchasing and other market processes.

Disillusion with the market reforms began as evidence spread that the buy-sell system, prospective payments for hospitals, Patient Choice, and the Family Doctor system were driving health expenditures upward, instead of reducing them. As implementation of the competitive reforms proceeded, policy analysts and politicians in CCs and the national government also began to fear that uncompromising pursuit of the logic of the market would destabilize Sweden's health system and undermine equal access to care. For example, the Patient Choice program and the productivity incentives included in Stockholm's contracts created the possibility that hospitals would cater to healthier and more mobile patients from outside their catchment area, at the expense of local patients. In like manner, purchasing decisions based on cost-effectiveness could lead to closing less popular or less efficient provider units and thereby reduce equality of access to care across geographical areas.

An even more fundamental concern was that reductions of health services in response to changes in market demand or performance would produce unemployment. Fearing losses of jobs and local services, CC members representing locales in which hospitals faced closure or reorganization joined with labor unions and municipal politicians to oppose these moves. With nationwide unemployment exceeding ten percent, politicians at all levels were wary of being accused of further aggravating an already difficult situation.[14]

During the run-up to the national and CC elections of 1994, these reservations about market ideologies and programs fed into a broad groundswell of public opinion and local political activity, which opposed further budget cuts and sought to preserve the generous and egalitarian benefits that Swedes had enjoyed for decades in employment, health, and welfare. The incumbent center and right parties became the targets of this opposition, even though the Social Democrats had also backed cost-containment in health throughout the 1980s and early 1990s and had supported the market reforms.

Rather than abandoning purchasing altogether, CC politicians sought new uses for it. Politicians in the CCs began to treat purchasing as a way to enhance coordination of services among caregivers – including ambulatory health care, geriatric, and social services. Throughout Sweden, contract periods were extended and efforts were made to enhance collaboration between purchasers and providers and among care sectors. Local purchasers pointed with pride to experiments with chains of care that encompassed all of the community and hospital services dealing with chronic conditions like heart disease and alcoholism (Int.).

At the same time, it became clear to most politicians that it was not politically feasible to rely heavily on market solutions to the problems facing Sweden's health care system. Politicians and planners recognized that competition would harm, rather than foster coordination within health sectors and weaken ties between health and social care. In like manner, the market seemed to hold little promise for enhancing the quality of care. Quality and care-coordination initiatives required cooperation and self-regulation of physicians and other health providers, rather than competition among them (Harrison, 1999).

As belt-tightening in the hospitals continued during the mid-1990s, responsiveness to these and other new health policy issues grew slowly. CC politicians and health and welfare professionals expressed concern that chronically ill patients, many of whom were aged, would suffer from cutbacks in services. To avoid this problem and reduce the tendency for contracting to fragment care, CC purchasers and administrators, along with some hospital managers and health care professionals, sought to develop networks that could link hospitals, primary care, and municipal services. In at least one county (Östergötland) this movement led to cooperation between the county purchaser and the university hospital to restructure care around broad diagnostic categories, thereby breaking down organizational boundaries between care sectors. Nonetheless by the late 1990s movement toward integration of care was still in its earliest stages. In like manner, calls for quality assurance had not produced much direct monitoring of the quality of hospital or community care. Nor had comparative data been distributed to patients or purchasers about the nature, quality, or efficiency of the services offered by specific providers.

Gradually market theories and terminology lost much of their appeal to decisionmakers in the CCs and the national government. In their place, there was renewed interest in regional planning and budgeting. Mergers among hospitals held out the prospect of attaining economies of scale. Both regionalization and hospital mergers reduced opportunities for market competition. Politicians and managers within CCs and the newly created regions gained further influence over health service configurations, while health professionals retained autonomy over practice.

CONCLUSION

Market experimentation emerged within the context of efforts by Sweden's national and county governments to further ambitious and conflicting objectives – including cost containment, reduction of waiting lists, and rendering the health services more responsive to the needs and preferences of their patients. When the reforms were implemented, public payers found fewer opportunities than expected for rational choice among providers, and providers showed less interest than anticipated in competition. As it became clear that market reform was costly and threatened important political values and interests, the political climate shifted rapidly from broad support for market solutions toward concern and skepticism about them. The chapter that follows examines the outcomes of market and non-market reforms and recent developments affecting private finance and delivery of health care.

NOTES

1 This divergence was evident in interviews conducted in 1993 by Twaddle (1999), in my interviews in 1994, and in numerous press reports and publications. See Harrison (1995a) and Twaddle (1999) for further references.

2 The right of center New Democratic Party, also supported market reform. It backed the Family Physician Program in 1993, but reversed its position in 1994 (Twaddle, 1999).

3 Swedes often use the term 'reform' to refer to actions that were defined in Chapter 1 as programs. In this chapter, I preserve this and other popular instances of Swedish usage.

4 For example, Blomqvist (1992); Enthoven, A. (1989). Management information and analysis for the Swedish health care system [IHE Working paper, No. 7]. Lund: Swedish Institute for Health Economics, as cited by Håkansson (1993); see also Twaddle (1999), Light (2000).

5 See Rehnberg (1995). According to Bergman and Dahlbäck (1995), by June of 1995 just one third of the CCs had introduced some type of purchaser-provider distinction.

6 Arrangements for regional health care developed as early as the 1960s (Bergman, 2002).

7 Both of these mergers have now been completed.

8 Between 1992 and 2000, the supply of hospital beds (of all types) dropped by 45%, with the steepest declines occurring between 1992 and 1996 (Federation of County Councils, 2002, diagram 4, p. 20). See Chapter 1, footnote 4 on reporting of changes over time.

9 The interviews in Brookside, which had pioneered the introduction of an American management information system, formed part of an in-depth case study based on 13 interviews, hospital documents, and statistics.

10 According to my informant, an official in the Stockholm County Council, one-quarter of patients self-referred to hospitals, one-quarter were referred by general practitioners in clinics, and half were referred by private specialists. Under Stockholm's market system, hospitals were paid per patient, a practice that was subsequently discontinued.

11 Except as noted, the analysis of CC purchasing that follows draws primarily on my interviews. Additional treatments of purchasing experiments appear in Bergman and Dahlbäck (1995); Harrison, (1995a), Federation of CCs (1990); and Saltman and von Otter (1992).

12 The following summary outlines major developments in Dalarna, rather than providing a detailed chronicle of the many changes that occurred in health finance and organization.

13 An important exception occurred in the Southern Region of Älvsborg County, where a new administrative director took a more strategic and proactive approach (Harrison, 1995a, pp. 128–130).

14 This figure includes both the officially unemployed (around eight percent) and another two to four percent who were enrolled in training programs and government-sponsored work programs aimed at the unemployed.

5

Reform Outcomes in Sweden and the Emerging Mix of Public and Private Care

This chapter examines the outcomes of Sweden's market reforms, and contrasts these outcomes to those of non-market reforms that were implemented during the same period. The first part of the chapter applies the administrative, bargaining, and interpretive frames. Then the second section applies the institutional frame to illuminate sources of institutional continuity in Sweden's health policies and contributions of the market reforms to institutional change. The chapter's concluding section examines recent trends toward market-based services that are producing a new mix of public and private care.

OUTCOMES

It is not easy to distinguish the effects of external forces and multiple change programs on Sweden's health system. Sweden's national government and County Councils (CCs) applied strict fiscal constraints on health expenditures before, during, and after the heyday of market experimentation. These resource constraints, along with rising demand for care and increasing costs of medical technology, joined in forcing ambulatory and hospital caregivers to learn to provide more medical care for less money – regardless of whether or not the providers had to compete with one another.

While holding down health costs, the national government and the CCs pursued other, potentially conflicting objectives: reducing waiting lists (by boosting hospital volumes); fostering patient choice of ambulatory and hospital providers; and devolving decisionmaking about health care to the CCs and their citizens. Assessment of program outcomes is further complicated by the diversity of programs formulated and implemented by the CCs and gradual changes in the goals and substance of these county-level programs. The implemented programs mobilized a range of change mechanisms – including caps on budgets and fees, direct fiscal incentives for production, market incentives for improvement of service and efficiency, and government-mandated reconfigurations and relocations of health and social services (e.g., movement of geriatric patients from CC-run hospitals to municipal facilities).

111

Powerful external forces also affected the health system during the period under study. These included population ageing, technological change, and changes in medical practice (Federation of CCs, 2002). Moreover, the economic downturn of the 1980s and the deep recession between 1991 and 1993 were accompanied by budget cuts and uncompensated currency devaluations, moves that weakened long-standing understandings between government, business, and labor. The economic decline indirectly contributed to compliance with reform programs and helped hold down health costs. As the recession deepened, concern over job losses and the very survival of public medicine in Sweden led medical staff unions to restrain their wage claims and exercise restraint in criticizing the reforms.

The *administrative frame* suggests two questions about the reforms' outcomes: First, how successful were national and CC governments in implementing their plans for quasi-market reform? At the broadest level both market and non-market reforms successfully continued prior moves to devolve responsibility for financing and providing health and social care to the counties and municipalities. Still, the national government retained its ability to oversee health finance and intervene in key decisions about the provision of health care.

Among nationally mandated programs, the Care Guarantee and Ädel reforms stand out. Rather than using market mechanisms, these two programs used the budgetary powers of the national government to foster change in hospitals and municipalities. Both programs were quickly implemented by the counties, hospitals, and municipalities (in the case of Ädel); as reported in Chapter 4, both operated much as expected. By 1994 the Ädel reform had reduced the proportion of elderly bed blockers in acute hospitals to 7.5%, as compared to around 20% in 1990. Further declines occurred through 1996 (Andersson and Karlberg, 2000).

Patient Choice of hospitals was the only national market reform that was implemented much as planned. This program created competition for elective patients but only led to movement of very small proportions of patients and resources. Moreover, Patient Choice increased financial uncertainties for CCs and eventually met with some resistance by them. In the mid-1990s the conditions of the Care Guarantee, on which patient choice depended, were changed to give patients the right to see a primary-care doctor for any condition within eight days and the right to all types of specialty care within three months. If these conditions are not met, patients are allowed to seek care outside of their CC (Federation of CCs, 2002).

As seen in Chapter 4, the Family Doctor program, which led to competition among primary providers, had a more checkered history, with many setbacks and revisions. Introduction of prospective payments, based on DRGs, was another national initiative that could contribute to public purchasing and foster more effective costing of hospital services. Despite the program's promise, by 2001 only six of 21 counties and regions were using DRG-based payment systems (Bergman, 2002).

The CCs' buy-sell experiments formed the heart of the market reforms. This set of policies and programs suffered from major implementation problems and did not diffuse widely among counties. In the CCs that did introduce purchaser-provider splits, very limited competition developed among acute hospitals, and this competition did not center on contracts from public purchasers. Instead, hospitals in counties with and without purchasing programs strove to attract individual elective surgery patients under the terms of the Care Guarantee and Patient Choice programs. Public purchasers lacked the opportunities, knowledge, tools, and power to influence the content, location, and quality of health services. Shortly after the experiments were launched, county politicians reasserted control over the very sources of power and authority that public purchasers needed if they were to influence health providers. Gradually the county politicians undermined the foundations of the original buy-sell system. They recentralized budget decisions – and in some areas regionalized them, cut hospital expenditures drastically, and enforced hospital restructuring.

The second question arising from the administrative frame concerns the degree to which the reforms attained their original objectives. At first glance, Sweden's market reforms seem to have produced many of the sought-for results (Bergman, 1997; Socialstyrelsen, 1995). But careful analysis is needed to uncover links between specific programs and outcomes. As noted earlier, Sweden's success in containing health costs began long before the reforms. Rather than reflecting market forces, cost containment during the 1980s and stability of national expenditures as a proportion of GDP during the early 1990s, mainly reflected strict enforcement of budget ceilings by the national and county governments (Calltorp, 1995).[1] The figures for per-capita health expenditure also seem to reflect the impact of budget ceilings more than market experiments. Per capita spending rose 17.4% in terms of Purchasing Power Parities (see Chapter 1, footnote 24) from 1987 though 1990, the years in which the market experiments flourished in the counties.[2] However, per capita expenditures stabilized after 1991, when tax ceilings were imposed by the national government and grew only one percent from 1991 through 1994 (OECD, 2001). The Ädel reform also helped hold down general hospital costs and resulting CC expenditures by giving the municipalities direct financial incentives to transfer geriatric patients out of general hospitals once medical treatment was completed. The reform also helped hospitals reduce lengths of hospitalization and increase patient throughputs.

The budget ceilings and hospital cutbacks also contributed to a gradual, but consistent, decline in reliance on hospitalization. Expenditures for in-patient care as a proportion of total public health expenditures declined by 3.6% between the start of 1987 and the end of 1991 and by 2.7% between 1992 and 1995 (OECD, 2001).[3] Similarly, there was an 8.5% reduction in inpatient care episodes between 1992 and 2000, while dramatic increases occurred in some common types of outpatient surgery (Federation of CCs, 2002). Nonetheless, inpatient care continued to absorb half of public health expenditures.

In contrast to the effects of the non-market programs, which used fiscal steering by central government, the most thorough reforms of CC health care along market lines failed to contain costs. In CCs like Dalarna and Bohus, which had local purchasing boards, the costs and complexities of administering purchasing proved to be much higher than anticipated, and the expected cost savings did not materialize. In like manner, Stockholm's program of hospital competition and productivity-based reimbursement produced rapid escalation of total hospital activity and costs (Håkansson, 1993).

The Family Doctor program generated competition among primary care-givers, but it too failed to reign in health costs. Advocates of the program had envisioned public purchasers substituting less costly primary-care services for hospital services (Twaddle, 1999, p. 93). Yet in Stockholm, and in a few other cities where this reform was most widely implemented, there was no significant substitution of primary care for hospital services (Int.). Moreover, expenditures for primary care rose, due to payments to independent practitioners (Ints.; Whitehead et al., 1997).

The market reforms in Stockholm and other CCs aimed more directly at increasing the health system's production levels and its efficiency than at controlling total costs. As hoped, ambulatory and hospital volumes rose dramatically during the market experiments, as did hospital productivity (Federation of CCs, 1993). According to one measure, which divides hospital outputs (discharges and consultations) by expenditures, productivity grew by eight percent in 1992, six percent in 1993, and two percent in 1994 (Anell and Svarvar, 1999). Volume of hospital production, as measured by turnover in acute hospitals, also rose dramatically during the reforms (10.3% in 1993 and 25.6% in 1994) – a jump in two years that was comparable to the 32% growth in turnover that had occurred during the entire decade of the 1980s.[4]

The question remains as to how much purchasing and hospital competition contributed to these productivity gains. Close examination of the available quantitative performance data raises doubts as to whether most of the observed system-level changes were produced by the market reforms and particularly whether the celebrated buy-sell system yielded the positive effects attributed to it. Although purchaser-provider experiments occurred in a minority of CCs, similar improvements in hospital productivity occurred throughout the country. Further evidence that generic forces were at work throughout Sweden – and even in Stockholm – comes from the finding that counties that ultimately introduced purchaser-provider splits experienced productivity gains and cost reduction *before* they introduced market mechanisms (Bergman, 1997). These data suggest that improvements in hospitals' performance mainly reflected pressure for productivity created by budget cuts, along with the effects of production incentives contained in the national Care Guarantee and Patient Choice reforms. Expansion of day surgery also contributed substantially to productivity gains (Federation of CCs, 2002). Although most evidence sustains the conclusion that the market reforms had little independent effect on hospital productivity, one study (Bruce and Jönsson, 1996) did show greater improvements in hospital productivity and throughput between 1990 and 1993 in Stockholm than in comparable counties that did not implement purchaser-provider splits.

The productivity gains of the early 1990s greatly advanced patient access to hospital care, which was a major objective of the market reforms. By the end of 1992, waiting lists for forms of elective surgery covered by the Care Guarantee had virtually disappeared (Hanning, 1996).[5] The Family Doctor program and patient choice of hospitals gave new freedom of choice to patients who were both able and willing to make these choices. However, this freedom came at a price: in an attempt to strengthen primary care, CCs raised co-payments on primary care visits and made payments higher for patients visiting hospitals without a referral by a primary care physician (Anell and Svarvar, 1999).

Unfortunately there are no systematic data available on changes in the quality of care. The available evidence suggests that the budget cuts and market reforms had mixed effects on care quality. On the one hand, many health professionals expressed concern that budget cuts and market reforms would pose risks to the clinical quality of care (Forsberg and Calltorp, 1993, 1994). On the other hand, neither my informants, nor expert analysts discerned concrete adverse effects of the reforms on hospital quality (Bergman, 1997; Ramström and Dahlström, 1995.) Hospital nurses suggested that the quality of nursing care may actually have improved in internal medicine during the reforms, because the Ädel reform relieved nurses of the heavy responsibility of caring for terminally ill geriatric patients (Ints.). In addition, service quality in hospitals, as indicated by waiting times, improved.

In contrast, the transfer of geriatric patients to municipal care ultimately resulted in poorer quality geriatric care. Although there were improvements in the standards of nursing care and growth in nursing staff after the reform (Andersson and Karlberg, 2000), the supply of nursing facilities did not keep pace with demand, and serious deficiencies occurred in the quality of care (Socialstyrelsen, 1993, 1998; Twaddle, 1999). Facing an ever-growing burden of geriatric care, the municipalities rationed care, rather than guaranteeing patient choice. What is more, they sometimes provided inadequate geriatric care. To reduce costs, many cities contracted with private providers in areas like food services. The result, according to the state-run body that oversees the health system, was that food quality deteriorated to the point where 30% of residents in municipal-care facilities were undernourished ('Crisis in...', 1997). The municipalities also encountered difficulties in assuring basic medical services for patients receiving home care (Federation of CCs, 2002).

The Family Doctor reform may also have harmed quality by contributing to the fragmentation of health services and reducing attention to preventive medicine and promotion of wellness. The reform reduced the influence of the polyclinic teams, where nurses and paramedics led efforts to prevent disease and promote health, rather than focusing on technology-intensive diagnoses and treatments of illness, as do most Swedish physicians.

The period of market reforms was marked by declines in equality of access to care, one of the fundamental values of Swedish health policy. Some of these changes can be traced to the market reforms, but much of the decline in access and equity in the 1990s reflects effects of other programs and simultaneous reductions in government spending. Most critical were the ways in which the Ädel Reform and changes in acute hospital practices disadvantaged the aged. Increasingly, elderly patients were sent home or to municipal facilities, where care was less adequate than in the acute hospitals.[6] Patient choice of both ambulatory and hospital care was more feasible for younger, healthier, urban, more geographically mobile, and higher income patients. Another development affecting equality was growing reliance within Stockholm and other large cities on private providers, who were reimbursed from public funds. The Family Doctor reform contributed directly to this trend, which made access to specialists easier in cities than elsewhere (Andersen et al., 2001). The system of flat rate co-payments for drugs and care in both ambulatory and hospital settings (Anell and Svarvar, 1999; Ljungkvist et al., 1997) also placed a greater burden on lower income and unemployed patients (Whitehead, Evandrou, Haglund and Diderichsen, 1997). A related development was curtailment during the 1990s of public dental insurance for adults. Together these developments made private payments increasingly important to Swedish health finance. After significant growth during the 1980s (from 7.5% to 10.4%), private payments as a percentage of all health expenditures rose steeply during the 1990s and reached 16.2% in 1998 (OECD, 2001). The result of these trends was some reduction in use of health care by lower income people and growing socio-economic inequality in access to care (Andersen et al., 2001; Burström, 2002). Private finance is likely to play an even greater role in the next few years, as government officials grow used to passing costs onto patients, and self-employed providers press for more private-sector funding. Both developments could further erode equal access to care.

An important question that fits within the *bargaining frame*, as well as the administrative frame, is whether the reforms empowered citizens by making health providers and politicians more responsive to the needs and preferences of individual patients and local communities. The reforms indeed continued a trend begun in the 1980s of devolving decisionmaking about health and social care from the national government to the CCs. Moreover, the CCs that experimented with purchasing, further devolved formal authority to local or area purchasers. However, in practice, these local boards gained very little influence over policies and priorities for health services. Purchasers at all levels – local, area, and county – struggled to cope with ever-stricter budgetary constraints and lacked the competence and power to shape hospital practices and policies (Bergman and Dahlbäck, 1995). Hence, purchasers had very limited opportunities for introducing new services or reconfiguring existing ones to fit community needs and desires. Most health budgets continued to be committed to maintaining long-standing commitments to providing accepted forms of hospital and community care.

Despite the government's decentralization policies, powerful centralizing trends emerged during the 1990s in decisionmaking about health. These trends further eroded the influence of patients, hospital staff, public purchasers, and local politicians. The national government and the Federation of CCs mandated major structural and fiscal changes in the counties. Within some CCs, elimination of political boards in hospitals reduced the influence of local politicians over hospitals and strengthened influence by CC officials. Moreover, there was widespread movement toward recentralization of decisions about hospital budgets and structures to the level of the CC and even to regions, where CCs cooperated and merged.

Although the reforms provided very limited opportunities for patients to exercise individual or collective 'voice' (Hirschman, 1970) over system practices, patient choice gave a minority of patients opportunities for exercising the 'exit' option. By linking hospital revenues to patient choice, the reforms gave hospital managers and physicians strong incentives to provide the types of services sought by patients and to make these services more appealing.

During the period of the market reforms, there were also changes in the standing of the health professions. For hospital nurses these changes stemmed primarily from the fiscal reforms and the Ädel reform, rather than the market reforms. Trained nurses gained operational and administrative control, even as they lost economic control. As CCs cut budgets, better trained nurses faced heavier patient loads and often had to handle additional tasks. The nurses were given most of the responsibility for facilitating patient treatment and discharge, so as to increase hospital throughputs. Nurses in the community lost some operational and administrative control, as GP-led practices competed for patients and funds with nurse-led polyclinics.

The budget cuts had little direct influence on the employment and remuneration of hospital physicians (Ints.; Anell and Svarvar, 1999.) On the other hand, there was some attenuation of the physicians' operational control, as they came under rising pressure to consider the cost implications of clinical decisions, speed up patient throughput, and expand outpatient treatment.

Neither the market reforms, nor top-down budgetary constraints produced direct challenges to the hospital physicians' clinical autonomy. Hospital managers typically sought to maintain the long-standing tradition of cooperating with senior physicians, rather than confronting them directly or attempting to intervene in their practices. Moreover, few hospitals developed management information systems capable of clinical practices among individual physicians. As concern deepened about clinical quality, national and CC politicians adopted a consensual approach to quality assurance and sought close cooperation with specialty organizations. These organizations led the development of quality assurance programs and practice standards (Harrison, 1999; Garpenby and Carlsson, 1994). CC purchasers and officials typically left it up to physicians to decide how to implement quality programs and report on clinical quality (Garpenby, 1997). Thus physicians and hospital departments participated in the quality activities of national specialty organizations on a voluntary basis without managerial intervention. In many hospitals, nurses and a few physicians also initiated programs to assess and assure quality, but these programs did not typically address issues of clinical practice.

The budgetary constraints and market reforms had very complex implications for department and division chiefs (Harrison, 1995a). On the one hand, clinical chiefs gained administrative control within their departments, as they were assigned responsibility for rationalizing services and meeting demand released by the Care Guarantee and Patient Choice programs. On the other hand, as budgets grew tighter and managerial supervision of departmental and divisional expenditures intensified, department and division heads lost some of their traditional influence over hospital administration and strategy.[7]

For community-based physicians, the Family Doctor reform brought enhanced economic control through self-employment, as opposed to salaried work in health clinics. Self-employment also gave the doctors more opportunities than did clinic teamwork for independent clinical and administrative control over work.

The reform period was marked by a further erosion of the strategic control of the SMA over health policy. Even prior to the reforms, the SMA had often been unable to influence the critical preparatory stage of policy formation, overcome the influence of other interest groups, or resist unpopular executive orders (Duffy, 1989; Immergut, 1989, 1992). Because the SMA was not well organized at the county or hospital level (Int.), its influence over policy eroded further, with the progressive decentralization of the health system.

The reforms also produced changes in the ways that health providers thought, felt, and talked about their work – developments that are best viewed through the *interpretive frame*. The discussion that follows illustrates these developments with statements from interviews with staff members from Brookside, a small general hospital in Western Sweden.[8] The findings from Brookside, while reflecting local conditions, are nonetheless largely consistent with my findings from other parts of Western Sweden and Stockholm; surveys conducted in Stockholm at the height of the market reforms (Forsberg and Calltorp, 1993, 1994); trends reported by local experts; and research on eight CCs that introduced purchaser-provider models (Bergman and Dahlbäck, 1995).

Perhaps the most immediate and widespread change in orientation among all hospital providers – including managers, physicians, and nurses – was growing awareness of considerations of cost and productivity and a feeling that their work was subject to more external constraints. These changes in orientations began with the budget constraints of the 1980s. Cost concerns among providers intensified as the recession deepened, whether or not CCs had introduced market experiments. As Dr. L, a veteran specialist in internal medicine at Brookside recalled:

In the 60s and 70s when I was a student, we never talked about costs, except for laboratory charges. You could keep patients in bed [as long as you wanted].

Along with cost-containment drives within hospitals came new ways of thinking about hospital services that originated in the world of business and industrial engineering. Particularly prominent was a production-efficiency frame that guided the drive to reduce length of stay (LOS). Concern with LOS preceded market experimentation and was virtually universal. Later, in some CCs, the introduction of DRG-based reimbursement gave further impetus to efforts to run hospitals in terms of what Mr. T, Brookside's Associate Director, called 'product-line management'.

> In a CC-backed project, Mr. T introduced an American management information system to Brookside. The system, which is based on DRG codes, allows the hospital's managers 'to compare results [costs and lengths of stay] for hospitals and treatments' and locate treatments that are 'DRG losers'. Mr. T views these comparisons as a powerful form of 'benchmarking'. The hospital management passes the data on to department chiefs and doctors responsible for specialties. They in turn strive to reduce length of stay and other costs for 'unprofitable' procedures. In addition, management has increased funding for operative procedures that the DRG system shows to be profitable.

This view of hospitals as 'a kind of industry', as Dr. J, a Brookside surgeon, put it, was widespread among top managers and departmental chiefs in Brookside and among surgeons in Stockholm, who also worked with DRG-based remuneration. For example, the chief of a surgical division in one of Stockholm's hospitals described how they created a unit for simple elective surgical cases that allowed for 'streamlining the production, improving timing, efficiency, and handling of patients'. Elsewhere, managers and clinical chiefs spoke of concerns about 'production levels' and 'efficiency', of departments, but they did not refer frequently to the costs or profitability of specific procedures or services. Along with the product-line orientation went enthusiasm for sophisticated management information systems that could generate data on comparative costs and revenues. At lower ranks, some physicians identified enthusiastically with the new way of viewing hospital services and the associated computer techniques. Take, for example, comments by Dr. J, an accomplished surgeon, who was hired to strengthen Brookside's surgery department:

> **MH:** Do you work with DRGs?
>
> **Dr. J:** Yes, I get the numbers from the administration... [from] Mr. T. on how many operations I do and the times. We can also look at patient flow for DRG number [gives DRG code]... and DRG number...
>
> **MH:** Are the data useful?
>
> **Dr. J:** Yes, of course, we have to compare ourselves all the time to other hospitals... (pulls sheet out of shirt pocket). Here are my latest statistics on [specific type of] operations... I did 80 this year – double last year's number.

In contrast, Dr. J and other enthusiasts reported that few of their colleagues actively analyze data on costs and LOS, although they are aware of the problems of efficiency and costs. Some physicians and nurses expressed doubts whether all these data on medical productivity contributed anything to their professional work. According to Dr. L:

The positive thing is you can see the costs of what you are doing and of how you handle patients..., but I feel that there are not so many doctors who use [the system]. We have a lot of information... about costs, but we can't use it. We have long lists about everything, but the doctors in the ward don't use it... We haven't caught on as to what we can use this enormous mass of information for... Much of the information is like rain off a goose's back. [DRGs might be all right for documenting length of treatment for myocardial infarction, with or without complications], but we have other diseases that are more complex and [their diagnosis and treatment] can't be measured on the [system's] scale. The work you've done as a doctor, the time spent with the patient and the nurse – it's not measured. This [computer system] is an economic [i.e. financial account-ing] system. It's difficult to describe what you do on the ward. You can handle a case professionally in many different ways.

When discussing inter-hospital comparisons on length of stay for specific diagnostic groups, Mr. T acknowledged the gap between himself and most of Brookside's physicians. Eight years after the launch of the first experiments in DRG-based remuneration at the hospital, Mr. T admitted:

It's easy to talk to the department chiefs. We understand each other. When they talk to their colleagues, it's not so easy. They are more focused on patients, as human beings. They say 'economic [i.e. financial] issues are not our interest [i.e. concern]'. It's getting better. As economic pressures increase, other physicians will take part [in these discussions].

Sometimes, department chiefs and other advocates of cost-driven change bridged the gap between physicians and management by legitimating cost reductions in medical terms. Dr. C, a department chief at Brookside, put it plainly as he described his success in convincing colleagues to cut LOS radically for a particular procedure:

Dr. C: My interest is economic. For my colleagues its other things.
MH: Like what?
Dr. C: As a physician you don't want to give worse care to a patient than your colleagues [would provide in another hospital]. A lot of writing in the medical literature shows that you can reduce length of stay without harming patients. I think this is more important than my explaining the economic need for reducing length of stay.

Some advocates of DRGs and other cost management techniques turned critic when they felt that politicians were dictating changes in reimbursement solely on the basis of financial considerations. This was the response of the Stockholm physician, who complained about how the CC suddenly stopped using DRGs as productivity incentives.[9] Generally, as was the case at Brookside Hospital, disaffection with DRG-based systems was greater among practitioners of internal medicine than among surgeons. Diagnosis and treatments in internal medicine often required cooperation between providers of community, hospital out-patient, and hospital inpatient care. By the mid-1990s dozens of internal medicine departments and primary care clinics throughout the country had adopted a locally developed computer program that was designed to track the entire chain of care for patients in fields like diabetes and anticoagulant therapy. This computer system allowed for recording of contributions to care by all caregivers in and out of hospitals. The system generated data that caregivers could use to assess their treatment of the patient. Practitioners could also discuss data on their patient's care program with the patient. The system also provided data that could be used to assess treatment outcomes, as well as costs. Dr. E, the origina-tor of this computer program, was a specialist in internal medicine at Brookside.

> Dr. E criticized Brookside's DRG-based system for failing to provide enough data on severity of illness and not supporting detailed follow-up of treatments and results. In his view, DRG-based management information systems were pushing physicians and managers to develop a 'cash orientation' and led them to miss many relevant questions: 'how can we work smarter, not harder? What do we do to link hospi-tals and primary care? How should we change the infra-structure [of care]?'

Another important interpretive development during the early 1990s was grow-ing awareness among politicians and health-providers of the importance of assuring clinical quality. Market forces were but one of several converging forces that facilitated the emergence of the Swedish quality movement. During the 1990s the National Board of Health and Welfare and most CCs backed quality activities, which spread far beyond those CCs with buy-sell experiments. This national health quality movement also drew inspiration from the international movement toward quality assurance in medical care (Garpenby, 1997).

The new emphasis on clinical quality in Swedish hospitals also came partly in reaction to growing stress on efficiency and throughputs among politicians and hospital managers. Some prominent physicians reported that they and their colleagues initiated programs for quality monitoring because they feared that the market reforms might compromise clinical quality. For example, in an inter-view in 1994, the head of a general surgical clinic in Stockholm recalled how two years earlier – at the same time that Stockholm implemented DRG payments for surgery – he initiated a database for recording common surgical practices and their outcomes:

> **Dr. U:** The systematic data gathering for Stockholm began in 1992. Previously we had local activities and irregular recording in the registry.
> **MH:** What was the background to the establishment of a systematic registry?
> **Dr. U:** There was agreement among eleven chairs [of departments of general surgery throughout the area]. When the [DRG] prepayment system started, we were worried about sudden changes in the amount of

surgery [or other procedures], and we wanted to monitor [possible developments]. In terms of ethical issues, [i.e., preference for procedures with more favorable DRGs], we have had very little problem.

In CCs that introduced purchaser-provider splits, the purchasing bodies lent their support to drives to improve quality. Purchasers required providers to take part in well-developed national quality registers in areas like orthopedics and required hospitals to develop local programs of quality assessment and improvement. The purchasers also sought to set service standards, which mainly focused on waiting times. Purchasing bodies typically left decisions about the nature of the hospital's quality assurance programs up to its doctors and nurses.

Attitudes toward patients also changed during the reform period. As hospital revenues and viability became more closely linked to patient flows, hospital managers and health professionals became more aware of the importance of attracting and satisfying patients. For example, the staff at Brookside Hospital were exposed to both market forces and threats of reorganization. According to the Director of Health Care in the CC, several proposals had been made over the past few years to close Brookside or merge it into one of the neighboring hospitals, while shutting down its surgical department. Local opposition, including demonstrations, had prevented the enactment of these plans, but discussion of restructuring continued. Here is how the resulting change in staff attitudes was described by the chief of Brookside's Department of Surgery:

MH: Have there been other major developments in the past few years, besides introduction of the new [DRG-based] costing system?

Dr. W: Yes, there is a different mentality among the people in the hospital. They are becoming more service minded. They know that the existence of the hospital depends on patient choice... The change in mentality is obvious. I really don't think that patient choice is so critical. Patients [typically] stay near home, but the staff are changing their approach. They are more concerned to be busy. Six or seven years ago people would say, 'The OR [operating room] session was done at noon. That's nice. Now I can relax'. Now if it's over at 2 pm, the people say, 'What's wrong?' People are nervous.

Recognizing that their hospital's operating environment was changing radically, physicians and nurses at Brookside and elsewhere accepted cutbacks, efficiency drives, and organizational changes designed to enhance patient flows – even when these changes created extra work for the staff.

Despite exposure to new forms of payment and threats of further budget cuts, few hospital managers or health professionals adopted very aggressive marketing orientations. Rather than actively courting patients or referrals, most hospital providers concentrated on providing elective services which were in high demand, while seeking to maintain a reputation for clinical quality among physicians in the community. For instance:

Dr. J viewed Brookside's recent expansion in orthopedic surgery as contributing directly to its survival, by warding off plans for reorganization or merger into a larger medical center. 'What counts is we can do the same high-tech surgery as is done 20 miles away [in a major city hospital]. If we can't, the patients won't come'.

Although Brookside Hospital received fees from patients from other CCs and obtained higher budget allocations after patient volume rose, Brookside's chief of surgery was still very cautious about actively recruiting patients. Dr. W's views became clear after he mentioned that waiting times were much lower in Brookside's emergency room than in two nearby hospitals located across CC boundaries:

Dr. W: I'm surprised that people don't drive here [instead of going to those hospitals].

MH: Do you try to let them know [about the shorter waiting times]?

Dr. W: No, we're a little scared of what will happen. We do try to develop good relations with primary care physicians in [our catchment area]. We're a little scared of attracting too many people... We have raised [our volume ceilings] a little. It's ambivalent. I'd like a little more, but I'm afraid of the ketchup bottle effect.

In areas like internal medicine, physicians at Brookside showed even less interest in actively marketing hospital services. They knew that most patients preferred their local hospital. Moreover, losses of patients to larger medical centers were balanced by inflows from rural areas lacking hospital facilities (Ints.).

Since physicians in community clinics were paid mainly on a salaried basis, their livelihood did not depend directly on patient flows. Nonetheless, in another community in Western Sweden, the head of the local polyclinic spoke of competition for patients with private physicians and among clinic physicians (Int.). Dependence on capitation fees or private, out-of-pocket payments gave private physicians even stronger incentives than salaried physicians to recruit and retain patients.[10] One private physician also justified his move to private practice in terms of his desire to devote more time to patient care and the prospect of greater autonomy in running his practice:

In my former job [in the clinic] you got a salary regardless of [your performance]. If you worked hard, you didn't get any response [from the system]... I couldn't stand it – meetings, meetings, meetings. Here [in private practice] we decide to buy something at 9:00, order it at 10:00, and it arrives at 11:00. There it took half a year!... I love to work with patients. All those meetings gave me a [pain]. Now we are independent.

Although providers recognized the importance of patient satisfaction, most hospital physicians and some nurses still viewed patients in terms that were more instrumental and pragmatic than humanistic or client-centered. Consider, for example, the following statement by Mr. G, a geriatric nurse in a suburban hospital in Western Sweden, whose job also included research:

> MH asked Mr. G to describe an activity that responded to pressure or demand from the outside community. Mr. G mentioned his work on pain relief and explained that patients suffering from Fibromyalgia created pressure for attention because 'as individuals they require a lot of time with the doctors... No one understands the illness, which mainly affects women. There was pressure from the local health clinics. These patients are time consuming and need a place... to be [taken care of]'.

Rather than showing concern for patient needs in their own right, Mr. G's statement focuses on the need to reduce patient demand on physicians. Dr. J's comments about orthopedic patients are also provider-centered:

> Dr. J said that his elderly patients 'are worried that we will send them home too early', but added immediately: 'We have to send the patient home, so we can bring another in. Otherwise it's not effective... You take one in and put another out as fast as possible'.

A young nurse who had worked just three years in internal medicine at Brookside expressed a more sympathetic and patient-centered view of the feelings of elderly patients, who were promptly transferred to municipal care under the terms of the Ädel reform:

> Sometimes its difficult for [their] relatives to understand that the patient can be taken care of elsewhere. In the past people stayed here. Now the system works that they stay a while and then go elsewhere. The old people sometimes feel thrown out. They don't feel well.

There was also new awareness among hospital professionals of the importance of ties to community-based medicine. Much of this reorientation reflected forces set off by local and national reforms. The Ädel reform led nurses to develop closer ties to municipal services (Ints.). CC purchasing experiments exposed hospital managers and professionals to the concerns of community representatives and practitioners. Reorientation towards community practitioners also stemmed from hospital physicians' desire to assure patient flows, as is clear from the comments above by Dr. W and other hospital physicians about their attempts to maintain good relations with primary-care physicians. Other illustrations of the emerging relations between hospitals and the community include the work of Dr. E and his colleagues on integrative computer systems and Mr. G's pain management project.

Despite these interpretive changes, there was little alteration during the market reforms in many of the fundamental beliefs, norms, values, and practices underlying the medical system and its occupational cultures. Hospital physicians continued to enjoy much greater prestige than community-based physicians in the eyes of both citizens and medical practitioners. There continued to be limited contact and cooperation between hospital physicians and their colleagues in the community. Here is how a GP, who headed a community clinic, described the situation:

MH: Have there been changes in the past few years in your relations to hospitals?

Dr. V: With the buy-sell system, each department pays for tests ordered, so we shove them back and forth between us. Both sides think this... The surgeons say that some GPs send their patients straight to the hospital without proper prior investigations. This throws a cog in the [hospital's] wheels.

MH: Have there been other changes in relation to hospitals? Do you see patients in the hospital?

Dr. V: No we didn't do it before [the reform], and we don't do so now. Sometimes we don't know that a patient was in the hospital. The patient is surprised [that we don't know]. Sometimes we have to see the patient after [the hospital stay]. The hospital notifies us, but we don't get the papers. We have been trying for 17 years to improve the situation. It may have improved slightly but not much.

As in the past, elite physicians retained control over medical training, ethics (see Rosenthal, 1995), technological innovation, and definition of practice standards. Most hospital physicians continued to identify strongly with their specialties and to defend its interests, rather than adapting a broader view of the hospital as an organization (Ints.; see also Ericson and Melin, 2000). Furthermore, physicians continued to put prompt treatment of patients ahead of cost containment or priority setting. For example, consider how Brookside's Dr. L cast herself as an advocate of her specialty and her patients' needs in heated debates over resource allocation with the hospital director and department chief:

'I'm there to argue for [my specialty within internal medicine]. When there are hot discussions, the colleagues with special interests in cardiology, diabetes, and so on are in contact with [the hospital director.] He is interested in hearing our opinions...' Dr. L then described how she sometimes tells the hospital director that he must authorize a procedure even if it costs extra money. In conclusion, she stated simply, 'you cannot deny an operation to a person suffering from [specific symptoms]'.

For the most part, hospital physicians also resisted proposals for patient-oriented services that bridged organizational and sectoral boundaries. Some integrative experiments took place in areas like cancer treatment, where care was provided by interdisciplinary teams. More typical was the cool reaction that many physicians at Brookside gave to Dr. E's call to reframe treatment regimes with the help of an integrated, patient-centered medical record.

Important innovations in professional practice continued to be anchored in traditional occupational norms and beliefs, rather than breaking out of accepted patterns of thought. Take, for example, physicians' responses to public pressure for more thorough quality assurance. Although many physicians acknowledged the growing pressure, few questioned the fundamental assumption that their own specialty organizations could and should provide the guidance needed to improve quality.

As shown in Chapter 4, Sweden's quasi-market reforms were legitimated to a substantial degree by academic and political discourse that viewed health and other public services through the lenses of neo-liberal economics. This radical departure from the rhetoric of governmental planning and budgeting shaped the discourse of politicians and providers for a few years. However, Sweden's politicians and health managers did not undergo as fundamental a change in orientations as did Britain's health system actors. Purchasers in Sweden said little about seeking value for money or assessing provider efficiency. Despite the talk of patient choice, neither government agencies, nor not-for-profit organizations, nor the press showed much interest in publicizing competitive rankings of providers on standards of quality and productivity, along the lines of Britain's league tables.

After a few years, much of the market rhetoric about health care fell into disuse. The terms of discourse gradually shifted towards a focus on collaboration among health system actors. Here, for example, is how Mr. T, the Assistant Director of Brookside Hospital, described his hospital's evolving relations with purchasers:

In the first years there were a lot of discussions about money and who is in charge, us or them. We were talking about the Psychiatric Department. They [the purchasers] said it costs too much and we should find another way to treat patients and reduce the number of in-patients... They had data from other buyers on the number of beds per 1,000 inhabitants. The buyers were making comparisons among themselves... Today we have a more constructive discussion. It's more friendly, with less conflict. They propose; we describe what will happen... I think they are not buyers but payers. They have to pay for what the patients choose.

As contract periods were extended beyond single budget years in CCs with public purchasing, negotiations and interactions between purchasers and providers took on a less confrontational tone. In negotiations and in descriptions of the contracting process, references to 'buying and selling' of services gave way to talk of 'consultation' and 'cooperation'. Although purchasers continued to be concerned about costs, they began to pay more attention to quality assurance, service quality, coordination among services, and relocating care in the community – all of which required cooperation. Within the CCs, politicians began to place their hopes for cost containment on consolidations and planning of services, rather than market mechanisms. At the same time the national health policy agenda shifted toward priority setting. This search for the best collective definition of priorities for health spending expressed distrust of the capacity of market forces to produce an effective and socially desirable mix of health services.

In conclusion, during the period of the market reforms – from the late 1980s through the mid-1990s – Sweden's hospitals grew more productive and efficient, and patient access to elective surgery improved dramatically. These outcomes did not result primarily from market forces that were set in motion by the competitive reforms. Instead, performance gains stemmed mainly from national programs that constrained and guided the behavior of health system actors. These included ever stricter ceilings on CC health budgets, restructured geriatric care, and earmarked funds for expansion of scarce surgical services. Public purchasing and Patient Choice, two of the most distinctive market programs, also boosted service production. But these two programs drove up total health expenditures, as did the Family Doctor program. The Family Doctor reforms, along with cuts in hospital capacities, contributed to increased use of primary care and may have contributed to an attendant drop in visits to specialists (Federation of CCs, 2002). On the other hand, these changes did not produce the expected reductions in hospital costs. Market reforms, along with increased co-payments, also contributed somewhat to growing inequality in access to care.

Despite these shortcomings, the market programs contributed to a shift in outlook and behavior among hospital managers and professionals, whose efforts were critical to sustaining improvements in efficiency and effectiveness. Increasingly, hospital providers recognized the necessity of cost containment and the importance of attracting and satisfying patients. However, few hospitals adopted broad marketing strategies. Neither the market reforms, nor hospital restructuring, seriously challenged the traditional occupational culture and professional dominance of hospital physicians. The market reforms also continued an ongoing process of devolution of authority to the CCs and within them to purchasing bodies and health-providers. However, by the mid-1990s counter trends emerged toward recentralizaiton of power at the regional and CC levels.

Just a few years after their start, Sweden's market reforms were transformed, and the market discourse that had accompanied them had largely disappeared. This rapid decline in market experimentation and rhetoric occurred in part because CCs and national politicians recognized that vigorous pursuit of market programs clashed with popular and deep commitments to the welfare state.

INSTITUTIONAL CONTINUITY AND CHANGE

After examining the institutional continuities that lay beneath this retreat from market policies, we will consider areas in which the market reforms nonetheless contributed to lasting, institutional change. Sweden's market reforms in health care formed part of a broader governmental challenge to the country's social welfare policies and institutions. Until the mid-1980s there had been few serious attempts to alter so fundamentally the principles of the Swedish model for the welfare state, which emerged after World War II. That model rested on the foundations of social solidarity, full employment, and labor-management cooperation. By the close of the 1980s, the national government had seriously cut back health and welfare spending, unemployment was rising, and experimentation was spreading with market solutions to health care delivery – and, to a lesser degree, health finance.

As the recession deepened and the market experiments expanded, politicians and voters saw a threat to universal and egalitarian health care and feared that unemployment would escalate. Opinion surveys (cited in Diderichsen, 1995, Table 2) and the results of the 1994 and 1998 elections showed how strongly the electorate felt about preserving Sweden's major health and welfare institutions – as promised by the Social Democrats. Public support rose between 1982 and 1992 for increased tax spending on health, pensions, and services for the elderly. In contrast, there were declines in approval of tax spending on means-tested social welfare programs, like those preferred by conservatives. Only a minority of citizens favored the strategy of the center and right-wing parties, which sought to achieve recovery by reducing government debt, taxes, and public employment. Sweden's citizens had grown more individualistic and more critical of state paternalism during the 1980s, but they still depended heavily on the state for work or welfare ('Too good...', 1999). What is more, they still believed in the Swedish model.

The fundamental beliefs and organizational arrangements underlying the Swedish model survived the challenges of the early 1990s. After a short period in which neo-liberal ideology flourished, Social Democratic policies and rhetoric quickly regained much of their former influence. In 1995, the newly elected Prime Minister announced plans to pour funds into the health, education, and welfare systems with the aim of boosting employment and using government spending as a lever for lifting Sweden out of recession. In a sharp reversal of its earlier policies, in 1995 the Stockholm CC guaranteed the continuing employment of all CC employees, including those in the health sector. The turnabout in political rhetoric was well illustrated by the response of Prime Minister Persson to revelations of problems in geriatric care after the Ädel reform ('Care review...', 1997):

In an attempt to cut costs, cash-pressed cities had been putting nursing home services out to private tender. In 1997 Swedish television reported that elderly patients in a private Stockholm nursing home were suffering from neglect. The Prime Minister blamed the market for patient neglect. He backed review of outsourcing practices among local authorities and stated that competition and the profit motive are inappropriate in welfare services.

Although the market reforms challenged some political values, institutions, and policies, they sustained others. Most importantly, the reforms continued the trend toward devolving authority for health-care finance and management to the CCs. Devolution of state authority to the counties continued after the demise of some market programs and the recasting of others. For example, beginning in 1998 the government capped drug budgets and passed responsibility for the cost of prescription drugs from the National Social Insurance Board to the CCs (Ljungkvist et al., 1997). As it had often done in the past, the national government relied on fiscal policy to influence health management and policy within the CCs.

Although long-term movement toward devolution to the counties remains strong, it is threatened by an institutional counter-trend. Regionalization of hospital care and CC mergers during the 1990s reflected efforts by CC politicians to cope with shrinking tax resources and growing economic interdependence among neighboring counties. Regionalization initiatives also partially reflected the difficulties encountered by CC's in managing and financing the movement of patients across county borders.

As a result of regionalization, many of the purchasing arrangements introduced by the CCs in the late 1980s and early 1990s are disappearing. Purchasers became payers, as county residents exercised their new rights of choice. In place of local and county purchasing, regional cooperation is leading to more centralized and hierarchical influence over health services. This trend is reshaping crucial areas within the health system – including the budgeting, planning and configuring of hospitals, community health care, technological innovation, and information systems.

The market reforms contributed to institutional change by making patient needs and desires central to health care and requiring providers to become more attuned to patient concerns. The reforms thus signaled a radical reduction in paternalism in the planning and delivery of health services. Patient Choice, the Care Guarantee, and the Family Doctor reforms were both a political response to public clamor for more responsive services and an impetus to change in the orientations of health care providers. In the wake of these reforms, providers sought for the first time to attract and retain patients and develop services in response to market forces.

The purchasing experiments also contributed to movement toward community-centered care. Purchasing enhanced the influence and legitimacy of those politicians and managers in CCs and local purchasing boards who sought to shift care from hospitals toward the community and encourage health-providers to foster citizens' health and wellbeing, instead of concentrating on disease intervention. However, resource constraints and the concentration of medical expertise among hospital specialists limited the ability of purchasers and local politicians to relocate care or alter service priorities.

Similarly, the Family Doctor reform increased activity and expenditures in community care, but failed to promote significant change in the way that patients and health professionals view health and illness. Instead of encouraging a comprehensive view of health care that includes patient education and preventive medicine, the Family Doctor reform led patients and practitioners away from the interdisciplinary polyclinics, which have traditionally given more attention to prevention and education than do independent doctors. Despite the market reforms, hospitals continue to receive the majority of health expenditures and still exercise a dominant influence over the ways that physicians and members of other health occupations think about and deliver care. Recently, CCs, municipalities, local clinics, and hospitals have begun to try to reduce the systems' fragmentation into uncoordinated, intervention-focused specialties by creating more integrated care networks. These networks link medical and social services and bridge between hospital and ambulatory care. In the long run, the development of chains of care and other forms of cooperation among caregivers should help promote care that is more focused on the entire spectrum of patients' medical needs and their wellbeing.

The market reforms also added momentum to the broad drive within Sweden toward greater accountability of hospitals and other health care providers. Movement in this direction appeared in CC purchasing, in public discussion of quality assurance, and decisions about priorities for health spending. On the other hand, the re-emergence of regionalization and the continuing dominance of quality assurance by physicians pose challenges to provider accountability and transparency.

The market reforms followed a trajectory that is characteristic of managerial and policy fashions (see Chapter 8). Nonetheless, they left their mark on fundamental structures and processes within Sweden's health system. Hospital administrators, who had previously administered predictable budgets, became active managers. They are now responsible to CC or regional payers for the hospital's financial status, levels of service production, and assuring that hospital staff engage in quality assurance.

The means of financing health care became more diversified during the reform period, as co-payments, private insurance, and out-of-pocket payments supplemented public budgets. Health care provision also became more diversified. Self-employed ambulatory physicians and private, for-profit providers of geriatric services took their place alongside the vast force of salaried health employees in the hospitals and clinics. New means of linking the finance and provision of health care also emerged. Besides using traditional forms of planning and budgeting, CCs signed contracts with hospitals and ambulatory physicians, while municipalities contracted with private firms. Providers formed networks and care chains, so as to focus on types of patients, instead of dividing services by specialty or organization.

CONCLUSION: MIXING PUBLIC AND PRIVATE CARE

From an administrative perspective, the market reforms of the early 1990s were a partial success. In reviewing their impact, it is useful to distinguish between two facets of the reforms: provider competition, which was the hallmark of market programs in Sweden, and the diffusion of business-like practices and thinking. In tandem with the imposition of strict budget ceilings, provider competition helped boost productivity and hospital efficiency. However, top-down regulation and government-mandated fiscal incentives had much more decisive impacts on these trends than did provider competition. Furthermore, provider competition failed to curtail health expenditures and even boosted some types of spending during a period when the governments could ill afford them. Thus top-down budget ceilings and regulation proved more effective mechanisms of cost control than did competitive incentives. The competitive reforms did succeed in making the health system more responsive to patient needs. In combination with the targeted funding that accompanied the Care Guarantee, Patient Choice helped eliminate waiting lists for elective surgery.

From the vantage point of the bargaining and interpretive perspectives, provider competition and diffusion of business practices together contributed to important incremental changes. The new financial arrangements that accompanied the competitive reforms contributed to an ongoing trend toward decentralization of authority in the health system. The new purchasing arrangements increased the voice of local politicians in health policy, but did not reverse the fundamental asymmetry in the power of providers versus payers. Nor did purchaser-provider splits or the family doctor program go far toward enhancing the power and centrality of primary care, as had been hoped. Patient Choice and the Family Doctor system did succeed in making hospital and primary-care providers more aware of patient preferences and more anxious to cater to them. The market reforms also made activities within the hospitals more transparent to public payers and enhanced managerial influence over hospital physicians.

Provider competition, together with other top-down programs – including the Ädel reform, the clinical chief reform, and budget caps – helped diffuse business-like practices, discourse, and thought among health-providers and public payers. Perhaps the most important change in this direction was that public payers, health managers, and a growing number of health professionals stopped viewing budgets as open-ended and learned to accept cash limits. Furthermore, payers and providers adopted quasi-industrial concepts and techniques that focused on boosting service production and throughputs. Yet another instance of the diffusion of market thinking was evident in the willingness of public officials to impose ever greater co-payments for health services. This approach rests on the assumption that it is reasonable to reduce the demand for health services by imposing higher costs to the consumer, just as one might do with any other commodity that people purchase in the market place.

Despite their great promise, the competitive reforms of the early 1990s rapidly lost momentum as policymakers faced the realities of shrinking resources, difficulties of program implementation, and widespread opposition to market restructuring of Sweden's medical and welfare systems. Politicians in the CCs and the national government curtailed the buy-sell system, the Family Doctor Reform, and even the popular Patient Choice program, because these reforms threatened to raise health costs and were politically risky. After just a few years of experimentation with market mechanisms, both county and national politicians fell back on budgeting and planning. Thus many politicians and analysts put their trust more in regionalization and mergers of hospitals than in provider competition. They assumed, despite a lack of convincing evidence, that increased hospital scale would save money and enhance clinical quality (Calltorp, 1999b). At the same time policy issues like patient empowerment and provider responsiveness, that had so concerned market reformers, lost ground to new issues, like quality assurance and coordination of care. Although they were short-lived, Sweden's competitive reforms complimented top-down moves to enhance provider efficiency and introduce industrial and business management practices to health provision. Moreover, the market reforms added complexity and flexibility to what had been a very monolithic system of financing and providing health services.

In these ways, the competitive reforms of the early 1990s paved the way for a new phase of market reform. These recent initiatives are further mixing public and private forms of financing and providing health services. The initiatives turn on competition among private and semi-private providers, rather than competition among publicly owned and managed providers, as did the reforms of the early 1990s. Moreover, the most recent and current experiments are not integrated within formal models for reform. For instance, in 1997 one hospital in Stockholm was reorganized as a publicly-owned company. After the 1998 elections brought liberal coalitions to power in Stockholm and several other counties, politicians renewed their efforts to launch programs for transforming hospitals into publicly-owned companies and privatizing their services (Calltorp, 1999a). Planners in Stockholm and the regions of Western Sweden and Skåne envisioned starting the privatization process with technical and hotel services, then moving to laboratories, and eventually privatizing some medical services. Over the last few years, there has been a gradual increase in the number of private physicians who entirely or partly own their medical facilities and contract with the public system to provide ambulatory services. By 2000, private, for-profit providers received nine percent of the CCs' total health expenditures (Federation of CCs, 2002, p. 11). In Stockholm, where this trend had gone farthest, private providers accounted for around a quarter of publicly financed health care (Bergman, 2002).

The trend toward diversification in finance and service provision is creating a more flexible system, which is more responsive to the needs and concerns of its citizens. But neither these recent initiatives, nor continuation of contracting by CC and regional purchasers seem likely to reduce total health costs or redirect most funds from hospitals to community care, as some advocates

131

of provider competition had originally hoped. Moreover, the growing diversification of health care provision and finance could fragment health care, making it harder to assure that all citizens receive comprehensive care and health promotion at a moderate cost. Rising co-payments and privatization of some types of care are also weakening the egalitarianism and solidarity of Swedish health finance.

In place of a rather monolithic public system, Sweden may gradually develop a very complex system that defies guidance and regulation at the national level. Such a system could reduce equality of access and raise costs, while failing to improve clinical care or health promotion. In fact diversification could create new barriers to integrating care across providers. These all-too-likely outcomes seem a high price to pay for increasing patient choice and satisfaction.

In the long run, Sweden's public health system faces the same threat to the principles of universal and equal access to care that looms over nearly all public systems in advanced nations: patient demand and costs of care are likely to outstrip the government's willingness to support health care. Such a development could lead to the emergence of a two-tiered system, consisting of a private sector for those able to pay with private insurance or out of pocket, alongside a larger, tax-supported sector serving less affluent citizens.

NOTES

1 Expenditures as a percent of GDP declined a little beginning in 1994 and reached 7.8% in 2000 (OECD, 2002, Federation of CCs, 2002, p. 4). Some of this change reflects economic growth, which resumed in 1994.

2 See Chapter 1, footnote 4 on reporting of changes over time.

3 The change for the entire period cannot be calculated because of the 1992 reclassification of geriatric inpatient care.

4 Acute turnover is the number of acute hospital admissions or discharges divided by available acute beds. Day treatment and beds are not included. Discontinuities in the data series rule out calculations for 1992. Occupancy rates for acute hospital beds, which are a crude efficiency measure, also rose slightly (four percent) in 1992–94 (OECD, 2001). In Stockholm, activity volume – including all types of outpatient visits and inpatient admissions, weighted for the relative costs of these services each year – began rising in 1989 and jumped dramatically between 1991 and 1993 (Whitehead et al., 1997, Figure 2).

5 Since then waiting lists have again increased, apparently because hospitals expanded their own services, and patients preferred to wait to undergo procedures in their local hospital, rather than moving to other hospitals (Andersen et al., 2001).

6 On the other hand, there were no indications that acute hospitals avoided treating elderly patients or others who might prove more difficult or costly to treat (Bergman, 1997).

7 Until the mid-1980s physicians had decisively shaped hospital policy by influencing resource allocation decisions and playing a prominent role in negotiations with county officials (Ham, 1987).

8 See Chapter 4, footnote 9.

9 See Chapter 4, p. 100

10 Unfortunately, there are no systematic data available on the orientations of physicians who entered private practice or the experiences of physicians under the various private practice arrangements.

133

6

Regulated Competition in the Netherlands

In the Netherlands broad support developed during the late 1980s for introducing 'regulated competition' among insurers and providers. Advocates of this approach sought to modify institutional traditions that had characterized Dutch health care for several preceding decades. After World War II the Netherlands developed a system that deftly balanced private delivery of health care with governmental finance and supervision of several distinct health insurance programs. Coalition partners from the political left, center, and right upheld the principle of solidarity in health care – universal and equal access to comprehensive services, regardless of ability to pay (Schrijvers and Kodner, 1997). Until the late 1980s an elaborate corporatist system of quasi-governmental advisory agencies regulated the financial operation of the health system. The participants in these agencies included representatives of major national interest groups in the health sector, along with government officials. During the 1980s, as the government struggled to curtail rising health expenditures in the face of recession, it introduced tighter and more direct state control of insurance fees and expenditures by providers, without dismantling the corporatist agencies. Although state regulation helped control costs, a broad movement developed in the late 1980s that favored reduction of state and corporatist involvement in health finance, while maintaining governmental commitments to solidarity.

The first part of this chapter uses the bargaining frame, along with the other three analytical frames, to account for the emergence and ultimate defeat of proposals to reorganize the health finance system so as to promote regulated competition. There follows an analysis of how incremental moves toward deregulation and encouragement of quasi-markets replaced the government's earlier plans for radical restructuring of the health system. The second part of the chapter blends administrative and bargaining frames in an examination of two parallel policy trends: First, continuation of control by state and quasi-governmental agencies; second, state support of initiatives by non-governmental actors, including patients' rights' groups and provider networks that integrate hospital and community care. Using similar frames, the third part of the chapter analyzes actions of hospitals and insurers that decisively affected regional and local implementation of regulated competition. The chapter concludes with a review of the anticipated and unanticipated forms of market behavior triggered by the reforms. Chapter 7 analyzes outcomes of the Dutch market reforms and recent policy developments that may lead toward a decentralized quasi-market in health insurance and care.

135

EMERGENCE OF PRO-MARKET REFORMS

Background: State Regulation during the 1970s and 1980s

The Dutch government's efforts to contain rapidly rising health costs began in the mid-1970s. At that time and throughout most of the 1980s the government relied on budget targets, regulation of hospital expansion, restrictions on acquisition of expensive technologies, and limits on fees and salaries.[1] As cost containment became a major health policy goal in the early 1980s, the government translated annual targets for the national health budget into prospective budgets. These provided the basis for negotiations with the national associations of providers and insurers. In addition, the Ministry of Health launched a complex system for planning the development of hospital facilities and the geographical distribution of health care specialists (Kirkman-Liff, Lapre, and Kirkman-Liff, 1988).[2] This system quickly proved unworkable, as providers, patient groups, and other stakeholders cooperated to find loopholes in planning regulations. Without formally abandoning the planning system, the government redirected its efforts toward creating financial incentives for hospital mergers and bed reductions. It also intensified its influence over the Central Agency for Health Care Tariffs, whose members came from the national associations of insurers, employers, hospitals, and physicians. This agency sets capitation fees for ambulatory physicians and approves fees negotiated between associations representing hospital specialists and insurers.

Direct state interventions dramatically curtailed increases in health expenditures during the early 1980s. As a result, total health expenditures as a percentage of GDP, which had grown by almost 17% between 1972 and 1982, began to decline and did not exceed the 1982 levels until 1990 (see Figure 1.1 on page 4).[3] Although hospitals proved more resistant to controls than other parts of the health system, general hospitals made substantial progress toward increasing outpatient care, lowering expenditures for inpatient stays, and reducing lengths of stay.[4] The main forces producing these developments in hospitals were government-imposed caps on hospital budgets; new technologies that supported less invasive forms of diagnosis and surgery; and government policies and budget incentives for hospital mergers and reduced bed capacities in general hospitals – but not in long-term care (Harrison, 1995a). In contrast expenditures generated by hospital specialists resisted control. Since insurers directly reimbursed specialists on a fee-for-service basis, the specialists' activities were not included in hospital budgets or controlled by budget ceilings.

Despite government-imposed cost controls, growing agitation by nurses and other salaried hospital employees and the rising volume of specialty care pushed hospital costs and total health expenditures upwards in the second half of the 1980s (Maarse, 1996; see also Figure 1.1 on page 4). The return of expenditure growth, along with other enduring problems, seemed, to many politicians and analysts to provide evidence for inherent limitations to the regulatory process. Chief among the other concerns were years of rancorous conflict between governmental officials and the medical specialists, domination of regulatory bodies by providers (Baakman et al., 1989), inequities in insurance arrangements, uneven geographic distribution of resources (de Roo, 1995), bypassing of regulations by hospital providers (Saltman and de Roo, 1989), and protests against curtailments of hospital services and facilities by patient and community groups (Ints.; de Roo and Maarse, 1990). Neither negotiation with stakeholders nor direct government intervention seemed sufficient to solve these problems and redirect expenditures toward community care and prevention – a move favored by the WHO and some Dutch politicians and health policy analysts.

Proposals for Regulated Competition

Dissatisfaction with attempts to regulate the health system from the top culminated in a proposal to restructure the insurance system so as to create competition among statutory health insurers.[5] This proposal was formulated by a government-appointed committee headed by W. Dekker, Chairman of the Board of Philips Corporation. Dekker was well-known for his 'orthodox' and 'uncompromising' market orientation (Int.). Although two successive governments accepted the committee's recommendations, only small parts of the original plan for regulated competition were enacted into law. Moreover, implementation of the policies enacted into law did not proceed as expected.

All four implementation frames help explain the character of the proposed market reforms and their limited implementation. Interpretive developments created support for the original reform proposals, through the spread of belief in the failure of government regulation and the corresponding advantages of deregulation and market competition. At the same time, divergence in values and interests prevented policy actors from agreeing about specific proposals for legislation, program details, and subsequent implementation of enacted programs. This divergence led to much bargaining within the institutional context of the coalition government. Bargaining processes were influenced by norms that encouraged a search for consensus among parties and stakeholders. This search for consensus gave dissenters substantial power to block governmental policies during their formulation and implementation. The result was that the government abandoned several controversial features of its original reform proposals as it sought to appeal to a wide spectrum of stakeholders. Political institutions also made it easier for successive Dutch governments to enact and implement incremental changes, instead of a radical program of reforms like that introduced by Britain's Conservative Party (Jacobs, 1998).

The market reforms proposed in the late 1980s by the Dekker Commission and elaborated upon by other government actors grew out of a major reorientation of political opinion that occurred in the Netherlands during the late 1970s and the early 1980s. During this period the Netherlands, and much of Europe, faced rising government debt combined with the worst economic downturn since the end of World War II. One response was a shift to the political right, which was evident in Holland's 1977 elections. Gradually critics of the welfare state became more outspoken. They vigorously promoted the view that cuts in government spending on social welfare benefits, deregulation, and privatization would help restore the nation's economic health and international competitiveness (Visser, 1990). Members of the governing center-right coalitions, employer representatives, many economists, and an Advisory Commission on Industrial Policy, all eventually endorsed this view. In consequence substantial privatization of public services took place. Even members of the opposition Social Democratic Party (Labor) advocated a 'new realism' in areas like welfare benefits and wage policies. For example, already in 1983 the Dutch trade-union confederation agreed to an end to wage indexation, in exchange for a promise by employers to create jobs. The confederation made this step under the leadership of Wim Kok, who was elected Prime Minister in 1994.

By the time the Dekker Committee convened in 1986, a broad spectrum of health policy actors, including both governing parties and the Social Democratic opposition, agreed that the traditional system of regulation and planning from the top had failed to constrain rising costs, coordinate disparate services, and reduce hospitalization. Moreover, these actors blamed the current regulatory system for the failings of health finance and service delivery. Advocates of reform argued that the existing maze of rules and regulatory bodies gave too much representation and power to providers (and particularly to physicians and hospital managers). Economists (e.g., van de Ven, 1987) pointed to perverse incentives that encouraged physicians to hospitalize patients and increase service volumes. Politicians and the media attacked the high fees earned by hospital-based specialists and the way that specialists – whose fees did not fall within hospital budgets – dictated hospital expenditures through their treatment decisions.

The neo-liberal approach to social policy both fed and framed this dissatisfaction with the prevailing system of regulation and planning in health. The reformers' proposed solutions to the health system's problems thus went hand in hand with their diagnosis. Taking their cues from the work of Alain Enthoven and other pro-market economists and policy analysts (e.g., Rutten and Freens, 1986; van de Ven, 1987), the Dekker committee members concluded that only deregulation and introduction of market incentives could contain costs and eliminate barriers to substituting community care for hospitalization. The committee assumed that competition among insurers and providers would create strong incentives for efficient use of resources by patients and providers, substitution of less costly community and ambulatory care for hospitalization, and better coordination of health services. A more market-oriented system was also expected to enhance patient choice and provide care that was 'tailored to the needs of the individual' (Ministry of Health, Welfare, and Cultural Affairs, 1988b, p. 15). Government regulation would be necessary to maintain solidarity and fairness and assure that providers, and particularly physicians, took responsibility for assuring the quality of care.

To make its ideas operational, the Dekker Committee recommended creating a single mandatory insurance system covering about 85% of the total costs of health and social care and merging the following separate funding streams (Ministry of Welfare, Health, and Cultural Affairs, 1988c):

1. Government funding for social care (family and institutionalized care for the aged, retarded, etc.)
2. Compulsory insurance provided under the Exceptional Medical Expenses Act (AWBZ) for long-term care, including nursing homes, and care for the retarded and mentally ill
3. Sickness fund insurance – compulsory health insurance funded by salary deductions for employees below a particular income level
4. Insurance for civil servants and other public employees
5. Optional private insurance for the self-employed and those earning above the income ceiling for sickness fund insurance.[6]

Both sickness funds and private insurers would offer statutory coverage under the new compulsory scheme. Both types of insurers could also provide optional supplementary insurance coverage for services like adult dental care and over-the-counter medications, which were not covered by compulsory insurance. Funding for the new, compulsory insurance program was to come from income-linked premiums, collected by a central agency and distributed to insurers on a capitation basis. The sickness funds, in turn, were permitted to contract with providers for services. In addition, insurers could directly collect flat-rate (or 'nominal') premiums. Furthermore, it was proposed that sickness funds no longer be assigned to a particular region, and that they be freed from regulations requiring them to contract with particular providers. To assure fairness, insurers would not be allowed to engage in risk selection.

These proposals prepared the foundations for patient choice among insurers who compete on quality and price (i.e. the level of 'flat' premium). According to the Dekker Committee, competition among insurers for clients and providers for contracts would release incentives for efficiency and change:

Insurers who were able to keep down costs by negotiating advantageous contracts with practitioners or institutions could pass the benefit on to policy-holders in the form of lower flat-rate premiums. The flat-rate element in the contributions is necessary to enable insured persons to bear part of the risk themselves (Ministry of Welfare, Health and Cultural Affairs, 1988c).

In fact the growing consensus about health system problems and solutions overstated the gravity of the problems (Lieverdink, 2001a) and the likelihood of solving them through market reform. The critics of regulation ignored its positive effects and – without much evidence – blamed bureaucratic planning and control for most of the system's ills. Moreover, there was not much historical basis or hard evidence for the Dekker Committee's optimism about the effects of releasing market forces. Instead, the committee members, like other advocates of market reform in the Netherlands and their colleagues in the UK, seemed to base their predictions on their own convictions and over-simplified models of market competition and rational choice (see Rice, 1998 for a critique). What is more, the adherents of market reform underestimated the difficulties of implementing their reform proposals.

139

The committee's recommendations appealed to a broad spectrum of parties and interest groups (Elsinga, 1989; van de Ven, 1991; Schut, 1995). The Christian Democrats, who led the coalition, particularly valued the reform's focus on cost containment, along with its preservation of solidarity and private provision of services. The Liberals, who were the right of center coalition partner, liked the idea of replacing planning with markets. The Social Democratic opposition was attracted by the elimination of the income-based distinction between statutory insurance through sickness funds and private coverage for upper income citizens. The Social Democrats anticipated that the Dekker reforms would put an end to the division in insurance coverage by introducing national health insurance – a proposal the Social Democrats had made during the 1970s.

The government endorsed the Dekker Committee's recommendations, and Parliament approved them in 1988 (Ministry of Welfare, Health and Cultural Affairs, 1988a). After the elections of 1989, the newly formed coalition of Social Democrats and the Christian Democrats continued the restructuring program. Plan Simons, named after the Secretary of Health, mapped out implementation steps that were very close to those envisioned by the Dekker Committee but further expanded the scope of compulsory insurance. Now the government proposed covering 96% of total spending under the expanded AWBZ program. This move would have promoted equity and avoided the possibility of risk selection in provision of supplementary insurance for medications and physical therapy. The new government framed the reform less in terms of regulated competition and competitive incentives. Instead it aimed at decentralization, consumer choice, reducing barriers between private insurers and sickness funds, and shared responsibility for health.

From Radical Reform to Incrementalism

Despite widespread initial support for the reform, opposition quickly surfaced in Parliament and among major stakeholders in the health system. The Liberals and the right wing of the Christian Democratic Party saw Plan Simons as disguised 'socialization' of the insurance system (Schut, 1995). At first most of the main non-parliamentary actors in the health system favored the plan; they apparently assumed that expenditures for health care would grow as a result of the government's extension of compulsory insurance coverage and its support for supplementary insurance. Once the financial and operational implications of Plan Simons became clear, the outlook changed for sickness funds, private insurers, and health providers. Most worrisome for them was the government's intention to hold down compulsory insurance premiums (Int.). Private insurers, along with the national employers' organization, spearheaded opposition to the plan. The employers feared that the reforms would lead to higher insurance premiums and labor costs (Int.). They faulted government policy for allowing the providers too much power, and doubted the market power of consumers (Lieverdink, 2001a). Representatives of the sickness fund also gradually turned against the reforms. In the past the funds had been reimbursed for their expenditures, held monopolistic or oligopolistic positions in their region, and enjoyed cooperative relations with providers. In contrast, the reform threatened to render the funds dependent on prospective payments and responsible for increasing portions of their budget overruns. These changes would force the funds to compete aggressively with one another and conduct tough negotiations with providers.

Service providers also grew hostile to the reforms. Hospital representatives balked at the prospect of competing for contracts on the basis of price and service quality. The hospital providers anticipated that increased competition among them would lead to further cutbacks in hospital facilities and tighter constraints on hospital expenditures. After initial support, the major physicians' organizations also joined the opposition to Plan Simons. In contrast, some younger specialists looked forward to employment opportunities that would result from development of new forms of practice, including health maintenance organizations and private, for-profit practice (de Roo, 1988).

Despite growing opposition by powerful policy actors, the government tried to lay the foundation for national health insurance by adding benefits to the existing AWBZ program, which was already universal and compulsory. But higher-income groups feared the effects of the income-related premiums of AWBZ, and private insurers objected to being subjected to complex, risk-adjusted capitation payments and being required to lower their premiums.

Faced with rising dissent in Parliament and upcoming elections, the government announced in 1993 that it would postpone implementing Plan Simons until 1996. After the 1994 elections, the members of the new coalition, which was again led by the Social Democrats, announced that they would abandon the Dekker-Simons program and make no more radical changes in the health system. Instead, the government intended to proceed cautiously and incrementally toward reforming the health system (Ministry of Welfare, Health, and Cultural Affairs, 1988a). It is ironic that forces on the right led the final, decisive attack on a reform plan that supporters had hailed as pro-market. The drive for reform was also weakened by the disappointing results of initial efforts to spur competition, which are reported later in this chapter and in Chapter 7.

True to its word, the new government enacted a series of small adjustments that moved the system toward deregulation and increased competition (Lieverdink, 2001a; van Het Loo et al., 1999). In place of national health insurance, the government created three distinct health insurance 'compartments' (i.e. components). The first, covering 52% of all health expenditures, includes long-term and catastrophic risks under the compulsory and universal AWBZ program, as was the case before the Dekker-Simons reform. The second compartment, covering 45% of expenditures, contains a compulsory statutory package of care that is uniform for members of sickness funds, public servants, and elderly and high-risk patients who are insured privately; this compartment also includes comparable packages offered by private insurers.[7] The third compartment includes services like cosmetic surgery, which are excluded from statutory coverage. These services, which comprise only 3% of total health expenditures, can be paid for out of pocket or insured through supplementary insurance policies marketed by private insurers.

According to this program, regulated competition is only planned for the second and third compartments. Competition and deregulation would be gradually phased in, and specific regulations governing services in the third compartment will be gradually eliminated. As services that had been included within AWBZ entitlements were shifted into the second compartment, income-related premiums were reduced. In addition income-linked cost sharing was extended, particularly for home care and regular care.

Although the government failed to implement national health insurance, which was central to Plan Simons, it did introduce many components of the original plan.[8] In 1989 and 1992 the government expanded the scope of treatments covered by the compulsory AWBZ program. Fixed (i.e. nationally standardized), income-dependent insurance premiums were mandated in 1992. A simple risk-adjusted capitation formula based on age and sex was applied in 1993. Insurers' 'flat fees', as envisioned by the Dekker Commission, were also introduced.[9] The government also canceled regulations that supported regional monopolies for the sickness funds and reduced barriers to entry into the insurance market. To allow for free choice of insurers and eliminate risk selection, private insurers were required to accept members on the basis of open enrollment.

Additional reforms aimed at fostering competition among health providers. General practitioners were no longer allowed to regulate the establishment of new general practices. Furthermore, the government allowed private, day-treatment centers to operate within the statutory insurance system. In 1992 the government and the central regulatory agencies stopped defining uniform rates to be charged by providers and began setting *maximum* rates.

The new regulations also strengthened the ability of sickness funds to negotiate with providers about fees and services – thus granting the funds freedoms that had previously been enjoyed only by private insurers. As of 1994, the funds were released from their legal obligation to contract with all licensed providers in a region and permitted to contract with providers outside of their traditional regional boundaries. Moreover, all insurers were permitted to cancel contracts with providers, if the cancellation reflected clear criteria and sufficient notice was given. Thus, for the first time all insurers could chose providers selectively, avoiding or breaking contracts with low-quality or very expensive providers.

The government also introduced a crucial change in financing of construction by hospitals and their acquisition of new technologies (Int.). Instead of guaranteeing bank loans to hospitals for these purposes, the government required hospitals to obtain loans from private banks. To do so hospital managers would have to convince the lender of the hospital's ability to repay the loan on time.

After 1995 the government permitted variations in the flat-rate premiums charged by sickness funds but did not permit fee differentials among enrollees in the same fund. To foster competition among providers and enhance individual choice, the government introduced personal care budgets – cash allocations for geriatric care and certain other community and home-based services. Parliament further ruled that ten percent of the growth in global budgets for geriatric care must be allocated to such personal care budgets (de Roo, 1999). The capitation formula was modified, with weightings for region (primarily indicative of urbanization) and employment status added to those for age and sex. At the same time the government gradually increased the financial risk born by sickness funds. Until 1997 the central fund that pays sickness funds reimbursed 95% of fund expenses in excess of revenues from capitation payments and other sources. Beginning in 1997 there was a cut of 50% in reimbursements for variable costs – which reflect per diem charges, outpatient fees, and other payments for services. Reimbursements for some variable payments were eliminated entirely in 1999 (Lieverdink, 2001a). By 2001, sickness funds were responsible for 75% of their costs for hospital services and 60% of payments to specialists (Lieverdink, 2001b).

There are several explanations for the government's ability to introduce these and other changes, despite their negative consequences for one or more stakeholders. First, the steps were modest, compared to the radical reforms envisioned by Plan Simons. Second, there was strong support across party lines for deregulation and increased competition within the health system. Third, the influence of corporate groups over health policy declined in the 80s and early 90s (Schut, 1995; van der Grinten, 1996). The government reduced the number and size of agencies in which interest groups were represented and substituted expert members for stakeholder representatives (Borst-Eilers, 1997). Moreover, the government began to bypass the hospital specialists when it formed policies, rather than soliciting their opinions, as it had done in the past (Harrison and Lieverdink, 2000). The specialists lost much of their power when they split into quarrelling factions in reaction to their organization's agreement in 1989 to cap the volumes of specialists' activities and redistribute earnings among specialty groups.

Fourth, the government's capacity to formulate and implement health policies grew with the appointment of Dr. Borst-Eilers, as Minister of Health, Welfare, and Sport in 1994 (Harrison and Lieverdink, 2000). Dr. Borst-Eilers took charge of the health portfolio herself, rather than delegating it to a Secretary for Health, as had been done under the two previous governments. This change meant that a minister who was knowledgeable and personally concerned with health affairs took part in all cabinet meetings. Previously the Secretary for Health would only have been invited to attend meetings when health issues were scheduled for discussion. A physician and experienced health manager with personal connections to prominent members of the medical community, Dr. Borst-Eilers also emerged as a capable negotiator and tactician. Eschewing the confrontational, all-or-nothing style of her predecessor, Health Secretary Simons, she reverted to a more incremental and consensual style. This approach harked back to less conflict-ridden periods in Dutch health politics. She and her staff relied on persuasion and classic carrot-and-stick techniques, plus strong governmental and parliamentary support, to convince the specialists and other powerful health system actors to implement her proposals.

STATE CONTROL AND SUPPORT FOR NON-GOVERNMENTAL INITIATIVES

At the same time that successive Dutch governments sought to enact market reforms, they pursued two additional routes to containing costs and reforming the health system. First, in support of regulated competition, they encouraged decentralized projects and activities among a range of national and local non-governmental actors, including physicians, insurers, providers, and patients. Second, in contradiction to the tenets of regulated competition, they maintained and even tightened top-down control over health expenditures. The following analysis of these conflicting policy thrusts blends administrative and bargaining perspectives. Moreover, in keeping with the institutional frame, the analysis shows how long-standing traditions of professional self-regulation influenced government policies in the 1990s.

Support for Initiatives by Non-Governmental Organizations

The governments elected in 1994 and 1998 pursued several policy objectives that developed independently of the proposed regulated competition reforms but were viewed by policy makers as compatible with deregulation and promotion of a more competitive health system. By devolving authority to non-governmental organizations, the government sought to promote integrated care networks, assure health quality, and help patients counterbalance the influence of providers and insurers.

Since the 1980s Dutch governments had encouraged integrated care, based on cooperation between primary-care practitioners in the community and medical specialists, who mostly work in hospitals (Mur-Veeman et al., 1999). Proponents of such 'transmural care' saw it as individualizing and improving care options. Advocates of regulated competition and other governmental policymakers assumed that substituting community care for hospitalization would save money – an assumption that has not always been supported by experience with home care of hospital patients (von Montfort, 1994). By 1999 transmural projects, which were also called 'health care chains' had become widespread in Dutch hospitals, but the nature and scope of projects varied widely (van der Linden et al., 2001). Most common were projects in which hospital nurses coordinated chronic care or engaged in hospital discharge planning, programs of home hospital care, and efforts to develop guidelines for transmural caregivers. Most projects linked individual practitioners in separate locales, rather than entire groups or organizations (Smit, 2000). The government did not earmark funds for transmural care. However, beginning in 1996 the Council for Sickness Funds permitted hospitals to transfer up to three percent of their budgets to home care. Cooperation across organizational boundaries also grew as rehabilitation hospitals, nursing homes, and home-care agencies developed working arrangements with one another or merged completely (Ints.).

These trends toward integration and cross-boundary cooperation faced serious barriers in the Netherlands, as in other countries. Sectoral funding arrangements often created disincentives for inter-sector cooperation. Moreover, there were many long-standing professional, structural, and occupational barriers to creating and sustaining integrated care networks (Hardy et al., 1999). Arrangements that stimulated provider competition, such as personal budgets for the elderly and chronically ill, also discouraged cooperation among providers (Mur-Veeman et al., 1999).

The government delegated most of the responsibility for assuring and improving the quality of medical services to the professionals who delivered these services. Until the late 1970s, in keeping with the traditions of corporatism, politicians and government administrators operated under the assumption that the professions defined good practice through medical research and education. Quality assurance was left up to individual practitioners. As cost pressures grew and the government introduced budgetary constraints, some members of the medical profession became concerned that cost considerations might endanger the quality of care (de Folter, 1997). In 1976 with the approval of the Ministry of Health, the physicians established a National Organization for Peer Review in Hospitals. In 1982 national specialist associations began to conduct consensus conferences, which developed practice guidelines (Dent, 1998).

Despite their belief in the efficacy of market forces, the Dekker commission did not challenge the country's long tradition of professional self-regulation. Instead, the commission's proposal for regulated competition assigned responsibility for assuring quality to providers, and particularly to the medical profession. The government's proposals for market reform also sustained medical control over clinical practice. In the wake of the Dekker report, the Royal Dutch Medical Association organized a series of government-sponsored conferences in which hospital managers, insurers, and representatives of patient associations participated. These conferences agreed with the views articulated by both the Dekker committee and a subsequent governmental committee on health care priorities: providers were to remain responsible for care quality by establishing protocols and care standards; insurers would make sure that quality assurance mechanisms were in place and operating effectively but would not actively assess quality (Klazinga, 1994). The specialists' organizations also responded to pressure for quality assurance and accountability by introducing re-registration requirements in 1991 (Swinkels, 1999) and developing a program of onsite assessment of specialty practices.

At the end of the 1990s, Parliament gave legal sanction to these emerging arrangements for quality assurance. It made recertification of specialists contingent on regular employment in a practice that is visited by the specialty association every five years. Moreover, a bill on the Quality of Health Care Organizations made hospital boards – and not just physicians – responsible for overseeing and supporting quality activities (de Folter, 1997) and required the boards to publish yearly reports on their care quality.

Although the specialists gradually accepted some inputs from insurers and patient representatives into their consensus conferences, they continued to dominate the development and use of practice guidelines. By the late 1990s more than 60 guidelines had been developed (Klazinga et al., 1998). The guidelines help physicians define normative standards for practice and contribute to the training of new physicians. Thus far, neither physicians nor hospital managers have used guidelines in the routine evaluation of the performance of individual doctors (Ints.). Nor do insurers or government regulators systematically use guidelines or other quality measures to evaluate physicians or institutions. The professionals' quality drive may help standardize medical practices and may shape the behavior of practitioners (Klazinga et al., 1998), but so far it has had very little effect on the practices of insurers or health managers. The impact of recent quality assurance efforts on clinical outcomes has not been systematically evaluated.

During the 1990s, the government's long-standing backing of patients' interests and rights developed in ways that strengthened policies favoring deregulation and provider competition. Most of the over 300 patient organizations were founded during the 1970s and 1980s (Blaauwbroek, 1997). Funded by governmental sources and contributions, many of these organizations concentrated on promoting the needs and interests of specific types of patients and their families. Others dealt more broadly with patients' rights and institutional responsiveness to patients. In the 1990s the government expanded its funding of patient organizations and passed a series of bills assuring rights like informed consent, privacy, and appeal through formal grievance procedures. The government also required all institutions to establish patients' councils, which can advise management on a broad range of issues.

In keeping with its pro-competitive policies, the government encouraged the development of patients' umbrella organizations, as a third party in health policy formation, alongside insurers and providers. These organizations were invited to take part in national policy deliberations, like the meetings on health quality and the consensus conferences just described. In addition, national and municipal governments supported patient and consumer organizations. These groups provide information about health care options, advocate patients' concerns, and help safeguard patient rights.

State Regulation and Control

Although each of the governmental coalitions of the 1990s declared their commitment to deregulation, all continued to control health expenditures through global budgets and centralized, quasi-governmental regulatory agencies

(Maarse, 1996; van Het Loo et al., 1999). Continuation of top-down control decisively shaped implementation of regulated competition policies and the operation of the health system as a whole. In 1994 the new government committed itself to limiting overall spending growth to 1.3% per annum and negotiated annual budget reductions on hospitals of around two to three percent (Ints.). The existing regulatory system remained in operation under the new government, and the government increased its influence over the representatives of providers and insurers in the regulatory agencies (Bjorkman and Okma, 1997).

During the second half of the 1990s, the government used its fiscal and regulatory powers to support cost reduction and movement of care out of hospitals. As it had done since the 1970s, the state distributed capital funds for hospital construction in ways that encouraged mergers and reductions in bed capacities (Boot, 1997). In addition to horizontal mergers between general hospitals, the government encouraged vertical integration – where general hospitals merged with nursing homes, and psychiatric hospitals merged with community mental health faculties (Konnen and Koning, 1998). At the same time, the government increased funding for home care and outpatient care (van Het Loo et al., 1999). Despite the policy of reducing hospitalization rates, for most of the decade, the official reimbursement rates for hospitals that were set by the Central Agency for Health Care Tariffs created disincentives for hospitals to shift inpatient care to outpatient settings (Int.). During the 1990s the government also weakened its own policies of health system decentralization and deregulation by retaining a planning regulation that required hospitals to get special approval before purchasing expensive new equipment and introducing certain high-cost subspecialties (Maarse, 1996). Although these regulations gave rise to rancorous negotiations and were sometimes bypassed by specialists, the government hesitated to eliminate them (Ints.).

In keeping with its regulatory drive, the Ministry of Health campaigned successfully to bring the fees paid to hospital specialists under control (Harrison and Lieverdink, 2000; Ints.). In 1994 the Ministry of Health, with parliamentary support, formalized its longstanding position that the specialists' earnings should be treated as an integral part of hospital budgets and be paid on a salary-like basis. The Minister of Health threatened further cuts in specialists' earnings unless the specialists agreed to negotiate prospective budgets for their earnings with hospitals and insurers. The resulting three-way agreements finally created fixed budgets for specialty care and in some instances helped equalize earnings among specialties. By 1997, nearly all general hospitals and the majority of self-employed specialists had entered into local or regional agreements of this sort (Kahn, 1997). In 1998, Parliament passed a law which required sickness funds as of 2000 to include physicians' services in contracts with hospitals, rather than making separate agreements with hospitals and physicians.

Integration of specialists' fees into hospital contracts and budgets removed one of the primary barriers to controlling hospital costs. For the first time insurers and hospital managers could sign prospective contracts in which both sides agreed to total expenditures for the fiscal year. Moreover, these agreements could now specify the share of outpatient care, rather than leaving decisions about the amount and location of care entirely up to the specialists. Contract terms could reflect global budget targets set by the government, cost competition among insurers, or some combination of regulatory and market pressures.

During this period the government also used regulation and legislation – rather than markets – to curtail pharmaceutical costs (van Andel and Brinkman, 1997). In the late 1980s and early 1990s the government negotiated voluntary price restraints with industry officials and imposed a reference price system that reduced reimbursement levels to insurers. The government also withdrew coverage for some items, including complimentary and over-the-counter medications. Dissatisfied with these efforts, the government passed an act in 1996 allowing for mandatory cost reductions if prices rise above a 'European average'.

As in Sweden and several other countries, some politicians and health analysts hoped that systematic priority setting would provide a fair and systematic way for the government to decide where to spend precious funds and how to ration care. In 1992 a government commission recommended that statutory insurance either cover or exclude services on the basis of their necessity, effectiveness, efficiency, and patients' responsibility for their own care in instances when costs are high and probable benefits low (van Het Loo et al., 1999). In practice the government was unable to make these priorities operational and act on them. Instead, priority setting and evidence-based medicine foundered on the shoals of provider opposition, broad entitlements to services, and political commitment to the principle of solidarity (Maarse, 1999; van der Grinten and Kasdorp, 1999). Plan Simons proposed putting nearly all services into the statutory package – without assessing their necessity, efficiency, or effectiveness. In like manner, the government elected in 1994 continued to assure coverage for nearly all services under either AWBZ or statutory insurance. The government made very marginal modifications to the statutory package by removing adult dental care and some physiotherapy (Schut, 1996; Int.). Even these modest changes met with protests and appeals to social solidarity. In the end, the government had to rescind its unpopular decision about dental coverage (Lieverdink, 2001a).

Other cost-containment moves met with substantial opposition by medical unions and sometimes aroused public protest. Nurses and other employee groups fought staffing cutbacks and in 1993 won concessions from the government in exchange for promises not to press for further wage gains (Ints.). Patients' groups, which sometimes allied with providers, proved themselves to be powerful interest groups. On several occasions, patient groups successfully appealed to the courts and lobbied members of Parliament to block hospital closures, patient co-payments to specialists, and limitations on the availability of services covered by insurance contracts (van de Ven, 1993; Maarse, 1993a; Paton, 2000).

The strongest opposition to governmental constraint came from hospital specialists. Throughout the 1980s and early 1990s the specialists used work stoppages, non-cooperation, and public-relations campaigns to fight successive governmental efforts to curtail their earnings and alter their status. Finally, in 1994 the specialists' wall of opposition to change began to crumble, as their national organizations lost power in the face of government cuts in the specialists' fees and growing support among politicians and other health-system actors for a change in the specialists' occupational status.

In summary, even as it encouraged decentralization of health markets and supported initiatives by voluntary groups, the Dutch government continued and even intensified its practice of regulating health expenditures from the top. Let us now examine how the implementation of market reforms affected regional and local actors.

IMPLEMENTATION OF MARKET POLICIES BY INSURERS AND PROVIDERS

Implementation of the government's regulated competition policies depended directly on the ways that insurers and providers viewed reform programs and acted in response to them. Although both groups of actors became more market oriented, they did not typically engage in the benign types of competition anticipated by proponents of regulated competition. The discussion that follows draws on my interviews to explore these and other aspects of policy implementation at the regional and local levels. All four of the analytic frames are used to explain why only some of the behavior expected by policymakers emerged and why insurers and providers responded to reforms in unanticipated ways.

Insurers

The insurers' most important response to proposals for regulated competition was to reduce the threat of competition by engaging in mergers and strategic alliances. The merger drive began during the mid-1980s in anticipation of the introduction of regulated competition and continued through the 1990s. The insurers reacted to the prospect of competition and to risks they would incur when the government reduced its retrospective reimbursement of insurers' payments to health providers. Of the 53 sickness funds operating in 1985 – just before the Dekker Committee was convened – 31 remained in 1998 (Lieverdink, 2001a article), and 25 were still operating in 2001 (Lieverdink, 2001b). In like manner, there were 69 private insurance firms operating in 1985, 59 in 1992, and 47 in 2002 (Maarse, 1993b; Vektis, 2002, p. 11). As a result of these mergers, many insurers developed regional monopolies. Moreover, most sickness funds came under the management of private, for-profit insurers (Int.). In accordance with the law, the sickness fund operations in these firms continued on an autonomous, not-for-profit basis.

As insurers strove to boost revenues, expand risk pools, and build market share in their regions and in the nation as a whole, they intensified their marketing and advertising activities and recruited more business-oriented managers (Ints.; Maarse, 1999; Lieverdink, 2001a). An important feature of the private insurers' marketing efforts was development of for-profit products and bundling of basic health insurance policies (which covered much the same conditions and services as did sickness funds) with other types of insurance, including supplementary health coverage. Sometimes insurers made strategic alliances with other companies in order to put together attractive packages (Int.). Many of these marketing ventures targeted lower risk clients; the capitation formula did not provide sufficient risk adjustment to create incentives for recruiting older and less healthy clients (van Doorslaer and Schut, 2000). Rather than engaging in outright rejection of high-risk individuals, insurers offered insurance packages to employees in large organizations, who were younger and healthier than the adult population as a whole. In addition, some firms arranged with hospitals and employers to set up clinics for the firms' employees, so as to provide faster hospital service than that available to other holders of statutory insurance (Ints.; Brouwer and Schut, 1999). This practice drew criticism from advocates of social solidarity, but the defenders of employee clinics saw them as a solution to growing waiting lists. In 1997, in response to the controversy, the government stated its opposition to employee clinics and began ear-marking funds for reduction of hospital waiting lists.

The financial mechanisms that were enacted to promote competition did not generate strong incentives for price or quality competition among insurers.[10] The sickness funds were supposed to compete over the level of the flat fees charged to all members of their fund. In fact, during the first half of the 1990s, the funds seemed to have reached a 'gentlemen's agreement' not to compete on price (de Roo and Boonekamp, 1994). Small variations in the flat fees charged by funds began to appear in the second half of the 1990s, but the differences were too small to motivate many people to switch funds. Nearly a quarter of respondents to a representative survey of Dutch households reported interest in switching funds between 1995 and 2000, but only 19% of these individuals (i.e. four percent of the total sample) cited differences in flat rates as a reason for wanting to switch. Just 6.6% actually switched funds (Gres et al., 2002). Price competition was also hindered by the failure of the government to inform people thoroughly about variations in fund charges and procedures for switching funds (de Roo, 1997b, November 12). In like manner, competition on quality was limited by lack of evidence and information about quality differences among sickness funds.

The reformers had expected insurers to use selective contracting and negotiation to reduce hospital charges and substitute less costly outpatient and community services for hospitalization. As the insurers began to be exposed to greater financial risk, they did strive to hold down hospital expenditures and contract for care substitution (Ints.), but they did not often use selective contracting or negotiate lower hospital charges below legal maximum levels.[11]

Several factors explain the failure of contracting to reduce hospital charges and costs. Hospital mergers effectively reduced the supply of services below that of demand, so insurers had few opportunities to switch providers (de Roo, 1995). Moreover, regulations that carried over from the pre-reform period limited the ability of sickness funds to negotiate vigorously with providers. For example, sickness funds were required to maintain contracts with hospitals in their region that were treating the sickness funds' members (Lieverdink, 2002). Furthermore, the government and central agencies like the Central Agency for Health Care Tariffs, continued to set hospital capacities, budgets, and service charges. A large part of hospital budgets continued to be set on an historical basis, over which insurers had no control. Moreover, insurers faced uncertainty about hospital charges, because the Central Agency for Health Care Tariffs retrospectively adjusted the fees charged by hospitals and physicians to bring total sectoral expenditures within macro-budget targets. Nor were insurers free to conduct independent negotiations with hospitals. Instead, the dominant sickness fund in a region, which had previously enjoyed a legal monopoly, still represented all insurers in negotiations with hospitals (Int.).[12] The result of these elaborate regulatory arrangements was that insurers never knew exactly what retrospective expenses they would face or how these expenditures related to their own costs and those of the providers.

Lack of sufficient data on their own costs and those of providers also contributed to the uncertainties surrounding insurers' negotiations with hospitals. Here is how Mr. L, the manager in charge of hospital purchasing for the largest insurer in his region, summarized the resulting situation:

> I am responsible for around half of the company's total expenditures. Cost awareness is growing, but we lack adequate information about how our budget arrangements with the hospital influence our company's results. For example, when – [as representatives for several insurers] – we make a contract with a hospital, we don't hold the entire contract. I don't know if the charges for particular services could be lower or higher. I don't know if I acted rightly or wrongly. The sickness fund budgeting system produces no clear outcomes [for the individual firm].

Insurers were in an even weaker position when it came to judging and influencing the content and quality of hospital services. In the absence of detailed data on procedures and case mix, insurers were unable to make systematic comparisons of the ways that hospitals handled particular procedures (Ints.). Insurers could include requirements for care substitution in contracts or press hospitals to bring their practices in line with those recommended by clinical guidelines. But the providers had the upper hand in these negotiations. Consider, for example, what happened in one hospital, here called Riverbend, when contract negotiations dealt with issues directly affecting specialists:

> When negotiations touched on length of stay, substitution of outpatient care for hospitalization, volume targets for a particular medical procedure, or other issues involving clinical judgments, Riverbend's managers consulted in advance with clinicians or invited them to take part in negotiations with insurers or consulted in advance with the clinicians. Then the managers explained specialists' views to the insurers. In such cases, insurers were reluctant to challenge the specialists' professional judgments.

In like manner, insurers generally did little about service quality, beyond requiring hospitals to report on quality assurance procedures. When I asked Mr. L what elements were contained in contracts with hospitals that did not take part in the new budget agreements with specialists, he mentioned service volume and amount of inpatient treatment versus outpatient treatment. Then he said:

> Of course you can say quality [is in the contracts], but that's a hollow phrase. We don't have the tools to control quality and don't want to. We consider the hospital responsible for quality and think that they can make appropriate arrangements for assuring quality.

Providers

During the market reforms, acute hospitals did not compete much for contracts with sickness funds. At the outset of the reforms, two thirds of Dutch hospitals enjoyed substantial control over their markets (Schut, 1992). Further mergers and bed reductions gave many general hospitals nearly monopolistic market positions (Maarse, 1999). Limitations on patient choice also reduced hospital competition. Hospital visits require referrals by general practitioners (de Melker, 1997), and patients are accustomed to visiting hospitals near home (Maarse, 1993a).

Although acute hospitals experienced few competitive incentives for cost reduction, insurers and governmental regulators put strong, direct pressure on hospital managers to contain costs (Ints.). Regulators billed hospitals and specialists retrospectively when they exceeded budget ceilings. In addition, insurers tried to get the hospitals to reduce their costs, because the insurers faced growing risk for any overruns of budgeted expenditures. To reduce costs, insurers urged hospital managers to reduce length of stay and favor outpatient procedures.

The regional agreements among insurers, specialists, and hospitals, which spread in the mid-1990s produced expenditure caps for each specialty. Decisions about how to allocate funds within agreed-upon specialty budgets were left up to the physicians (Ints.). These agreements thus eliminated the strong production incentives contained in the older fee-for-service system. An unintended consequence of this change was that many specialists reduced their pace of activity as their units approached or even exceeded their budget ceilings. As a result, waiting lists grew rapidly (Ints.).

When demand for services rose, hospital managers could join insurers in appealing to government regulators for budgetary exceptions. But these appeals involved 'an uphill battle', as one experienced management consultant put it (Int.). The most prominent exception to the pattern of shrinking resources was the influx of government funds for hospital programs that could reduce waits for specific procedures (Ints.).

In response to current and anticipated cost pressures, hospital managers began to change decision processes and structures. For example, they appointed care managers, who were responsible for reducing costs in nursing and ward operations. Top managers also sought to enlist physicians in cost-containment efforts and reconfiguration of hospital services. Most large hospitals created decentralized structures and delegated responsibility for containing expenditures to physicians managing clinical units (Pool, 1992; de Folter, 1997; Ong and

Schepers, 1999). In some cases, savings attained by decentralized 'care units' could be spent within the unit (Int.), thereby creating incentives for cost-containment by the medical managers heading these units. In addition some hospital set up joint physician-management decision forums. Discussions in these forums focused mainly on hospital policies, rather than on day-to-day administration (Versluis, 1993).

Throughout the 1980s the specialists had been almost universally antagonistic to overtures to involve them in budgetary and managerial decision processes. However, by the early 1990s, some specialists had developed a more pragmatic orientation toward hospital directors and managerial tasks (Ints.). These specialists began to take part in decisions about areas such as staffing, introduction of cost savings, and treatment priorities. Physicians also shared in managerial decisions when they acted as coordinators of several specialty groups or units. These leading physicians also represented their clinical units in negotiations between hospitals and insurers. In many hospitals, managers and specialists also cooperated in the development and promotion of additional hospital services, such as employee clinics and community-based services. These entrepreneurial ventures in ambulatory care boosted hospital revenues and physicians' income. Moreover, they responded to pressure from insurers and the Ministry of Health to substitute ambulatory care for inpatient care and develop integrated care packages (van der Grinten et al., 1998).

Despite the trend toward physician involvement in managerial decisions, major differences remain among hospitals in the degree and nature of professional involvement. The following description of two large hospitals illustrates the range of possible relations between managers and the medical staff:

> Physician involvement in St. George Hospital began shortly after the hospital board began to construct a new hospital in the early 1990s. The board appointed new General and Managing Directors, who then tried hard to 'restore the confidence' of the medical staff in management. In cooperation with the physicians, the board and top management developed a management structure that gave physician managers responsibility over two major divisions and sub-functions within these divisions. These 'medical coordinators', who are chosen by the medical staff, have autonomy over decisions about para-medical personnel and resource allocation within budgetary limits set by top management. Each month top management meets with the medical coordinators, as well as with members of the medical staff board, who are elected by the physicians.[13]

Participation in these new structures ensures two-way communication between physicians and managers. Physicians gain opportunities to explain clinical considerations to top managers and share in setting budget priorities. At the same time, the physicians' involvement in management exposes them to top management's own change agenda and creates pressure for cooperation in the drive for cost containment.

Although William Hospital introduced similar structures to those in St. George Hospital, cooperation between managers and physicians has been limited:

> At William Hospital, the general and medical directors meet weekly with one medical staff committee to discuss strategic questions and meet with another medical staff committee to review budget allocations to care units and departments. The hospital recently created a divisional structure, based on care units, each of which is managed by a nursing manager and a medical specialist manager. The specialist manager, who continues to be an active member of the medical staff, is recruited from the largest specialty group in the care unit and chosen in consultation with staff members. The care units receive budgets covering nursing staff, internal costs, and equipment and can use budget savings within the unit. Despite these structural changes, top management has not been very successful in its effort to introduce efficiencies into medical work. So far management has worked mainly with nurse managers, who address issues like length of stay and patient flows. The specialist managers and their colleagues have not cooperated in these discussions. As one member of top management put it, 'We want to make changes in the medical management of the care units'. 'But' – he added with a nervous laugh – 'that'll take a long time'.

At William Hospital and elsewhere (Ong and Schepers, 1999) medical managers who cooperated with top management challenged traditions of professional autonomy and risked conflicts with colleagues. Here is how Dr. T, the head of the William's medical staff board and a militant advocate of physicians' interests, explained the conflicts facing medical managers:

Dr. T: The specialist care manager is responsible to the medical staff as a primus inter pares [chief among equals], but the hospital management sees him as a member of a line organization. From the medical professionals' viewpoint, there is no hierarchy [among physicians in a specialty group].

MH: So what happens? ...

Mr. G: There can be collisions. In the hierarchy [i.e., as a manager] you have to work constructively with the hospital director. If you change the organization of the outpatient clinic or nursing care, you directly interfere with the doctors' professional and business interests. For example, the number of beds in the unit affects the doctors' income ... It's a struggle between the doctors, who own their practices, versus the hospital... As the head of one care unit, I cannot change things [that I used to control]. These have now become the responsibility of the medical care manager.

Along with continuing physician resistance, several other factors limited the ability of hospital managers to cut costs. Managers had almost no control over demand for services, which came from the patients, who in turn were responding to clinical decisions. The hospitals were bound by law to provide medically necessary care.

Lack of adequate management information systems also hindered hospital control over expenditures (Ints.). Despite growing investments in this area, hospital managers still lacked data on the real costs of medical procedures – as opposed to the official charges for procedures. This situation was well illustrated by Dr. G, a hospital Medical Director. After explaining the complex procedures through which hospitals and specialists are billed retrospectively for expenditures that exceed global budget allocations, Dr. G commented:

Dr. G: The whole thing cries out for something simpler – a way to put specialty fees and other hospital costs together.

MH: You mean something like a DRG?

Dr. G: Yes, but the surgeons tried this and ended up with around 150 different categories. It's too complex!

Although there was little competition among hospitals over statutory insurance contracts, competition did develop over patient referrals and revenue flows from private insurance. In cities with more than one hospital, for example, hospital managers sought to assure patient referrals by encouraging their specialists to cultivate strong relations with general practitioners (Int.). The establishment of special employee clinics, as described above, was another form of competition over patients and insurance fees. Some hospitals went even further and established purely private clinics on their premises (Maarse, 1999). Hospitals also competed for revenues and market share by establishing alliances or even merging with community care providers in areas like rehabilitation and nursing care. These developments were accompanied by growing entrepreneurialism, strategic thinking, and marketing among hospital managers and by involvement of some physicians in market-oriented ventures (Ints.).

In ambulatory care, as in acute hospitals, there was a wide range of responses to regulated competition. The first test of plans for deregulation and provider competition occurred in the rehabilitation sector. In that instance, providers and their insurers joined forces to block regulated competition (Ints.; Wiggers, 1994). Prior to the market reforms a limited number of hospitals and clinics held licenses that made providers eligible for reimbursement for rehabilitation services by the statutory health insurance system. Under the reform all providers meeting minimum standards – including private, for-profit clinics – were allowed to compete for contracts with insurers. When the Ministry of Health announced its plans to allow insurers to contract with all providers, the licensed providers protested, arguing that they had not yet developed a pricing system suitable for competitive contracting. The Ministry ignored the objections and announced that open contracting would go into force on 1 January 1994. The licensed clinics and practitioners quickly reached an informal agreement with the insurers that averted the implementation of open contracting. By reaffirming contracting arrangements that predated the reform, the parties prevented additional individual practitioners and provider organizations from entering the field. In addition providers and insurers avoided having to calculate and charge real (i.e., market-determined) costs for rehabilitation services.

Opposition to regulated competition and criticism of its appropriateness also developed in fields like mental health and retardation. Critics pointed out that patients in these areas, like those requiring rehabilitation, could not readily defend their own interests or choose rationally among competing providers. In response, in 1994, Minister Borst-Eilers restored these services to their former non-competitive status within the first (AWBZ) compartment of her revised, three-compartment plan (Paton, 2000).

Although rehabilitation providers beat back competition, other ambulatory providers welcomed it. For example, some medical specialists set up private clinics in anticipation of deregulation and demand for services (van de Ven, 1993; Maarse, 1999). As these entrepreneurs had hoped, the government rescinded the ban on social insurance reimbursement of for-profit providers. Private provision also expanded rapidly in home care and geriatrics (Ints., de Roo, 1999; Paton, 2000). These enterprises offer choices to patients and families receiving funds under personal care budgets, as well as to clients with private or supplementary insurance. Yet another area of entrepreneurial initiative involves the establishment of private mental health clinics, which serve both individuals and employees of companies (Maarse, 1999).

CONCLUSION: INCREMENTAL REFORMS AND UNANTICIPATED MARKET BEHAVIOR

In conclusion, the original proposals for regulated competition were only partially implemented. What is more, the market reforms that were introduced led to a wide range of unanticipated actions on the part of insurers and providers, including unanticipated forms of market behavior. Conflicts and negotiations among health policy actors and coalition partners led government reformers to abandon their original plans for radical market reforms. Instead, the government took a set of incremental steps toward deregulation, encouraging competition among insurers and raising their responsibility for cost overruns. At the same time, the national government continued to cap spending by hospitals and insurers, retained pre-reform regulatory agencies, and strengthened state influence over these agencies. As managers in hospitals and insurance companies encountered greater financial risk and ever-tighter expenditure limits, they learned to view their work in more business-like terms. Moreover, managers in both sectors actively sought to improve their organizations' financial positions. The insurers pressed hospitals to reduce costs. Hospital managers, in turn, reduced expenses and introduced programs that could generate additional revenues. After years of resistance, hospital specialists gradually began to co-operate with managerial efforts to run hospitals more like businesses.

In contrast to these expected developments, the insurers engaged in a form of market behavior that was not anticipated by reformers and seriously undermined prospects for competition: instead of competing on the price or quality of statutory care, insurers mainly endeavored to increase their market share and avoid competition and risk. To these ends insurance companies engaged in mergers and targeted their marketing at healthier people. Hospital managers also responded to direct government intervention and growing financial risk by merging and developing alliances with community-based providers. There was substantial entrepreneurial activity among some community-based providers, such as those in geriatrics and home health care (Ints.; Paton, 2000). However, practitioners in other sectors, like rehabilitation and mental health, actively resisted competition and deregulation.

Anticompetitive actions by providers and insurers were quite rational from a business standpoint and could have been anticipated from experience with health markets in other countries (Light, 2000). In like manner, incentives in the capitation formula led to the tendency of insurers toward some risk selection – by avoiding or getting rid of poor insurance risks and marketing intensively to healthier clients (Schut, 1992; de Roo, 1997b, November 12).

Another unanticipated development was that the reforms failed to empower patients to chose insurers or providers on the basis of cost and quality. Although the government championed patients' rights and autonomy, it did not disseminate information about insurance charges, provider performance (e.g., waiting lists), and clinical quality. Data on these dimensions could have informed and stimulated patient choice. Nor did insurers actively seek to monitor or improve quality. The failure of both government agencies and the insurers to assess and report on quality partly reflected the difficulties of gathering adequate data about quality and performance. More fundamentally, the treatment of quality by government officials and insurers provided a way of avoiding conflict with the medical profession; few officials and managers dared challenge the tradition of leaving clinical quality assurance up to the physicians.

NOTES

1 For details on global budgeting and other cost-containment measures during the 1970s and 1980s see Baakman et al. (1989); Bishop et al. (1994); Harrison (1995a); Kirkman-Liff (1989).

2 The name of the ministry dealing with the health system was changed by successive coalition governments. For simplicity I use the term Ministry of Health.

3 See Chapter 1, footnote 4 on reporting of changes over time.

4 Acute beds declined by 6.4% between 1980 and 1985, 5.7% between 1985–90, and 8.7% between 1990–95. Dutch figures for acute hospital beds include day beds. The decline in overnight beds in general hospitals was undoubtedly higher. Total inpatient beds (in absolute numbers) remained constant between 1980–1989 and rose by 1.3% between the start of 1990 and the end of 1995 (OECD, 2001).

5 This discussion draws on interviews I conducted with Dutch policy analysts in 1994 and 1997, as well as on published and unpublished documents (see Harrison, 1995a). For helpful analyses of the politics of the reform proposals see Schut (1995), van de Ven (1997), and Lieverdink (2001a).

6 Around one-third of the population fell into this category.

7 Private insurers are allowed to engage in underwriting but must provide high-risk individuals and those over 65 with a standard policy at a reasonable fee. The private insurers are compensated for resulting deficits by mandatory cross-subsidization from other private insurers (van Doorslaer and Schut, 2000).

8 The following discussion draws on my interviews, the sources cited in footnote 5, and van Etten and Okma (1992); Directorate-General for Health (1993); Groenewegen (1993); Lieverdink and van der Made (1997); and van de Ven (1993).

9 Compensation for flat premiums was given to low-income people, thus reducing the salience for them of sickness fund fee levels.

10 This conclusion is supported by my interviews and is shared by Lieverdink, (2001a) and Paton (2000). In contrast, van Doorslaer and Schut (2000) maintain that there has been 'significant' price competition among sickness funds since 1997.

11 Ziekenfondsraad [Sickness Fund Council] (1995). Evaluatie overeenkomstenstelsel Ziekenfondswet en Algemene Wet Bijzondere Ziektekosten [Evaluation of the contracting system of the Sickness Fund Act and the Exceptional Medical Expenses Act] Report 673. Amstelveen: ZFR. Cited in Schut (1996) p. 284.

12 After 1997 a single representative of all smaller sickness funds was added to the negotiating team (Int.).

13 Medical staff boards (or committees) formally represent physicians in Dutch hospitals. I add the word 'boards' to distinguish these formal representative bodies from the hospital's entire medical staff.

7

Reform Outcomes and New Policy
Trends in the Netherlands

Even though the market reforms proposed in the Netherlands during the late 1980s were not fully implemented, they triggered important developments in the health system. The first part of this chapter analyzes administrative, bargaining, and interpretive outcomes of the market reforms. The second part assesses their long-term, institutional consequences. The chapter's conclusion describes recent policy developments that may lead the Netherlands toward a national health insurance reform much like the one envisioned in the original proposals for regulated competition.

As was true for Sweden and the United Kingdom, it is hard to separate the effects of the Dutch government's market reforms from more powerful effects of top-down, budgetary and regulatory control. During the period of market reform, national politicians and officials continued to limit hospital expenditures through direct and indirect means, provided strong budgetary incentives for hospital mergers and reductions in bed capacities, and fought long and hard to bring specialists' fees into hospital budgets. Moreover, as in other countries, an uninterrupted stream of technological innovations made it possible to shorten many hospital stays or replace them with day surgery or ambulatory care in the community. At the same time, medical innovation fuelled demand for expensive new procedures.

A further difficulty in assessing the impact of regulated competition is that very limited competition developed among Dutch insurers and hospitals. Hence, it is not plausible that market forces were the main cause of improvements in hospital productivity and other related developments that fit the expectations of market reformers (Paton, 2000). Nonetheless, the initial formulation of market policies and moves toward deregulation of the health system led insurers and providers to anticipate major changes in their operating environments and act accordingly. Thus the combination of government-driven fiscal restraint and incremental deregulation did produce important outcomes.

The *administrative* frame focuses on the extent of policy implementation and attainment of the reforms' original objectives. Here we concentrate mainly on the second of these issues, since the first was examined in Chapter 6. By the late 1990s, it was clear that the Dekker-Simmons policies had not led to the hoped-for transformation of the health system. There was progress toward many of the specific objectives of the market reformers, but this progress owed more to top-down government regulation than to the release of market forces. The advocates of regulated competition viewed deregulation both as an end in itself and as a step toward reducing costs, increasing provider efficiency, and substituting ambulatory care for hospital care. Progress toward fiscal deregulation occurred in the gradual shifting of financial risk onto insurers and in new types of funding of ambulatory care. However, the existing quasi-governmental mechanisms for setting fees and budgets remained in place, as did most regulations governing the operation of sickness funds and hospitals.

The complexities of evaluating the effects of market and non-market forces are well illustrated by changes in the nature and settings of medical care. Market reforms encouraged efforts to relocate care: as the government increased the insurers' financial risk, insurers sought to save money by shifting costs out of hospitals and into the community (Ints.). In practice, considerable substitution of ambulatory care for hospitalization occurred during the 1990s. For example, between 1994 and 1999 short-term, day treatments jumped by 30% in general hospitals. Initial outpatient visits to hospitals rose by four percent, but return visits fell by five percent (Prismat, 2000). The drop in return visits suggests that hospitals returned patients to community care more quickly than in the past. Yet market forces seem to have played a minor role in driving these changes in treatment patterns. Instead, the developments reflect the availability of new medical technologies, growth of day surgery, and reduction in the length of hospital stays. As hospitals reduced length of stay, patients had to rely more on ambulatory care. The trend toward reduction of lengths of stay occurred throughout the industrial world during the 1980s and 1990s (see Chapter 1). In the Netherlands, average length of stay in acute care declined steadily at a rate of around 20% per decade from 1966 through to 1998 (OECD, 2001). This trend was fuelled by government-imposed budget caps and later by direct financial incentives for community care, as well as by new technologies (Ints.).

The reforms also aimed directly at increasing hospital efficiency and thereby reducing health expenditures. The Dekker Committee defined efficiency in terms of reduced wastage and enhanced cost-awareness among hospital staff. Thus hospitals were expected to reduce unnecessary care. One indication that hospitals moved in the expected direction is their reduction in length of hospital stay. Turnover in acute care, a productivity measure that is closely related to length of stay, also rose steadily and grew by 20% between the end of 1987 and 1996 (OECD, 2001).[1] Despite these attainments and substantial consolidation of hospital facilities, considerable slack resources remained in acute hospitals. Occupancy rates in these facilities fell during the 1980s but then remained around 73% during most of the 1990s (OECD, 2001). Moreover, length of stay in acute hospitals remained much higher in the Netherlands than in many other industrial countries.

Unfortunately, there are no data with which to conduct systematic pre-reform and post-reform comparisons of productivity over expenditures for hospitals or for the health system as a whole. Trend data and comparisons based on indicators like turnover and length of stay must be interpreted with caution. In addition to suffering from artifacts in data gathering and reporting, aggregate data like these can mask local variations. Moreover, the data do not include case mix and quality – which should be controlled statistically in calculations of hospital productivity and efficiency.

As the market reformers hoped, hospital staff did become much more aware of cost considerations. However, the growth in cost-awareness reflected state-driven constraints on capacities and budgets, as well as anticipation of more market-like conditions. Contrary to the hopes of the Dekker Committee, insurers and providers did not make systematic efforts to enhance efficiency: they did not ordinarily use best practice protocols and other forms of evidence-based medicine. Nor did hospitals or insurers systematically examine the costs and outcomes of specific practices (Ints.). Instead, insurers and hospital managers urged general policies of cost reduction; lower-level managers, physicians, and nurses responded to these cost pressures by modifying their activities and consolidating facilities in ways that seemed likely to reduce costs without harming patients or evoking opposition by internal and external stakeholders.

Perhaps even more frustrating for advocates of regulated competition was the failure of deregulation to curb health costs. The available macro-economic data make it clear that the drift toward de-regulation and marketization did not yield a dramatic curtailment of total health expenditures, like that produced by tight global budgets in the early 1980s.[2] Instead, health expenditures rose steadily in real terms from 1986 through to 1999, when they stood 40% higher than they had been a decade earlier (OECD, 2001). Expenditure as a percent of GDP rose from eight percent in 1986 to a peak of nine percent in 1993. Then, thanks to the return of economic prosperity, they stabilized at 8.7% between 1997 and 1999 (see Figure 1.1 on page 4).

Nor was there any evidence that the market reforms directly curtailed expenditures on hospital care. There was some progress toward this goal during the late 1980s, thanks to government fiscal incentives for reducing inpatient capacities and preferring ambulatory care. The proportion of total public health expenditures devoted to all types of inpatient care fell by 8.6% between 1986 and 1990; public expenditures for acute care dropped 12.5% in this same period. However, there were no further reductions in the burden of hospital expenditures after 1990.[3] Throughout the 1990s the government had to devote around 60% of its total health expenditures to all types of inpatient care. As the reforms progressed, many participants and analysts concluded that a more active market for health care might even increase total health expenditures. Entrepreneurial behavior by providers and pharmacists appeared to drive demand and costs, rather than curtaining them (in t'Veld, 1999). A further concern was that insurer and provider competition could generate new transaction costs, which could exceed productivity gains.[4]

The architects of Holland's market reforms assumed that insurers would compete on the quality of the services provided, and to a lesser degree on their price. In particular, the Dekker Committee expected competition to lead insurers and providers to become more responsive to the needs and preferences of divergent types of patients. Moreover, the emerging market was supposed to give patients more choice among insurers and providers. Deregulation of the insurance system did enhance patient choice, since sickness funds no longer enjoyed regional monopolies. Deregulation also encouraged the spread of private clinics and emergence of new types of ambulatory care. One of the most noteworthy market developments that enhanced patient choice involved patient budgets for a small portion of geriatric and rehabilitation care. At the same time, government policies and incentives that were not directly related to regulated competition also helped enhance patient rights and autonomy (Blaauwbroek, 1997). Despite progress toward patient choice, there was little change in the conditions governing patients' choice of physicians. General practitioners continued to serve as gate-keepers to specialized care. Moreover, the insurance packages of sickness funds remained virtually identical, and cost differences among insurers remained small. Neither the government, nor any other health system player systematically assessed provider or insurer quality or distributed information that could help patients make informed choices of providers and insurers.

Reduction of waiting times was not a prominent objective of the Dekker-Simons reform policies. However, during the 1990s waits for orthopedics and other types of hospital care became a political issue, because the government capped hospital budgets and specialists' fees. In 1998, rather than allowing market forces to respond to the shortage of hospital care, the government earmarked funds for specialties with long waiting lines (Sheldon, 1998). These direct budgetary interventions did not reduce the overall waiting list, but they quickly produced substantial improvements in waiting times for orthopedics and ophthalmology (Sheldon, 2000a).

The advocates of market reform did not explicitly target improvements in clinical quality as a reform objective, but they did acknowledge the need for the government to assure that clinical outcomes were not adversely affected by reform. Concern about the impact of the reforms was one of several forces that led to increased public and governmental attention to quality assurance. In keeping with this trend, health insurers began to require hospitals to report on quality assurance efforts – but the content of these activities was left to the providers. In response to the implicit threat of intervention by insurers or government regulators, hospital specialists took steps toward self-regulation. These steps included periodic re-registration, intensification of existing peer review practices (Swinkels, 1999), and introduction of other quality assurance activities. Physicians in hospitals did not typically share findings from their quality activities with managers or insurers.

The market reformers assumed that market forces would produce better coordination of care than that provided by the existing welter of divergent agencies, regulations, and budget systems. During the 1990s, awareness of the need for coordinating care grew in response to governmental support and local initiatives by professionals in health and social services. Although collaborative care projects multiplied, there is little reason to credit competitive incentives with these developments. On the contrary, competition created financial uncertainties among providers and encouraged opportunism, both of which added to the many difficulties of bridging sectoral, organizational, budgetary, and occupational barriers to cooperation.

Social solidarity and equal access to health care were not goals of the market reforms, but critics judged the reforms in terms of their likely impact on these principles. Several broad effects of the reforms can now be discerned. First, inadequate risk adjustment in the capitation formula gave insurers incentives for risk selection (van de Ven et al., 1994; Lamers, 1999). The most important expression of the insurers' preference for lower-risk clients was marketing services to employees of large organizations, who were better insurance risks. Second, deregulation of mental health and long-term care – a move that was eventually rescinded – placed patients and their families at a disadvantage: These new health care consumers had to chose providers and negotiate terms of service, yet they often lacked the information, knowledge, and skills needed to make informed choices. Third, solidarity and the comprehensiveness of care were threatened by the government's attempts to remove statutory coverage for low-priority services and require patients to pay for them out of pocket or through private, supplementary insurance. In practice, because of popular opposition, very few services were removed from statutory coverage. Fourth, in the view of the Social Democrats, provision of health insurance by both private firms and sickness funds threatened social solidarity. Yet efforts to implement a single insurance package for all types of care repeatedly failed to muster the needed political support. In fact, the damage to solidarity from this division within the insurance system does not appear to have been great: for the most part insurers offered their privately insured clients the same basket of health services that the companies provided under law to sickness fund members (de Roo, 1999).

Analysis of the market reforms from a *bargaining* perspective shows important changes in the power of health system actors. The most important trends were declines in the power of physicians at both the national and hospital levels and the rise of professional managers within insurance companies and provider organizations. In addition, national corporate bodies lost influence in health policy, as they did in other areas of government. Particularly significant for the health system was the reduction of influence of providers and insurers within regulatory agencies.

Ironically, the trend toward deregulation did not weaken the state. Instead, the national government actually enhanced its capacity to regulate the health system through budgetary controls. Government pressure and the new local and regional agreements between physicians and hospital managers undermined the power of the National Association of Medical Specialists (LSV in Dutch), which for years had spearheaded the specialists' opposition to fee regulation and managerial influence. The new agreements for setting physicians' fees subjected hospital physicians to economic control by managers, who faced tight budget caps on total expenditures. As the LSV declined and concern with medical quality grew, associations representing particular medical specializations (e.g., cardiology), assumed a greater national role in establishing treatment protocols and conducting peer reviews of clinical activities within hospitals. Thus at the national level, the medical profession lost economic and strategic control but retained operational control over clinical practice.

In theory the reforms should have empowered consumers and subjected insurers to market discipline. However, only a small proportion of people switched funds (see Chapter 6), and few chose insurers outside of their own region. Moreover, mergers gave insurers oligopolistic control over emerging regional and metropolitan markets. Mergers and strategic alliances among providers also reduced opportunities for patient choice and other forms of patient influence.

Within health insurance firms, managers handling for-profit products gained influence over the activities of the firm's not-for-profit (sickness fund) insurance (Int.). Although the insurance companies continued to recruit managers from the pool of experienced health insurance managers (Int.), the companies appointed more sickness fund managers with strong marketing orientations.

Parallel developments occurred among hospital managers. Changes in bylaws and accepted practices during the 1980s and 1990s gradually shifted power from the hospital board to the director, who was a professional manager (Ints.). Top management also included a Medical Director, who remained dependent on the 'good will' of the medical staff (Int.), while striving to contribute to the financial viability of the hospital. In many hospitals the top management team seized the strategic initiative in developing new programs and forging alliances with other providers.

The new contracts gave top management far more influence over the specialists' working conditions, their terms of remuneration, and their total earnings, than had been the case when specialists received fee-for-service payments. Moreover, new hierarchical structures, in which physicians and nurses took on managerial roles, reduced the managerial autonomy of the specialty groups (maatshcapen). These developments were strengthened by the report of Biesheuval Commission of 1994, which proposed subordinating physicians to management in an 'integrated' organizational structure. Although the new structures created opportunities for enhanced managerial supervision and control over specialists' activities, they did not attain the level of integration envisioned by Biesheuval and his colleagues. Instead, the new managerial hierarchies operated side by side with the physicians' traditional forms of organization and representation. Thus specialists could muster substantial countervailing power to managerial initiatives through their elected medical staff boards and through forums originally created to foster management-professional cooperation. In practice, top managers rarely infringe on clinical autonomy within specialty groups. However, specialty groups face increasingly tight budgetary constraints, which limit practice options. These specialty groups and the national specialty associations with which they are affiliated enjoy a free hand in quality assessment and assurance (van Herk et al., 2001).

It is too soon to judge whether relations between managers and physicians have reached a new equilibrium. The structural and political changes taking place within the hospitals may ultimately lead to the demise of independent specialist groups. Indicators of this trend include growing managerial control over departmental budgets and the tendency of members of specialty groups to shift to salaried employment. Furthermore, physician participation in management could lead to the cooptation of physicians by managers. On the other hand, hospital specialists may use participation to influence managerial decisions and sustain their struggle for control over clinical practice and administration. It is also possible that in some hospitals both managers and physicians will gain power by expanding entrepreneurial activities (van der Grinten et al., 1998).

Neither the market reforms, nor legislation on patients' rights, enabled patients to act as a countervailing force to providers and insurers in acute and primary care. In the acute hospital sector patient groups lobby and occasionally support legal actions designed to assure coverage of care, but these groups do not usually exercise much direct influence over hospital management or treatment (Ints.). The influence of patients' organizations in general hospitals is limited, because the patients' groups depend on government funding, represent divergent subgroups of patients, and pursue separate agendas (Blaauwbroek, 1997). In addition, the volunteers and paid staff in these groups – like patients and patients' representatives in other countries – often lack the expertise, status, and power needed to negotiate effectively with insurers and providers. Furthermore, to shape policy and provide effective guidance for patients, patient groups in Holland and elsewhere in Europe need much better information than that currently available about health quality and health treatment options.

In contrast, patients did gain power in home care and in non-acute institutions for psychiatric, retarded, and geriatric patients. In these areas legislation and government funding supported representation of well-organized groups, which championed patient interests (Ints.). Empowerment of patients and citizens came at the expense of health professionals in one functional area: in the late 1990s a new law assigned responsibility to independent regional centers for assessing need for community-based treatments among most patients. This law eliminated exclusive control over needs assessment by physicians and health providers; instead assessment boards were required to include representatives of insurers, patient organizations, and local communities (de Roo, 1997a, May). Non-acute care providers were required by law to publish information on the extent to which they provided patient-oriented care. However, the Ministry of Health did not require systematic evaluations of the quality of mental health or geriatric care.

Interpretive developments during the 1990s were even more dramatic than the changes in power and political alliances. The interpretive changes resulted from the combined effects of the original market proposals, incremental deregulation of health markets, and continuing governmental enforcement of tight budget ceilings on providers and insurers. Together these reforms led to a radical transformation of the ways that health system actors thought and spoke about their work and the health system as a whole. The shift in orientations among health managers and professionals fit the expectations of regulated competition but was influenced more powerfully by governmental requirements for fiscal accountability than by market competition. As managers in provider and insurance organizations strove to conform to new budget requirements and find sources of private revenue, they infused their organizations with the language and paradigms of commercial business management. The growing influence of professional managers, and particularly of those trained in business, contributed directly to this interpretive shift. The transformation in managerial thought and discourse was so dramatic that one knowledgeable health-system consultant observed that 'the most pervasive effects of the Dekker-Simons reforms were cultural, not structural' (Int.).

There were several facets to this transformation (Ints.; Harrison, 1995a, van de Ven, 1993). First, managers in both hospitals and insurance companies became more aggressive in their pursuit of cost savings and efficiency improvements. This shift from reactive budget management to active cost control in sickness funds and hospitals found expression in increased investment in staff and equipment for computerized information management. Second, sickness fund managers and managers of not-for-profit health providers – including hospitals, community nursing, and geriatrics – began to adopt more aggressive business orientations. In particular, they emphasized marketing and development of workable business strategies, including development of strategic alliances that could help them enhance market share. Third, there was an upsurge of entrepreneurialism and marketing of services by for-profit insurers and providers.

Comments by Mr. L, the sickness fund manager quoted in Chapter 6, provide an illustration of the ways that managers adopted business concepts and frames:

> Mr. L said that he worried about the impacts of hospital contracts on 'the company's results'. He took a strictly commercial approach to his firm's decisions on coverage provided in its 'high-priced' supplementary insurance package, remarking, 'We don't believe in alternative medicine, but we sell it'. He described glowingly a marketing campaign that focused on 'employers as customers', and a 'strategic alliance' with another insurer that allowed the sickness fund to bundle statutory insurance with for-profit insurance products.

When I asked whether the use of such marketing and strategic approaches were new to the sickness funds, Mr. L stressed how thoroughly and rapidly private-sector thinking and techniques had suffused the not-for-profit sickness funds:

> Until three or four years ago the sickness funds and the private insurers were divided on everything – the way they operated, the way they defined issues. We have now integrated the two sectors. Commercial thinking now infuses sickness fund thinking, and this holds for all sickness funds.

This radical shift toward aggressive business management resulted in part from the exposure of sickness fund managers to financial risk (de Roo, 1997a, May). In addition, this transformation resulted from mergers between sickness funds and private companies and emerging cooperation with private-sector managers in areas like contracting, marketing, and management-information systems. In fact, a study released in 1997 revealed that 18 out of 25 sickness funds studied had become 'hollow' institutions, consisting simply of boards that contracted out virtually all of their activities to private agencies – most of which were part of the commercial insurance agencies with which the funds were affiliated (Maarse, 1997; Lieverdink, 2001b). Thus structural ties between commercial and non-commercial (public) insurers became so extensive that the two sectors 'can hardly be disentangled anymore' (Maarse, 1999). Managers in not-for-profit hospitals also faced greater financial risk and became more accountable to insurers and government regulators for attaining production levels and staying within budget limits. Some hospital managers forged entrepreneurial ties with for-profit insurers and with other not-for-profit and for-profit providers. Other managers concentrated mainly on cost containment and enhancing hospital efficiency.

Hospital physicians, as well, began to interpret management's budgetary and business concerns very differently than they had a few years earlier (Harrison, 1995a). In the 1980s most specialists had resisted acknowledging the cost implications of their clinical activities for hospital costs. Many resented and sought to block attempts by the Ministry of Health to curtail their earnings. Physicians often became hostile to hospital directors or physicians' representatives who sought to implement budgetary limits on medical production. In contrast, by the mid-1990s most specialists had abandoned active resistance to the new contracts and other forms of cost constraint. These physicians became more willing to recognize the impact of their clinical decisions on hospital expenditures and the need for cost containment. For example, the head of the medical staff board in Riverbend Hospital, who works closely with top management on planning and cost containment, commented, 'The doctors are more aware than in the past. Everyone knows – especially as their budgets shrink – that there are budget limits'.

The change in the specialists' orientations reflected failure of their national campaign against cost limits on their earnings. In addition, participation in joint management-physician forums directly exposed specialists to the tight fiscal limits facing their managers. Through formal and informal contact with management some physicians learned to view hospital activities through business frames, as opposed to strictly professional ones.

Although cost consciousness spread widely among specialists, far fewer were willing to work actively with management to achieve budget constraints and enhance efficiency. Even in St. George's Hospital, which had pioneered physician involvement in managerial decisions, physicians expressed a wide range of views on participation.[5] Dr. R, a specialist in internal medicine, described himself as active in his specialty association, but not in hospital management. He explained his stance this way:

In general I choose just to do medical work. More [physicians] are expected to think about management problems than in the past. I agree to ten to fifteen percent involvement in this, but doing more than that leads directly to your professional worth being diminished. I chose my job for patient content and for research in pharmacology. More meetings is not my cup of tea, not the way its being done now… On the other hand, there must be participation by medicine in management. I don't deny its importance.

Even physicians who actively worked with management retained much of the oppositional thinking of the past and felt the tension between practice and management, as described by Dr. R. Consider the response of Dr. Q, a surgeon and head of St. George's medical staff board, to a question about whether changes had occurred in his attitudes toward management and those of his colleagues:

Dr. Q: Ten years ago you were not bothered by management. You just did your work. We felt freer then. Now we feel we have to fight management – for example, they turn down requests for [a new medical device], because they cost too much money.

MH: What's your feeling about that?

Dr. Q: A little bit ambivalent. It's good for us to realize that you cannot just be a doctor but have to consider the costs of treatments and health care in general. On the other hand, it takes too much time from you. Sometimes you feel you're spending time on discussions, meetings, and so on, instead of seeing patients.

Medical quality was another area in which changes occurred in prevailing orientations. Discussions about quality assurance among regulators and managers surged during the late 1980s and early 1990s. In the acute sector, where general hospitals and medical specialists dominate, the main emphasis was on clinical quality. Among the sources for the new interest in quality assurance and assessment was concern that deregulation of health markets and price competition among insurers might harm quality. Hospital physicians shared these concerns. Few physicians adopted substantially new understandings of the nature of clinical quality. For a while, in the early 1990s, physicians began to treat quality assurance as an interdisciplinary, hospital-wide issue – an approach shared by many nurses and health consultants. But by the mid-1990s, the specialty organizations had taken over most of the responsibility for defining and assuring quality. These organizations focused mainly on quality issues within separate specialty areas (van Herk et al., 2001) – rather than examining issues that spanned departments or encompassed networks of physicians and paramedical professions.

Rather than reconceptualizing clinical quality and quality assurance, most regulators, insurers, and hospital managers accepted the medical profession's own standards of clinical practice and did not question the appropriateness or efficacy of collegial supervision of professional behavior. For example, when the new contracts were introduced in the mid-1990s, the Ministry of Health required the contract signers (physicians, hospitals, and insurers) to introduce projects to promote quality or enhance transmural care. However, the nature of the new projects was left up to each hospital, and hospitals were not required to file progress reports on their projects (Ints.). A few years later, researchers found that 80% of hospitals were conducting projects designed to enhance care across organizational boundaries, promote quality, or enhance efficiency, with about half of the projects focused on transmural activities (Ninerood-Bare, 1997). However, many of the reported projects had apparently been in operation *before* the introduction of the new physician contracts. Hospital managers and physicians simply re-labelled existing activities to conform to government regulations. For example, physicians had long conducted problem-focused peer review committees; now they began to call them 'quality committees'. Like hospital quality projects, the system of quality assessment through visits by external specialists was not new. It had existed since the 1970s (Klazinga et al., 1998). Neither regulators, insurers, or managers took significant steps toward direct monitoring of clinical quality. Instead, Ministry officials agreed that quality assurance would rely on recertification and visitations by medical peers (Int.).

INSTITUTIONAL TRENDS IN DUTCH HEALTH CARE

Did the changes triggered by the market reforms help transform Dutch health care institutions or were those changes just part of a passing wave of policy fashion? In response to this question, let us recall fundamental features of the Dutch system that remained intact after the implementation of the market reforms. Then we can examine areas in which the reforms helped reconfigure institutionalized patterns of health care delivery, finance, and regulation.

Despite the reforms, there are strong resemblances between many current features of health finance and those that prevailed before the reforms. Chief among these is the split between sickness fund insurance for the lower two-thirds of income earners and private insurance for the highest third. In their original form, the Dekker-Simmons reforms would have eliminated this fundamental distinction. However, the split among insurers survived, because powerful stakeholders opposed absorbing the private insurers into the statutory system, and other equally powerful forces objected to forcing sickness funds to compete with private insurers. No less important is the government's continuing commitment to insure all its citizens against critical illness and cover costs of long-term care. Thus the AWBZ insurance system survived the market reforms, and providers of services covered by AWBZ were not exposed to competition, as the market reformers had proposed. In addition, the government has remained active in regulating health finance. In fact, central government involvement in the national agencies that regulate health tariffs and budgets actually grew during the late 1980s and early 1990s. The state also continues to regulate entry of individuals to professional training and still tries to restrict providers' acquisition of expensive technologies.

Two important political values lie beneath these continuities in Dutch health finance and regulation. One is the principle of subsidiarity, whereby the government entrusts most health delivery and insurance to private, mainly not-for-profit agencies (Schut, 1995). The other is the principle of solidarity. In keeping with this second principle, wealthier and lower-risk individuals continue to pay premiums and taxes that subsidize treatment and insurance for poorer and sicker individuals. Moreover, the statutory health system continues to provide very compressive care; public resistance to rationing is strong. The quality of care provided under this insurance system appears to remain good, but systematic quality data are sorely lacking.

Despite the market reforms, individuals still have fairly limited choice of health insurers. Regional monopolies among sickness funds were eliminated by the reforms, but mergers quickly led to insurance oligopolies in most areas. Furthermore, sickness funds must provide identical coverage, and the basic policies offered by private firms provide very similar coverage to the sickness funds. Price differences among sickness funds and even private insurers are small. Differences among insurers in service and clinical quality are not widely publicized. These limits on patient choice reflect a lack of commitment among successive governments to fostering insurer and provider competition. During the late 1980s and the 1990s, Dutch governments tolerated mergers among insurers, restricted their autonomy over policies and charges, actively encouraged hospital mergers, and gradually withdrew types of care from the competitive arena.

The structure of health care provision also retains many features that predate the market reforms. Like the systems of other advanced countries, health care delivery is highly differentiated and segmented. In each subsector, organizations operate according to different occupational and practice norms, management systems, and funding arrangements. Providers face continuing difficulties in coordinating operations across sectors. For example, contact between general practitioners in the community and hospital specialists continues to be very limited, despite experiments at integrating care and providing functional, rather than sectoral funding.

Hospitals still continue to dominate most health care sectors, despite efforts to shift care to the community. Inpatient care absorbs more than 50% of the country's total health expenditures and over 60% of its public health expenditures (OECD, 2001). Hospital physicians continue to form the elite of their professions. They dominate medical innovation, training, and the definition of care standards for the health system as a whole. Despite growing managerial control, hospital specialists enjoy autonomy over their clinical practices. Public pressure for quality assurance is growing. Nonetheless, so far the traditional unwritten contract between the state and the physicians remains intact: The medical profession retains responsibility for supervising its members, defining practice standards, and assuring conformity to them.

Nonetheless, the health system is changing rapidly and stretching the limits set by long-standing institutions. The market reforms contributed directly to these institutional changes, even if the reforms did not always constitute the sole or primary force for change. There has been significant decentralization of the system and some deregulation. The national government abandoned or relaxed most of its programs for planning health system development, including state controls over capital construction in the health sector (de Roo 2001). Furthermore, the national government is using fiscal controls to force insurers and providers to accept greater responsibility for assuring that expenditures do not exceed revenues. Decentralization and changes in the funding of ambulatory care have encouraged considerable market activity, including new types of contracts and alliances among insurance companies, among providers, and between insurers, providers, and employers.

Closely related is the weakening of the neo-corporatist system of national representation and negotiation among interest groups (van der Grinten, 1996). National corporatist agencies still operate, but their influence is declining, as health care and insurance become more differentiated and diversified at the local and regional levels. Two indications of this trend are the declining power of the national specialists' association and the drift toward privatization and private-sector influence among insurers, hospitals, and community care providers. The trend toward commercial initiative and private, for-profit ownership in health runs parallel to developments in fields like public transit, social insurance, and telecommunications (Maarse, 1999) and fits with the Dutch version of the third way – between open market and state control ('Crumbs...', 1999). Still, caution is required in interpreting the implications of these trends. Since the market reforms, there has not been much change in the overall proportions of care funded by the private sector or paid for out of pocket.[6]

Diffusion of business thinking and practice throughout the health system is perhaps the most influential institutional change triggered by the market reforms and by tight government control over health budgets. Cost management, marketing, and strategic thinking are now widespread among managers in insurance firms, hospitals, and other provider agencies. Sickness funds now receive many of their services from the commercial divisions of the insurance companies that run the sickness funds. As a result, the practices and outlooks of sickness fund management are becoming hard to distinguish from those of commercial insurers. Forthcoming improvements in the risk adjustment formula in capitation payments and improvements in other governmental fiscal tools will accelerate the tendency for insurers and providers to manage their finances carefully, market them aggressively, and pay close attention to the cost implications of attracting different types of clientele (de Roo, 2001). Gradually, and with considerable reluctance, physicians and other health care professionals are accommodating themselves to the shift that has occurred in insurance and health care provision from passive budget administration to active business management.

CONCLUSION

In summary, the health system moved toward decentralization and partial deregulation during the 1990s, but there was only limited implementation of the most fundamental features of the market reforms envisioned by the

Dekker-Simons policies: the coherent quasi-market envisioned by the reformers never emerged. Instead, only limited competition developed among insurers and hospitals, and the contracting process provided very limited stimulus for improvements in hospital efficiency and quality. Productivity improvements in hospitals during the late 1980s and the 1990s stemmed from much broader and more enduring forces than those triggered by the market reforms. Chief among these forces were new medical technologies, the expansion of day surgery, government-led reductions in bed capacities in general hospitals, budget ceilings, and reductions in government reimbursements to insurers. Other sought-for developments that occurred during the reforms – including shifting of care to the community, enhanced patient choice, and incorporation of the work of hospital specialists into hospital budgets – also owed more to governmental initiatives and changes in prevailing medical practice than to the workings of the market.

Nonetheless, the trend toward decentralization and deregulation and the spread of market discourse profoundly affected the behavior and outlook of managers and practitioners throughout the health system. The market reforms stimulated many new entrepreneurial ventures and strategic alliances in health provision and finance. Moreover, by the end of the 1990s, health care practitioners were far more aware of considerations of cost and efficiency than they had been a decade earlier. Managers in health provision and insurance thought and acted in more market-oriented and strategic terms and tried to apply conventional business techniques to attain efficiencies and hold down costs within their organizations. In addition, the reforms contributed to loss of power among national corporatist groups. The reforms also helped foster greater managerial and political control over physicians in hospitals.

For decades the Dutch health system successfully balanced governmental commitments to high quality, universal care, and social solidarity with reliance on private insurers and providers. The market reforms threatened to upset that balance. Yet so far the growing commercialization of the health system does not appear to have seriously undermined solidarity. Instead, traditional rules remain intact to assure that healthier and wealthier citizens subsidize the costs of insurance and care for poorer and sicker individuals.

Despite the system's attainments, support is growing in government and Parliament for creation of a single, national system of statutory insurance, which would incorporate regulated competition along the lines envisioned by the market reformers of the 1980s (Sheldon, 2001a). The Social Democrats have favored such a move for decades. In the late 1990s the Minister of Health submitted a plan for insurance restructuring, as part of her drive to reduce inequalities in health care and assure equal access to services (Sheldon, 2001b). Creation of a unified national insurance system may also be necessary if the Dutch are to bring their system into line with requirements laid down by the European Court (Court of Justice, 2001; Sheldon, 2000b; Hermans, 2001). Failure to do so could lead to court restrictions on the ability of private insurers to use requirements for prior authorization as a way of rationing care. The court rulings could also affect government programs that regulate the numbers of physicians who are trained and licensed.

Although promoted as encouraging competition and enhancing individual choice, a national insurance system could actually reduce competition among private insurers, reduce choices for individual citizens, and intensify government regulation of insurers. If the past is a reliable guide, such developments would not necessarily affect the quality of care, which remains largely in the hands of health professionals and does not currently depend on patient choice or provider competition. Nor would these trends affect governmental commitments to universal health care and solidarity. However, the revival of proposals for national health insurance could well curtail current trends toward decentralization, increasing system complexity, and commercialization of health care.

NOTES

1 Acute care turnover includes day beds in the Netherlands.

2 Total health expenditures had risen by 42.7% in real terms (1995 prices) between 1972 and 1982. Between 1982 and 1985 they were virtually stable.

3 In 1990 expenditures for *all* types of inpatient care were 61.4% of total public health expenditures; in 1999 they were 62.5% of total expenditures. Acute care absorbed 32.7% of total public expenditures for health in 1986; 28.6% in 1990; and 29.9% in 1999 (OECD, 2001).

4 See Vienonen (1997). Unfortunately, no data are available on management costs, nor would it be possible to distinguish between costs of handling regulations and those incurred through market activity (Paton, 2000).

5 See Chapter 6, p. 152.

6 The proportion of total health expenditures coming from private sources was 30.8% in 1980, 31.9% in 1986, and 31.5% in 1999 (OECD, 2001). The figures for out-of-pocket expenditures as a percent of total expenditures are available only for 1996–98 (OECD, 2001). They show a rise from 7.7 to eight percent. In 1998 the Dutch figure was the second lowest among ten European Union countries for which data are available.

8

Conclusion

Chapters 2 through 7 through analyzed three of the boldest attempts by politicians in developed nations to implement market reforms of their publicly funded and government-regulated health systems. This chapter examines similarities among the reforms of the United Kingdom, Sweden, and the Netherlands, as well as some of their major differences. The in-depth studies showed how policymakers in each country developed new ideas about reforming health systems and public management. Some of these ideas extended or reacted to previous health policies. Some were imported from abroad or from fields other than health and then adapted to the country's health system. Among the most important forces shaping policy formulation and implementation were power distributions in the health and political systems; accepted decision processes in health and politics; previous policies; and established political values. Policy formulation and implementation in each country were further affected by dynamic social, economic, and political developments – such as electoral results and economic downturns.

The market reforms of the 1980s and 1990s promoted competition among publicly regulated providers or payers.[1] Competition among public agencies or between them and private ones was to focus mainly on the availability of services and their quality, and to a lesser degree on their price. This competition would take place in highly regulated quasi-markets. Capitated payments to public purchasers in Sweden and the UK and to statutory insurers in the Netherlands would give these payers incentives to reduce costs and assure the health of patients. Competition among providers for contracts from payers or for patients would create incentives to become more efficient so as to reduce costs and improve access to care – for example by reducing waiting lists. Competition would also release incentives for providers to improve service and clinical quality. The reforms also encouraged managers in provider and payer organizations to apply business practices and concepts from the realm of mass production and mass-marketing.[2] Many of these practices figured prominently in New Public

Management. They included decentralized budgeting and management, systems for increasing managerial control and accountability, assessments of organizational efficiency based on input-output comparisons, and productivity-linked rewards and financing.[3]

Although many politicians and policy analysts advocated quasi-market competition during the 1990s, continuing governmental regulation, as well as actions by both payers and providers, curtailed opportunities for competition among public purchasers in the UK and Sweden, insurers in the Netherlands, and providers in all three countries. In consequence, tight budgetary constraints and other governmental mandates more decisively shaped the behavior of health-system actors and had greater impacts on health system outcomes than did market forces. After a few years, politicians and health system actors in all three nations backed away from advocacy of vigorous market competition among providers or payers. Instead, decisionmakers promoted cooperation between public providers and payers and integration among health services.

To help bring together the findings from the three case studies and link them to broader discussions of policy implementation and health system change, this chapter addresses the three research questions presented in Chapter 1:

1. What forces affected implementation of market reforms?
2. What were the main outcomes of the market reforms?
3. Did the rapid rise and decline of political support for market reforms in health care reflect the dynamics of policy fashion?

After examining each of these issues, the chapter's conclusion discusses critical processes in implementation of market reform and assesses the capacity of market reforms to revitalize national systems of health care and other types of public services. It then outlines a decentralized, learning-focused approach to health system change that seems to hold more promise than market reform or top-down reforms of entire health systems. Also discussed are current developments in the countries studied and implications of the research for future studies of policy implementation and system-wide change.

IMPLEMENTATION OF MARKET REFORMS

The cases examined in the preceding chapters shed light on a central concern of research on planned change in complex systems: what forces affect the implementation of policies and programs that aim at system-wide change? Politicians and managers can also benefit from examining this issue before launching ambitious change programs.[4] Four types of forces shaped the ability of policymakers in the UK, Sweden, and the Netherlands to implement quasi-markets in health care and diffuse business practices within the health sector. In most instances these forces blocked progress toward managed competition. The same types of forces are likely to come into play during market reform of other public sectors.

First, as expected from past research on policy networks, interactions among powerful policy actors greatly influenced implementation of market reforms.[5] In each country, the course of these reforms depended greatly on the ability of state actors to develop and sustain a broad coalition in support of market reform and overcome opposition to proposed changes. Second, long-standing political values and institutions helped define the rules of the policy formulation and implementation games. These political traditions affected the ability of policy actors to mobilize support or opposition for market reforms and attain the upper hand in ensuing policy struggles. As indicated in Chapter 1, these two sets of forces also play a major role in system-wide transformations that do not rely on market mechanisms. Let us briefly review the combined effects of these two types of forces for each of the countries studied.

In the UK, the Thatcher government could drive through radical, internal-market restructuring, because it enjoyed strong electoral support and tight control over Parliament. Institutional conditions that helped sustain the regime's power included the two-party system and England's tradition of central government control over the National Health System.[6] Despite the success of market restructuring, the national government did not really rely on market forces to produce improvements in NHS services. Instead, the government drew on its centralized power and hierarchical control over the health system in its efforts to create tangible improvements in the NHS and win support for its market policies. The government poured money into the NHS, while praising the ability of the market to enhance efficiency among providers and the system as a whole. As the Conservatives' electoral support eroded during the 1990s, the Thatcher and Major Governments retreated from allowing market forces to force hospital closures in London or produce other controversial reconfigurations of services.

In Sweden during the late 1980s, a broad coalition of parties and policy analysts within the counties and the national government supported market reform. Although parties of the right and center were the strongest supporters, many Social Democratic politicians and analysts also favored market experimentation. Those supporting experimentation hoped that competition among providers for patients and funds would reduce waiting times and make the health system more responsive to patients' needs and preferences. Decentralization of health finance and management, along with a tradition of seeking consensus on public policy, prevented the national government from radically overhauling the health system. Still the government did introduce the Family Doctor and Patient Choice programs, both of which encouraged provider competition. At the same time the national government retained fiscal control over county council expenditures, most of which went to health care. Within the counties there was wide variation in the nature and degree of experimentation with market mechanisms.

Sweden's market reforms quickly foundered on the shoals of budgetary realities. As recession deepened at the start of the 1990s, health and welfare costs posed an ever-growing burden on county council budgets. What is more, expansion of private medical practice and productivity-based financing in Stockholm actually increased health expenditures. In response, county politicians began to express doubts about the expensive Family Doctor reform, the buy-sell experiments in hospital finance, and Stockholm's famed use of productivity incentives for hospitals. In addition, the reforms ran aground on long-standing political commitments to social solidarity, government support for employment, and generous welfare benefits. These foundations of the Swedish model had endured without challenge from the 1950s to the late 1980s. Unions, politicians, and voters across the political spectrum withdrew support for market experimentation and neo-liberal ideologies once they began to view market reform as a threat: They feared that introduction of markets into public services like health would weaken Sweden's social welfare system, reduce public employment, and weaken the country's historic commitment to social equality. In place of market forces, politicians and health managers began to back cooperation between public purchasers and providers. To hold down costs, decisionmakers supported regionalization of health finance and hospital mergers. They also turned to new policy issues, including quality of care, priority setting, and evidence-based medicine.

The Dutch system of coalitional governments, along with its tradition of seeking consensus across parties, toned down the drive for market reform from its onset. In the late 1980s a broad spectrum of health policy actors, including both governing parties and many members of the Social Democratic opposition, favored decentralization, competition among insurers, and greater financial responsibility for insurers and providers, along with preservation and even extension of statutory health insurance. It was hoped that these moves would control costs, increase the health system's efficiency and flexibility, and reduce emphasis on hospitalization.

After the Social Democrats regained control over the government in 1989, they continued the restructuring program that the Christian Democrats had initiated. However, the newly elected government sought to broaden health benefits, extend public insurance coverage to the entire population, and cap health expenditures – proposals that alienated the center and right parties and nearly all the interest groups that had initially supported reform. As a result, by 1994 the government was forced to abandon its comprehensive reform plan and proceed more cautiously and incrementally toward decentralization, managed competition among insurers, and increased fiscal responsibility for insurers and providers.

To implement system-wide change, policymakers in all three countries needed to gain the support of the physicians or at least avoid direct confrontations over the new policies. Nonetheless, national politicians broke traditions of consultation with the medical profession and allowed very little input from the medical profession during the formulation of the original proposals for market reform. In the UK the Thatcher government's strong parliamentary backing and its rapid reorganization of the NHS forced the British Medical Association to adopt a more conciliatory stance toward market reform. As the internal market reforms progressed, it became evident that the UK's general practitioners provided the key to developing a system of managed care that could loosen the hegemony of the country's hospitals over the health system as a whole. To promote a primary-care led NHS, government and NHS officials gave general practitioners generous incentives for entering the fundholding program. Moreover, both Conservative and Labour governments consulted closely with the general practitioners in their efforts to give primary care organizations central roles in NHS purchasing.

In Sweden the national government steered clear of confrontation with physicians and took steps that directly benefited them. The Clinical Chief reform (which put physicians – rather than nurses or managers – in charge of departmental finance) and the Family Doctor reform, increased opportunities and earnings for doctors. As budgets grew tighter, county politicians and health managers avoided cutting jobs for doctors. Instead, they concentrated on reducing the number of non-academic nurses and recently hired, non-tenured employees. Resistance to these moves by hospital staff unions was reduced by the depth of the recession and the employees' concerns that failure to moderate costs would threaten the survival of the entire Swedish social welfare system.

The most direct confrontation between physicians and national government officials occurred in the Netherlands. Here too, coalition politics and institutional arrangements proved critical to health system change. Dutch hospital physicians enjoyed legal and financial independence from hospital management. Until the mid-1990s this arrangement posed a major barrier to implementation of hospital budget ceilings and extension of managerial control over physicians. The government only succeeded in overcoming the specialists' opposition to change in hospital finance and management when a broad coalition of actors, including the parliament, allied against the hospital physicians. In addition, the specialists' national organization fragmented into disputing factions, which could not mobilize enough power to resist government pressure. At that juncture Health Minister Borst-Eilers successfully negotiated a change in the physicians' status.

The governments of the UK and Sweden were more able than the Dutch to regulate hospital budgeting and reorganize the structure of hospital finance in the late 80s and early 90s. In both the UK and Sweden, hospital physicians were salaried employees. Moreover, the UK had already tightened managerial control over hospital budgets and set up a system of clinical directors during the reforms of the 1980s, when the Thatcher government was at the peak of its power. Sweden had moved in a similar direction during the 1980s. In 1991 when Sweden's government followed the British example and unified managerial and clinical authority under a single physician, the move was supported by the Swedish Medical Association.

Although government actors in all three countries eventually succeeded in implementing structural changes in health finance and management, they were far less successful in their efforts to gather necessary data about the quality of provider services and clinical practices. Nor did they lead public payers and hospital managers to engage in effective forms of quality assessment and assurance. Long-standing traditions of professional self-regulation over clinical practice helped block progress toward non-medical control over quality. These traditions were rooted in institutional arrangements that assured the specialists' autonomy over training, supervision of their peer's activities, discipline of errant colleagues

(Rosenthal, 1995), and review of clinical irregularities or errors. In Sweden and the Netherlands, neither government officials nor health managers made concerted efforts to exercise direct supervision or influence over clinical practices in the hospitals and clinics. Nor did they press payers to assign high priority to clinical quality assessment in the contracting process. Instead, Dutch and Swedish politicians left clinical quality assurance up to peer control and the specialty associations, which undertook voluntary programs of quality enhancement and development of protocols for clinical practice.

In contrast, the UK's government tried unsuccessfully to enforce managerial monitoring of clinical practice within the hospitals and make hospitals accountable for clinical performance. The physicians successfully resisted the government's call for comprehensive and compulsory clinical audits. Instead, the hospital specialists encapsulated audit as a form of professional education and conducted highly circumscribed investigations that robbed medical audits of their potential as a source of clinical information and managerial control. Under Prime Minister Blair the Clinical Governance program sought again to tighten political and managerial supervision of clinical work. It is too soon to judge whether these formal governance programs will ultimately overcome deeply entrenched professional norms and lead to managerial control over clinical work.

Despite resistance among physicians to inroads into their clinical autonomy, governments in all three countries did exercise influence over service-related dimensions of care, like waiting times. Officials and managers could monitor service more readily than clinical quality. Physicians and managers seeking to meet official service standards could more easily change their practices or take steps to look good on paper. Change also occurred in the managerial involvement of physicians. In all three countries, hospital physicians who served as heads of departments and divisions took on more managerial and budgetary responsibility. These physician managers continued to draw their legitimacy from their peers and depended heavily on their colleagues' expertise and cooperation. Still, as medical managers participated more in managerial decisions and undertook greater fiscal responsibilities, they began to identify more with management and internalize managerial beliefs and norms. Moreover, these department and division heads introduced cost awareness and other business concepts into the clinical realm and began to exercise influence over their colleagues' clinical practices.

A third set of conditions influenced opportunities for competition among payers or providers. For the most part, the reforms did not change statutory entitlements to broad packages of care and standard formulae for reimbursing providers. In consequence, providers in all three countries and insurers in Holland could not compete much on the price or mix of statutory services. Geographic conditions and the behavior of both patients and providers further limited provider competition. Areas that were not heavily populated often had only one hospital within reasonable travelling distance. In Sweden some younger and healthier patients took advantage of possibilities for choice among urban hospitals. But elderly patients, and even most younger ones, typically remained loyal to their local hospital and resisted travelling long distances to speed up or improve treatment.

Even in the cities of Sweden, the UK, and the Netherlands, contracts between hospitals and payers turned out to be less contestable than had been expected.[7] Purchasers and insurers often could not find any alternative hospital capable of providing the large volume of required emergency and elective care. The tendency of urban hospitals to specialize in particular types of treatments and populations further restricted the ability of payers to shift contracts among hospitals. What is more, powerful political forces prevented public payers in Sweden or the United Kingdom from withdrawing major contracts with local hospitals. Dutch insurers faced legal and practical constraints to removing contracts from hospitals. Professionals in ambulatory care who had developed long-term working relations with one another also resisted attempts to introduce competitive bidding and other forms of provider competition.

Hospital mergers further reduced opportunities for competition in all three countries. Despite the anti-competitive effects of consolidation, governments tried to reduce costs by merging units or entire hospitals. Furthermore, Dutch insurers averted competition among themselves through a wave of mergers before and during the competitive reforms. Hence, even after introduction of managed competition, insurance companies continued to dominate the regions where they had previously held legal monopolies.

As a result of the above conditions, Swedish and British hospitals did not compete much for contracts from major public purchasers, and Dutch hospitals did not really compete for major contracts from sickness funds. However, Swedish hospitals did compete for patients seeking more accessible and better quality elective procedures. British hospitals competed for contracts with General Practitioner Fundholders. This competition focused on prices, accessibility of services, and quality of service. Dutch hospitals competed on the mix and prices of services offered to privately insured patients. Dutch insurers competed for private customers by bundling different insurance packages and offering attractive services. The minimal competition that emerged among the statutory sickness funds mainly concerned perceived quality of service.

A fourth barrier to implementing market reform came from limitations on the managerial capacities of public payers and providers. Managers in both types of organizations often had too little knowledge, experience, and power to develop and implement the business procedures and systems needed to sustain effective contracting, marketing, or operational control. Purchasing contracts did not give payers much leverage over providers. At the start of the reforms public purchasers in the UK and Sweden and statutory insurance managers in the Netherlands had very limited experience executing the management functions required for operating under market conditions. Gradually, recruitment of managers from commercial backgrounds altered this situation in the UK and the Netherlands. Less change occurred in purchaser recruitment in Sweden, where elected politicians or their nominees served as purchasers. In the Netherlands, practices from the for-profit divisions of insurance companies spread rapidly to the firms' not-for-profit (sickness fund) divisions. Despite adoption of norms and practices from business, purchasing contracts in all three countries remained service agreements based on publicly regulated forms of prospective budgeting, rather than legally binding agreements. The contracts lacked the specificity and enforcement mechanisms that characterize legal contracts. Moreover, much of their content was set by governmental or quasi-governmental agencies, rather than being negotiated between autonomous parties.

Throughout the decade, inadequate management information systems also made it hard to carry out basic managerial functions. For instance, available data typically did not allow providers or payers to compare costs and production rates for specific procedures or units. Even where data were available, controls for severity of illness and patient case mix were usually missing or inadequate. Often payers and providers used available data less effectively than they might have, because they were distracted by more urgent obligations, they faced resistance by physicians, or they lacked experience in data analysis. Physician resistance and technical difficulties posed particularly high barriers to attaining data on clinical quality. Yet without agreed-upon quality measures, government officials and health managers could not tell whether production increases signalled genuine efficiency gains or had been accompanied by reductions in the quality of care.

Similar problems arose when government officials or health managers tried to decide which medical practices were preferable clinically and provided the most value for money. For the most part, these decisionmakers lacked the expertise and clinical knowledge needed for such exercises in evidence-based medicine and technology assessment. Gradually the medical specialty associations responded to government and public pressure for quality assurance. The associations developed best practice standards, but these standards, and available scientific evidence, usually provided only limited guidance to decisionmakers as to which procedures and technologies were most cost effective (Drummond et al., 1997; Harrison, S., 1998; U. S. Congress, 1995; Woolf et al., 1999).

Technical limitations in important financial tools formed still another hurdle to market reform. In the Netherlands, for example, the capitation formula created incentives for cream skimming. All three countries encountered difficulties in developing effective systems for prospective payment to hospitals and assessing patient case mix. Moreover, governmental caps on hospital budgets often hampered full implementation of prospective budgeting.

OUTCOMES OF MARKET REFORMS

This book examined the outcomes of policy implementation through four analytic frames. First, the administrative frame focuses on the extent of top-down implementation of policies and attainment of policy objectives. The other three frames direct attention to outcomes that policymakers less often discuss in public. The second frame examines changes in bargaining and power relations among health system actors. The third assesses changes in actors' interpretations – their thoughts, norms, and discourse about their work and the health system as a whole. The fourth frame draws attention to ways in which the reforms affected institutions underlying health politics, finance, and service delivery and created precedents for later health policies. Let us review the most prominent outcomes of the market reforms from the vantage point of each of these four frames.

Administrative Change

The reforms led directly and indirectly to important changes in the structuring of health care provision and finance within all three countries. During the same period, other structural changes took place that were independent of market policies and in some cases contrary to them. In the UK, the most prominent and enduring market-directed changes were separation of public purchasers (Health Authorities) and providers, and introduction of contracting between purchasers and providers. Closely related was the transformation of former district hospitals into semi-autonomous trusts. General practitioner (GP) fundholding did not survive the return of Labour to power but still set an important precedent by assigning purchasing power and responsibility for managed care to primary care practices. The Blair government built on this foundation when it introduced Primary Care Groups and Trusts, which are assuming the purchasing functions previously assigned to Health Authorities. During the 1990s power became more centralized within the British health system, a trend that contradicted the letter and spirit of market-oriented reform.

During the main years of market reform in Sweden, only a minority of county councils introduced purchaser-provider splits and public contracting for health care. However, by the end of the 1990s, most counties had adopted some form of centralized purchasing of hospital services. As in the UK, Sweden's state-owned hospitals gained substantially more managerial and budgetary autonomy during the market reforms. Two other influential structural changes, which were unrelated to the market reforms, were transfer of responsibility for non-medical geriatric care to the municipalities and regionalization in government and health services. The geriatric care reform complemented the goals of the market reforms by making general hospitals responsible primarily for 'curative' medical treatments to which industrial-style standards of efficiency could be more readily applied. In contrast, regionalization reduced opportunities for hospital competition and contracting by payers within counties or municipalities. At the start of the reforms these types of devolved contracting had been thought to hold the keys to empowering citizens and their representatives.

In the Netherlands, not-for-profit, statutory insurers (sickness funds) obtained somewhat more managerial autonomy and fiscal responsibility and were permitted to compete for clients outside of their previously assigned regions. However, mergers among insurers substantially reduced opportunities for competition. Mergers among hospitals had a similar effect. The incorporation of hospital specialists' pay into hospital budgets contained far-reaching implications for Dutch health care, but this development was not directly related to the government's programs for regulated competition.

Although the reforms in all three countries generated some of the structural preconditions for quasi-markets in health care, they were less successful in generating the necessary market and managerial processes. As noted in the first part of this chapter, many organizational, legal, and political forces limited competition among providers and payers. Moreover, powerful technical, political, and organizational forces undermined rational choice of services by public payers and limited the development of explicit and effective forms of contracting.

Relocation of care in the community was less central to market reform but was anticipated as a byproduct and facilitant of reform in all three countries. In practice, the locus of care changed slowly and incrementally. Moreover, rather than flowing from strong market forces, the drift toward ambulatory and community care mainly reflected the influence of new medical technologies and government-mandated reductions in hospital facilities.

Although reform objectives varied between countries, market reformers in all three countries sought tangible improvements in hospital efficiency and moderation of growth in total health costs. In the end, only Sweden succeeded in restraining total costs during the 1990s. Total health expenditures rose substantially in both the UK and the Netherlands during the years of market reform. On the other hand, during the period of market reform, hospitals in all three countries boosted their production and efficiency, as measured by throughput rates or outputs per expenditures.

In fact, market mechanisms contributed very little to these attainments in hospital productivity. Instead, the observed changes mainly reflected powerful impacts of *non-market forces* in health finance and management. Along with a torrent of market rhetoric, each country experienced an intensification of top-down, state control over health budgets and direct governmental pressure on providers to attain cost-savings. Sweden had used global budgeting to reduce health costs in the 1980s and continued to apply them in the 1990s to enforce cost stability. Thanks to these policies and hospital mergers, bed capacities dropped substantially. In the UK, the Thatcher and Major governments enforced tight global budgets and hospital cutbacks. At the same time they generously funded hospital programs to reduce waiting lists, management and information systems, and supported GP fundholding. The Dutch governments used global budgeting throughout the 1980s and 1990s and obtained reductions in acute hospital beds during the 1980s and the first half of the 1990s.

The explanations for the hospitals' productivity gains are similar to those for cost trends. In the UK, governmental requirements that health managers show annual efficiency gains were particularly direct and draconian. In all countries, patient demand for services rose, while budget caps often reduced spending per patient. Thus hospital managers and their staffs were forced to learn to provide more services at lower marginal expenditures. At the same time, new technologies facilitated shorter hospitalization periods, substitution of ambulatory treatment for overnight hospitalization, and other improvements in hospital throughput. Other non-market developments, such as the shift of geriatric care to municipalities in Sweden and incorporation of Dutch hospital physicians' pay into hospital budgets, also contributed to improvements in hospital performance.

Changes in national hospital capacity and productivity began before the market reforms and were largely unrelated to the intensity of these reforms. For example, productivity gains were as prominent in Swedish counties that did *not* introduce purchaser-provider splits as they were in counties that experimented with public purchasing. Moreover, there is reason for doubting the impact of market processes on hospital performance in all three nations studied. The level of competition that emerged among hospitals in the UK and Sweden and among Dutch insurers was so modest that it seems unreasonable to attribute changes in provider performance mainly to competitive incentives. What is more, parallel reductions in length of hospital stay, which is one indication of productivity, took place in other Western European nations that did not implement market reforms.[8] Hospital capacities also declined during the 1980s and 1990s throughout the industrial world – with or without market reforms (OECD, 2001).

In contrast to competitive incentives, one business-like practice stands out for its contribution to hospital productivity: targeted productivity incentives, in the form of extra governmental payments for high-demand services, produced rapid improvements in hospital production in the UK and Sweden. More generally, as noted below, the market reforms, in tandem with budget ceilings, sharpened awareness of health providers of the need to cut costs and boost production. Thus market reform may have indirectly contributed to productivity gains.

It is hard to determine how, if at all, the market reforms affected the quality of health services. There are a paucity of good data on quality and serious challenges to disentangling the forces affecting quality. Consider service quality, an area where the reforms are widely thought to have had some beneficial effects. In all three countries small, but organizationally important portions of hospital revenues became dependent on patient choices or provider referrals. This type of competition sharpened staff awareness of the patient as consumer. Providers in all three countries sought to attract and satisfy patients and referring physicians. Similarly, insurers in the Netherlands actively marketed private insurance policies and sought to attract clients by improving their image as service providers.

However, insurers and providers aimed most of their marketing efforts at the high end of the market. Dutch insurers, for example, sought to attract low-risk clients and worked harder to sell private insurance than to expand their sickness fund membership. In like manner, providers in the UK sought contracts from fundholding GPs but did not compete very intensely for contracts with Health Authorities – which held budgets for most patients and had responsibility for more poor and aged patients than did fundholders. In the Netherlands, providers sought to attract healthier and wealthier patients, who were privately insured. Swedish hospitals competed over geographically mobile candidates for elective surgery, but made no special efforts to attract older, less mobile patients or those needing emergency or chronic care. It is possible that awareness of the patient as consumer and client spread to staff providing services that were not exposed to competitive incentives and even affected staff members who provided services to less desirable clients and patients. Nonetheless, it is clear that hospital managers and professionals sometimes diverted energy and resources to serving the minority of patients who brought in extra revenues.

The market reforms had no demonstrable direct effects on clinical quality. Clinical quality in hospitals does not appear to have changed much in the Netherlands or Sweden during the market reforms. However, Swedish geriatric care suffered when a non-market reform shifted most nursing care to municipalities, which were subject to tight budgets. Clinical quality in British general hospitals may have declined the market reform period. Many observers argued that cuts in hospital beds and services and increasingly rapid turnover of patients reduced care quality in the NHS. However, these potentially harmful hospital developments mainly reflected government-imposed budget ceilings. Market forces played a lesser role, but the government's heavy-handed reliance on production models of efficiency certainly encouraged hospitals to push patients out faster than in the past.

The UK's internal market reorganizations had more direct and deleterious effects on service coordination, which is crucial to quality. Contrary to the hopes of market reformers, contracting, competition, and other market processes did not assure continuity of care for the chronically and mentally ill. Nor did market mechanisms help integrate social and medical care. Instead, the purchaser-provider split and fundholding deepened existing structural, financial, and occupational divisions within and between primary care, the hospital sector, and social care. The spread of contracting and other market practices discouraged cooperation among health actors and encouraged rivalry and self-interested behavior. Fiscal and reporting techniques encouraged providers and payers to conceive of care in terms of narrowly-defined services. Fragmentation and self-interested behavior also occurred among Swedish and Dutch providers. These forces, along with traditional barriers to cooperation, made it hard for health and social care providers in both countries to implement interdisciplinary and inter-agency coordination.

Policymakers in all three nations expected market reform to shift care to the community and promote a reorientation toward prevention, health education, and population-based services. In the UK, general practitioner fundholding created a precedent for involving family doctors in decisions about the entire spectrum of services provided to their patients. In the Netherlands, as well, market reforms and changes in hospital budgeting encouraged cooperation between hospitals and community-based providers. Growth of day treatments in all three countries helped keep patients in the community, while reductions in the length of hospital stays speeded the return of patients to their homes or to non-acute facilities. Nonetheless, the hoped-for reorientation of caregivers toward health promotion did not occur. Nor did spending patterns and service priorities of public payers change much. In the UK, budgeting and contracting processes often diverted the attention of public payers and other actors from broader objectives, such as promoting public health. In Sweden and the Netherlands, as well, providers were largely occupied with the struggle to maintain current types of services under ever-tighter budgets.

The market reforms also strengthened movement toward privatization of health care. This development was most evident in the UK, where the government maintained pre-reform policies of limiting NHS coverage. Pro-market forces in the Netherlands tried to move in the same direction but met much opposition. Selective marketing by Dutch insurers also posed threats to solidarity. In Sweden, development of private ambulatory care in the large cities reduced equality of access, while growth in co-payments weakened solidarity.

Changes in Bargaining and Power Relations

In concert with tighter health budgets, the market reforms provided opportunities for shifts in alliances and power distributions among health system actors. Despite decentralization policies, national health officials and politicians in the UK and the Netherlands gained strategic, administrative, and economic control over providers[9]; similar developments occurred among county council officials and politicians in Sweden. Among the sources of growing external control over hospital providers was the assignment of more financial responsibility to hospital managers and improvements in the transparency of financial and operational reporting by the hospitals. This trend began in the UK and Sweden with structural reorganizations during the 1980s, but in the Netherlands it emerged mainly during the 1990s.

National policy actors also gained power over physicians. The national governments avoided early consultations with physicians about health system reforms and then decentralized portions of enacted reforms. This process of decentralization made changes affecting physicians less visible and less vulnerable to pressure from national medical bodies. In all three countries, national and local politicians also divided the medical community by providing selective incentives for groups of physicians to cooperate with reform. For example, the British government generously supported fundholding, while some Swedish counties encouraged expansion of private ambulatory practices. In all countries, hospital consolidations brought benefits to elite physicians in more advanced hospitals at the expense of other medical practitioners.

Market reform in the Netherlands strengthened the financial influence of statutory insurers and for-profit insurance managers over hospitals. However, insurers were unable to exercise much direct influence over hospital policies, internal management practices, or clinical activity. The reforms had a similar, but even weaker influence on relations between public purchasers and hospitals in Sweden and the United Kingdom. In no country were payers able to fundamentally restructure the mix of hospital services or systematically monitor the quality of services.

Reformers in all three countries anticipated that patients would be empowered by the release of market forces. In Sweden, patient choice of settings for elective surgery and the Family Doctor program gave healthier and more mobile patients the ability to chose providers. Neither program increased patients' influence over clinical decisionmaking, but the programs did promote responsiveness to patients' concerns among health managers and physicians. In England, GP fundholders acted as advocates for patients within the hospital system. However, patients had no choice over the hospitals to which fundholders referred them. Changes in the procedures for appointing members of Health Authorities reduced the influence of patients and their representatives within the NHS. British programs designed to solicit the views of community residents on health policy and involve them in decisions were usually superficial and involved narrow sets of participants. In none of the countries studied did patients receive information needed to make rational choices of providers.

Choice of insurers in the Netherlands was also supposed to empower patients. However, neither the Ministry of Health nor any other agency gave patients the information needed to compare the charges and quality of insurers. In practice, insurers put more emphasis on marketing bundles of for-profit and not-for-profit services to consumers than on soliciting patient concerns and transmitting them to health providers. In contrast, the Dutch government encouraged patient representation within provider organizations, a process that met with some success in non-acute care settings.

There was an important, and largely unanticipated shift in power alignments within the British medical profession. The GP fundholding program moderately enhanced the influence of primary care physicians on hospital clinicians. The Blair government sought to broaden and deepen the empowerment of primary care physicians by granting them the purchasing authority previously vested in Health Authorities. Neither of these structural innovations eliminated fundamental asymmetries of power and professional status between the two groups of physicians. In the Netherlands and Sweden relations between hospital and community physicians remained much as they had been before the market reforms.

During the market reforms, hospital managers in all three countries also obtained greater economic, strategic, administrative, and operational control over health professionals. The market reforms acted in concert with government controls over hospitals to increase the ability of hospital managers to monitor and control the work of physicians. For example, in the UK, publication of ratings of hospital performance and public criticism of poorly rated hospitals increased the leverage that managers exercised over physicians. During the height of the market reforms, these ratings concentrated on crude measures of costs and performance; later the Blair government began rating hospital quality on a wide spectrum of measures and publicizing the ratings. Participation of Dutch clinicians in hospital management and inclusion of their pay in hospital budgets also gave insurers and hospital managers new – and as yet largely unrealized – opportunities to oversee medical practices. Despite these developments, hospital clinicians continued to defend their control over clinical decisions and resisted attempts by medical and non-medical managers to monitor and influence clinical practice.

As information systems improve in European nations, insurers, public purchasers, and managers in provider organizations will develop new capacities to assess medical performance in terms of best practice standards and compare practices of provider agencies and individual physicians. Insurers and public purchasers will then be able to choose better performing or less costly hospitals and give priority to more cost-effective procedures. Developments like these have already occurred in the United States (Gold et al., 1995) and are emerging elsewhere (Berg, 1996; Rappolt, 1997; Harrison and Shalom, 2002; Shadmi, 2002).

Patients are also beginning to choose hospitals, practitioners, and insurers on the basis of quality ratings (e.g., HealthScope, 2003). As they progress, the trends toward choice and monitoring of professional practices will further erode the occupational and clinical autonomy of hospital specialists and community practitioners.

Interpretive Change

In the UK and the Netherlands, and to a somewhat lesser degree in Sweden, market reform helped undermine established forms of discourse, thinking, and practice among health managers and professionals. Gradually the administrative and professional mind-sets that dominated health care from the 1960s through the early 1980s began to give way to more business and market-oriented discourse and thinking. Decentralization of budgetary responsibility to local or regional payers and providers, combined with government-imposed budget ceilings, radically altered the working assumptions upon which medical activity rested. Previously, health professionals could provide services based solely on their medical value. Now they became aware of the cost implications of their decisions and encountered fiscal constraints on their practices. Moreover, as managers in provider organizations became directly responsible for cost overruns, they pressed health professionals to play an active role in reductions in hospital capacities and other cost control programs.

The transformation of thinking and talking about health care was most dramatic and extensive among Britain's public payers and hospital managers. There business rhetoric and concepts from industrial management and mass marketing supplanted much former administrative discourse. A more moderate move in this direction occurred in the Netherlands. Diffusion of market discourse and thinking also occurred in Sweden, but was less extensive and was often short-lived. Even in Sweden, it became commonplace to concentrate attention on the efficiency of hospital units and to define efficiency in terms of patient throughput.[10]

Within a few years of the start of market reform, talk of purchasing and provider competition declined rapidly in all three countries, while other popular concepts gained ground. Many of these new ideas and techniques also came from the world of business. Instead of stressing the ability of the market to pit providers or payers against one another, politicians, analysts, and managers talked more of quality assurance, improving relations among providers through networking, consultation between providers and public payers, systematic priority setting by government, and cost-benefit analysis.

In contrast to developments among health managers and public officials, the occupational subcultures of health professionals changed less dramatically during the market reforms. Besides fostering cost consciousness among physicians and nurses, the reforms strengthened a trend toward making nurses responsible for managing or reporting on efficiency drives and cost-containment. However, the market reforms had very little impact on many important features of subcultures of hospital and ambulatory physicians. Professional norms, assumptions, and practices remained largely unchanged in crucial fields like specialty training, clinical practice, peer supervision, professional ethics, research, and relations among specialties. For instance, hospital physicians continued to resist giving information about their practices to managers or even to members of other medical specialties. Furthermore, most hospital physicians continued to devote their energy and attention to clinical practice within their specialty. In doing so, these physicians distanced themselves from senior managers, who adopted organizational and systemic approaches to hospital operations. In like manner, hospital physicians showed little enthusiasm for efforts by health managers, purchasers, politicians, and some primary care physicians to link hospitals more closely to providers of medical and social services in the community. Nor did most physicians show increased interest in preventive medicine and health promotion.

Finally, mention should be made of broader interpretive drifts that affected attitudes toward government health policies. In the UK during the 1990s, the public, along with many NHS employees, grew increasingly dissatisfied with the government's treatment of the NHS. Successive reorganizations and chronic shortages of funds led many people in and outside the NHS to lose trust in the government's capacity and commitment to revitalize the NHS. In particular many NHS physicians grew cynical and even embittered about prospects for the NHS. Public concern over the future of the NHS was an important cause of the defeats of the Conservatives in local and national elections in the mid-1990s. In the Netherlands and Sweden there were few signs of such a widespread shift in sentiments toward the national health system or the government's handling of the market reforms. However, in Sweden the election campaign and results in 1994 demonstrated widespread public concern over entrusting Sweden's health system and its other social welfare institutions to pro-market parties.

Institutional Change

To what extent did the market reforms contribute to lasting transformations of institutions that shape the finance, delivery, and politics of health care? First, consider the impacts of the reforms on health finance. Basic features of health finance remained unchanged in all three countries. Nonetheless, there were major moves toward decentralization of the allocation of public funds to providers. Another fundamental change in the UK and Sweden involved distribution of public budgets for health care to public purchasers, who had varying degrees of contact with local patients and agencies. In the Netherlands the market reforms used capitation to distribute funds from statutory insurance fees to private, not-for-profit insurers. This procedure increased the insurers' autonomy and contracting responsibilities.

Despite these moves toward decentralization, national governments continued to play a major role in regulating health finance as they sought to curtail total health spending. In the UK and the Netherlands central state bodies actually tightened their control over health finance during the market reforms. The

Swedish government placed ceilings on county council taxation. Along with cost concerns, the growing intervention of state actors in the UK reflected attempts to assure the success of the market programs and reduce opposition by local politicians and physicians.[11] Ironically, in none of the countries studied did government agencies or other powerful actors act to assure the fairness of competition among providers or payers, as envisioned by advocates of managed competition.[12] Nor did the states or other organizations make much progress toward gathering and disseminating quality information, which could guide rational choice of health services by purchasers and individual consumers.

Second, the atmosphere generated by the market reforms provided fertile ground for narrowing the scope of statutory care, allowing some growth in private funding of health care, and expanding provision of medical and social care by private, for-profit agencies. In the UK the Conservative governments drove substantial movement in these directions. The government effectively privatized nursing care for the elderly, and led to the gradual privatization of several other types of care, including dental care. The government also fostered outsourcing of municipal social services to private providers, encouraged tendering of hospital support services to private contractors, and mandated private financing of hospital construction – a program that sometimes led to private operation of newly built hospital facilities. In the Netherlands, provision of statutory ambulatory care by private entrepreneurs and bundling of private, for-profit and statutory insurance packages led to a blurring of the boundary between for-profit and not-for-profit insurance and care. In Sweden, patients' co-payments for services rose substantially, and public payers increased their reliance on private providers of ambulatory care. The UK also increased co-payments for several types of treatments and for pharmaceuticals, while the Dutch continued to debate the merits of such moves.

Despite this changing mix of public and private (for-profit and not-for-profit) finance and provision, neither the public nor their political representatives abandoned their long-standing commitments to the values of universal access to care and solidarity in health finance. In all three countries coalitions of patients, local politicians, opposition parties in parliament, and medical and non-medical unions fought governmental moves to curtail hospital services. Elections in the UK and Sweden also demonstrated the public's desire to retain broad entitlements to health and social care. Commitment to universal health care, along with divergence of stakeholder priorities, also hampered forays by governmental bodies and public payers into evidence-based medicine and systematic priority setting. At the outset both techniques had seemed to provide rational, non-politicized grounds for allocating scarce public funds.

Third, the market reforms contributed to the spread of industrial and business practices throughout the health system. In all three countries, hospital managers gained autonomy and responsibility for boosting productivity and operating within tight budget limits. In response, managers strove to reduce costs, speed throughput, and market revenue-generating services. Hospital managers mobilized nurses to document and support this efficiency drive, recruited some senior physicians into clinical management roles, and involved others in discussions of managerial issues.

For the most part, both medical and non-medical managers refrained from exercising direct control over clinical practice or applying production standards to individual practitioners. After the market reforms peaked, political pressure grew for hospitals to become more accountable for the quality of care. National medical specialty organizations reacted by developing and diffusing voluntary practice guidelines. In response to direct pressure by central government – as opposed to market forces – British physicians reluctantly cooperated with governmental monitoring of hospital quality and agreed to recertification of physicians.

Fourth, market reforms in each country complimented other more powerful forces that reduced the centrality of general hospitals within the health system. Among the non-market forces were government-mandated mergers and cutbacks in hospital capacities, new technologies that supported ambulatory care, shorter hospital stays, and growing belief in the benefits of community-based care. In the UK, primary care practitioners gained some influence over public contracting, while payers in all three countries sought to shift care to the community. So far hospitals continue to provide most ambulatory surgery and advanced diagnosis. Moreover, major hospital centers continue to play leading roles in medical research, innovation, and training.

Although specific types of care were rarely removed from hospitals, there was considerable growth in treatment, diagnosis, and post-hospital care within the communities. Especially in the UK and the Netherlands, a wide range of for-profit and not-for-profit organizations offered these new and expanded services. The national governments explicitly encouraged these developments, while established providers sometimes resisted them. The rapid expansion and differentiation of community care weakened inter-unit and inter-organizational ties and working relations among professionals and agencies for health and social care. In place of these ties, a web of contracts link practitioners, provider agencies, payers, and sectors. These new contractual ties make possible patient or problem-focused cooperation across occupations and agencies. However, the new linkages – with their focus on costs – often disrupt older working relations that rested on norms of trust and reciprocity among professions.

Fifth, the market reforms contributed to important institutional changes in the health politics of all three countries. Chief among these was growth in the importance of national health policy within domestic affairs. Issues of health finance and delivery became subject to debate in many governmental and non-governmental forums and formed important electoral issues. At the same time, the central government gained power as a national health policy actor, while the medical profession grew weaker. Nonetheless, most governments continued to avoid direct confrontations with the physicians' national organizations.

Adoption of the language and standards of business management also helped redefine the rules of health politics and place interest groups at a disadvantage. Casting decisions about health finance and service configurations in rationalistic terms gave power to health economists and other technical experts and reduced the ability of physicians and other stakeholders to challenge policy decisions. Market reforms thus helped erode constellations of power that had shaped health politics and the delivery of health services for several decades.

As contracting replaced budgeting, relations among health system actors became more complex and disaggregated. Proponents of this centrifugal thrust of market reform point to its contribution to health system functioning: reduced politicization of health finance and management, greater provider efficiency, and direction of resources toward areas of high demand. On the other hand, the trend toward disaggregation of finance and delivery reduced equality of access to care and rendered health care more fragmented and less amenable to integration. Service fragmentation was one force blocking movement toward important policy objectives, including health promotion, coordinating services for growing numbers of chronically ill patients, and linking medical care to social care and other public services.

In summary, the market reforms did not generate vigorous quasi-markets, could not hold down health costs, made only modest contributions to hospital efficiency, and failed to attain other outcomes that had been envisioned by the reforms' promoters. Hospital efficiency gains owed more to top-down fiscal controls and government-led reductions in hospital capacity than to market forces. On the other hand, the market reforms helped diffuse cost consciousness and business-like practices and orientations among payers and managers in provider organizations. The reforms enhanced patient choice somewhat, but they only provided choice for a minority of patients and did not empower them in other ways. At the same time, the market reforms had substantial impacts that were less often anticipated or acknowledged by reform advocates and planners: Decentralization and marketization helped strengthen management, weaken physicians, and produce other power realignments. Furthermore, the reforms contributed to growing inequality in access to health care and payment for it.

MARKET REFORM AS POLICY FASHION

During the 1980s and early 1990s, market reform of health services aroused the interest and enthusiasm of many health system decisionmakers throughout the developed world. In all three of the countries examined here and in several other nations, policymakers quickly enacted ambitious reforms based on quasi-market principles. Within a few years market reforms lost favor among politicians and large sectors of the electorate. In the UK, Sweden, and the Netherlands political support for market reform declined even before the original programs were fully implemented. Many practices and ideas associated with the reform survived this decline in support, but policymakers gradually abandoned their broad campaign to reform the health systems through market forces.

Other types of health care policies also waxed and waned in popularity in industrial countries during the 1990s. These included evidence-based medicine (Brown, 1995), rationalistic priority setting (Holm, 1998; van der Grinten and Kasdorp, 1999) public participation in decisionmaking (Calnan et al., 1998), and state action to promote clinical quality (Becher and Chasin, 2001). Over the last few decades many policies and practices in education, public administration, and social services also experienced rapid surges and declines in popularity and political backing (e.g., Birnbaum, 2000, Calhoun and Joyce, 1998; Etzioni, 1975; March and Olsen, 1983; Mossberger, 2000, Sarason, 1971). Many new management techniques also underwent cycles of popularity and rapid diffusion, that were soon followed by periods of decline and criticism (Abrahamson and Fairchild, 1999; Cole, 1999; Gibson and Tesone, 2001).

As often occurs with management innovations, the rapid rise and decline of market reforms reflect underlying dynamics in a fashion life cycle.[13] A model of this life cycle is proposed here to account for the rise and decline of market reforms and to stimulate further research on policy fashions. The term fashion is used in an analytic and non-pejorative sense to describe shifts in support for policies that reflect an underlying process of fashion-setting, formulation, and implementation. No judgment is implied about the impacts of policies that go through fashion cycles. Some managerial and policy fashions leave their mark on organizations and institutions, as did the market reforms in health care. Other fashions have little lasting impact. Fashion setting is but one route to policy change (Wilson, 2000). Others include realignments in governing coalitions, new initiatives by policy actors, and responses to critical events, like the attack on the World Trade Center.

Policymakers and government officials in the West often search for new ways to improve the organizations and systems over which they exercise authority. This search rests on taken-for-granted norms and beliefs: Progress is positive in its own right and rationalized, organized action can produce progress toward almost any goal (Meyer and Rowan, 1977). Reward systems in management and politics bring benefits to those who embody these norms of progress and purposive action. Managers and politicians therefore imitate practices that seem to have produced progress and success in other organizations or systems (DiMaggio and Powell, 1983). Policymakers are especially likely to endorse new ideas and programs when these innovations are promoted by policy entrepreneurs or have already been adopted by prestigious organizations or governments.

Despite their divergent content, policy fashions typically pass through four main life-cycle stages:

- Fashion setting
- Policy formulation
- Implementation
- Decline and search for alternative policies.

Let us briefly examine how developments in each life-cycle stage contribute to the distinctive path followed by policy fashions. Figure 8.1 presents the main stages in the fashion life cycle and interactions among them. Forces leading to policy decline are represented in the figure as negative feedback flowing from the implementation stage.

Policy fashions originally develop and circulate through a *fashion-setting* process that is initiated by policy entrepreneurs. Influential academics, consultants, policy analysts, stakeholder representatives, and non-governmental agencies such as foundations, fill this entrepreneurial function when they promote new – or newly discovered – ideas and practices. They publicize these new views

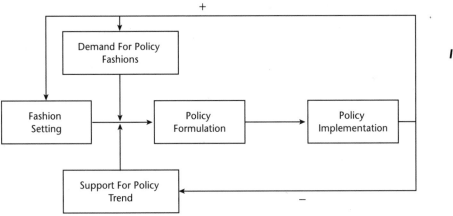

Figure 8.1 *Dynamics of policy fashions*

and techniques through specialty publications, consultations, and the mass media. Early adopters of new ideas and programs, including foreign governments and non-governmental organizations, also contribute to fashion setting when they serve as exemplars of a new policy trend. Policy entrepreneurs and the mass media frequently attribute much of the success of these early adopters to their use of newly fashionable techniques or policies.

As described in Chapter 1, Professor Alain Enthoven of Stanford University in California acted as one of the most prominent promoters of market reform of health systems. He urged European policymakers to learn from the example set by America's new system of competing health maintenance organizations. Professor Enthoven and other American advocates of managed competition consulted directly to governmental agencies and policy groups in the UK, Sweden, and the Netherlands. Their ideas were endorsed and diffused by local policy analysts in all three countries, along with other consultants from abroad. Advocates of the broader New Public Management movement in English speaking countries and parts of Europe, including many for-profit consultants, (Saint-Martin, 1998), played a complimentary role in legitimating and spreading neo-liberal solutions for public service reform. As in many instances of a new policy fashion, the early advocates of market reform and more broadly of the New Public Management, defined their proposals as innovative and progressive – not as a return to 'old-fashioned' market or management principles. The credibility of the proponents' claims were reinforced by popular stereotypes that view public bureaucracies as unadaptive and inefficient, while attributing the opposite tendencies to businesses. Although market reform in health increases the financial burden on lower income families and reduces equality of access to care, advocates of market solutions nonetheless presented them as if they provided rational and non-political techniques for financing and delivering health care (Evans, 1997). This presentation appealed to the popular belief that Western nations can and should search for technical, non-ideological solutions to challenges facing public administration and the social welfare system.

Initial discourse about market reforms was remarkably enthusiastic and uncritical. As such it closely resembled discourse about management fashions (Abrahamson and Fairchild, 1999, Birnbaum, 2000) and policy fashions outside of the health area (e.g., Czarniawska-Joerges, 1989).[14] Policy entrepreneurs, local adopters, and politicians supporting market reforms typically continued to use expansive rhetoric well into the policy formulation stage. Advocates of market reform envisioned great benefits from the new policies, such as enhancement of producer efficiency, empowerment of patients, and containment of growth in national health expenditures. However, these proponents of reform often gave vague and unrealistic explanations about *how* market forces would produce these desirable outcomes. Nor did reform advocates adequately acknowledge the probable costs and difficulties of implementing the proposed changes. The enthusiastic rhetoric about market reforms that prevailed during the fashion setting and formulation stages is well illustrated by formative policy documents like the UK's *Working for Patients* (Secretary of State for Health, 1989) and the report of Holland's Dekker Commission (Ministry of Welfare, Health, and Cultural Affairs, 1988c).

During the *policy formulation* stage, national and local advocates within government and related agencies urge development and governmental support for policies based on ideas and practices promoted by high-status fashion setters or previously adopted by high-status organizations or sectors. By promoting the new fashion, politicians, interest-group spokespersons, government officials, managers, and experts aim to resolve recurring dilemmas in public policy or cope with pressing issues – or at least appear to do so. By endorsing the new fashion, its supporters present themselves as progressive and rational. Moreover, by backing a new policy fashion and diffusing it, the supporters of the fashion build their personal reputations for being innovative and activist and identify their organization with these same values.[15] The organizational and normative forces just reviewed boost demand for many types of policy fashions, as shown by the uppermost box in Figure 8.1.

In addition, many forces shape demand for policy trends having a particular content or ideological thrust. For example, groups and individuals may expect adoption of a particular policy to enhance their political influence or provide access to valued resources. Other forces affecting support for substantive policy trends include changing political ideologies and values, social and cultural developments, electoral politics, interactions among policy actors, organizational and technical conditions, and past policy precedents and institutional commitments. These forces are depicted in the lowest box in Figure 8.1 but are not elaborated upon in the following discussion.

To facilitate adoption, experts and decisionmakers often propose borrowing techniques and ideas from one institutional area for use in another. Thus health reformers throughout Europe followed the American lead in adopting definitions and measures of organizational efficiency that came from manufacturing and commerce. As they import fashions from other countries or sectors, policymakers modify the policies and associated programs to fit local conditions. For instance, the Dekker Commission adopted the ideas of Enthoven and other Americans about insurer competition to fit the legal and institutional context of Dutch statutory health insurance.

To move ideas toward policy formulation and official approval, their backers must put the new ideas on the public agenda and build political coalitions in support of them. To get attention and appeal to diverse stakeholders, policy advocates often promise attainment of divergent and even conflicting policy outcomes. An early advocate of market experiments in Sweden described the process this way:

> We sold it [the buy-sell model] with different arguments: we told the doctors [that] there would be more autonomy for the hospitals and [that] the hospitals would get paid based on their performance [i.e., production volume]. We made the opposite appeal to the politicians: We said, 'you'll get control over the doctors'.

To gain support for new policies, their advocates also minimize discussion of probable costs and risks. Sometimes to avoid opposition or conflict among stakeholders, policy supporters deliberately provide only broad outlines of the new approach, leaving their substance to be worked out during implementation.

The types, breadth, and strength of coalitions needed to enact new policies vary greatly by issue, policy sector, and country. In Sweden and the Netherlands, political norms and institutions made support by multiple parties and interest groups necessary for market reform; reform stalled when these coalitions began to break up. In contrast, the electoral system in England and the cabinet's tight control over the NHS allowed the Conservative Party to enact sweeping structural changes without support from Labour and with only limited cooperation by other powerful health system actors.

Once new policies enter the *implementation* stage, struggles among affected stakeholders intensify. Participants in implementation discover internal contradictions within policies and conflicts between the policies and other widely held values. There are two reasons why struggles over policies intensify during implementation. First, many implications of the policies only become clear to stakeholders during implementation. For example, county politicians in Sweden did not anticipate the escalation of health expenditures that resulted from subjecting local hospitals to competition for productivity-linked reimbursements and expanding the Family Doctor system. Second, actors become involved in implementation who did not take part in the initial policy formulation process. These additional actors include officials and politicians in national government and many members of lower levels of government. Also included for the first time are managers and staff members in organizations responsible for implementing policies at the local or regional level. Non-participating stakeholders, such as recipients of services and local politicians, also become active during implementation. The newly involved actors often have very different orientations and interests than the people who originally formulated and enacted the policy. For instance, physicians in local hospitals, who were not consulted during formulation of market policies, were expected to implement programs that sometimes contradicted their values and interests. It is not surprising that many physicians resisted or reinterpreted these programs. In a similar fashion, when the purchaser-provider split was implemented in the UK, Health Authority managers were told to treat hospitals that they had formerly directly managed as if the hospitals were anonymous bidders for purchasing contracts. Naturally many of the new Health Authority managers balked at doing so and were reluctant to make changes that would put hospital staff out of work or disrupt local health services.

As implementation progresses, technical and organizational barriers also become more prominent. For instance, in all three nations studied here, governments, payers, and health managers encountered serious barriers to obtaining adequate data on the quality and efficiency of health providers. Yet this information was crucial to rational choice by payers and systematic efforts to improve provision of health care. No less fundamental to implementation were forces that limited the potential scope of competition among insurers or providers.

Sometimes, participants and policymakers learn to overcome or avoid technical barriers encountered during implementation. Dutch sickness funds, for example, quickly responded to market reforms by upgrading their management information systems and recruiting managers from the commercial insurance sector. County council politicians in Western Sweden decided not to link hospital payments directly to production, because this technique had produced rapid cost escalation in Stockholm.

More often growing implementation difficulties and widening conflict among stakeholders weaken support for new policies and programs. As experience with implementation accumulates, participants and policy analysts develop a more critical approach to the policy. They begin to discover many contingencies affecting attainment of policy objectives and recognize that more time and resources will be required for implementation than had previously been thought. The contrast between these unfolding realities of implementation and the rhetoric used to launch and enact new policies often leads to the policy's rapid undoing: documented policy benefits fall short of those promised, while implementation costs are greater. What is more, stakeholders gradually discover threats to their interests in policies that had previously seemed to offer benefits for all.

Policy *decline* begins with the spread of skepticism and even hostility to policies that previously enjoyed wide popularity. Previous supporters of the policy start to rethink the political and material costs of the policy or program and the risks of continuing to support them. As a result, the coalitions that supported the original formulation and adoption of the policy fashion grow weaker and more fragmented.

Even though the outcomes of implementation disappoint policymakers and other stakeholders, these outcomes can still have lasting implications for the systems and organizations affected by them. As was the case for the market reforms, even short-lived policies can shift power relations among key policy actors, alter actors' interpretations and discourse, and promote change in basic institutional arrangements. These transformations restructure the contexts in which future policies are developed and applied.[16]

As support for implemented policies dwindles, politicians, policy analysts, and other stakeholders seek other ways of solving their enduring problems. Sometimes policy actors revive programs and policy options that had been rejected in the past. To demonstrate that they have not lost the capacity for effective action, policy actors also look for newly fashionable ideas and proposals. These ideas can lead to new definitions of pressing problems and pursuit of new policy goals.

As policy actors absorb fashionable new ideas and proposals, they initiate another fashion cycle. Figure 8.1 depicts these processes as positive feedback from the implementation stage to Demand for Policy Fashions and the Fashion Setting stage. This hunt for new policy issues and solutions was evident in all the countries studied. For instance, as Swedish decisionmakers grew disillusioned with market reform, they turned to priority setting and regionalization to contain costs. They encouraged networking across health care settings to foster the kind of coordination that the hidden hand of the market had not sustained. At the same time, they discovered new policy concerns, like health quality, that had not been on the policy agenda when the market policies were first fashioned.

Policy fashion appears to be an unavoidable feature of contemporary political life. The fashion cycle brings the benefits of experimentation and the challenge of new ideas. However, fashion leads policymakers and users to neglect analysis of the feasibility and implications of new policies and programs. Nor does the policy fashion cycle provide much opportunity for learning and improvement of programs during implementation. Thus rapid adoption and abandonment of programs wastes resources, often leads to failure to achieve worthwhile policy objectives, burdens those responsible for implementation, and leaves them cynical about the prospects for meaningful system improvement.

CONCLUSION

This section begins with an assessment of the capacity of market reforms to revitalize health care systems. Then it presents a decentralized learning-focused approach to policy implementation. This approach should also help policymakers avoid some of the consequences of rapidly launching and abandoning policy fashions. Moreover, the principles of planned change proposed here provide an alternative to both quasi-market restructuring of health systems and highly centralized reforms, like some of those introduced in the UK by Prime Minister Blair.

Although the health market reforms of the late 1980s and early 1990s failed to deliver the results anticipated by their advocates, policy debate continues over the potential contribution of markets to renewing national health systems and other types of public services. The following comments illustrate the range of views:

There are two ways of reforming public services. Change can be ordered from above or it can be allowed to happen from below by giving consumers choice and freeing producers to respond to these choices... The big disadvantage of central control is that it stifles local initiative, preventing those delivering the services from responding to the demands of those they serve... Creating a market in public services, in effect – is difficult... but these difficulties have to be faced because introducing choice and competition into public services is the only way to improve them. ('Tougher than the Taliban' [editorial], *Economist*, November 24, 2001, p. 13).

Market forces may indeed have a prominent place in health care organization, but... economic theory does not show them to be necessarily a superior approach to health care policy (Rice, 1997, p. 423).

In this book I tried to contribute to this debate on the merits of quasi-market reform. Unlike the editors of the *Economist*, I do not see Western governments as facing an either or choice. Instead, they increasingly rely on a mix of market and regulatory mechanisms to promote health system change. Unlike many proponents of market reform (e.g., Enthoven, 1993) and some critics (e.g., Rice, 1997; Evans, 1997), I did not assess the merits of market mechanisms primarily on the basis of theoretical or normative arguments. Instead, I joined the researchers cited throughout the book who explored what *actually happened* when governments tried to create quasi-markets within national health systems. In this spirit, I examined in detail how pro-market policies evolved and market-driven changes were implemented in three European nations, all of which were leaders in market reform. I also asked what system changes could plausibly be attributed to the market reforms, rather than to parallel developments in health policy, technology, demography, and political economy.

There are evident risks in generalizing from the case studies reported here. The market reforms of the UK, Sweden, and the Netherlands diverged from one another and from those of other nations in policy objectives, substance, and implementation processes. Each country developed and implemented its reform policies within the framework of its unique national health system and its distinctive political institutions. In addition, in Sweden there were major variations among policies and practices among county councils, which form a middle level of government between the state and the municipalities.[17] The timing of the reforms further complicates cross-national comparisons and generalizations about market reform. In each country a distinctive mix of currents in politics, economy, and society came together during the reform period and shaped policy formulation, implementation, and outcomes. These rapidly changing currents are not likely to converge in the same way in the near future. Nor is it likely that social, political, and economic currents will come together in identical ways in other nations.

The case analyses nonetheless pointed to critical processes in implementation of quasi-markets in health. These processes are likely to shape market reform in most nations with strong social-democratic traditions and institutions. From an administrative perspective, the following processes are crucial:

- Specification of the nature of competition among providers, public purchasers, and publicly regulated insurers
- Creation of conditions supporting competition

- Gathering and disseminating information about the performance of providers and public payers
- Contracting with providers by public purchasers or insurers
- Decisionmaking and management control within payer and provider organizations
- Implementation by managers and health professionals of officially mandated changes in the volumes and nature of clinical practices.

From a bargaining perspective, the critical processes include moves by policy actors that influence policy formation and sustain, oppose, or redefine top-down policy directives and programmatic mandates. For example, bargaining among Dutch coalition partners and other stakeholders decisively shaped the formulation of regulated competition policies and reduced chances for radical reform. Resistance to bureaucratic monitoring of clinical quality by British hospital physicians and mergers among Dutch insurers blocked implementation of important features of government policies. From an interpretive standpoint, the most important processes concern the ways that actors at various levels define and act on pressures and constraints flowing from reform policies and programs. For example, in the Netherlands and the UK, and to a lesser degree in Sweden, hospital managers quickly adopted business and industrial concepts. The institutional perspective points to traditions, policy precedents, norms, and structures within health and political systems that shape crucial administrative, bargaining, and interpretive processes. For instance, Britain's GP fundholding program drew strength from the country's strong tradition of patient reliance on general practice.

As reviewed in the first part of this chapter, the case analyses uncovered powerful forces limiting the ability of health system actors to behave like rational actors in a health market. These included constraints on provider and insurer competition, professional and political opposition to service reconfigurations, legal entitlements to services, and limited capacities for assessing and managing the costs, productivity, and quality of health providers and insurers. It is very likely that these same forces will pose barriers to implementation of quasi-market systems in the health sectors of other countries, as well as in sectors like education and social welfare.

The case studies also pointed to important commonalities in the outcomes of market reforms. Some of these outcomes are quite similar to those found in other countries that have experimented with market reform.[18] Providers did respond to patient preferences and movement when these were tied directly to payments. More broadly, hospitals boosted efficiency and production in response to direct budgetary incentives, caps on expenditures, a new climate of cost awareness, and diffusion of industrial and business thinking into hospital management. On the other hand, hospital physicians responded very slowly, and with significant resistance, to market pressures and imposition of operational controls by managers or politicians.

In summary, the country studies reported in this book make a two-fold contribution to the debate about markets in public services: they help uncover the main processes affecting implementation of quasi-markets, and they point to probable impacts of this type of reform. These studies of leaders in market reform of health systems provide little room for optimism about the capacity of quasi-markets to reform public sector services: market reforms are very hard to implement in countries with strong social-democratic traditions. Moreover, competition in quasi-market reforms provides little or no help to countries seeking to contain total health costs. Nor do quasi-markets yield many of the other benefits envisioned by their champions.

Some analysts (e.g., Le Grand, 1999; Enthoven, 2000) argue that reforms like the ones examined in this book were a poor test of market solutions in health, because contracting and competition were highly constrained and information about performance by providers and payers was too limited. Under the circumstances neither payers nor providers experienced powerful market incentives for improvement. That argument has considerable empirical merit. However, it assumes that release of market forces would have desirable effects and would not produce less desirable ones (Light, 2000). Moreover, the argument that European governments didn't give markets a fair chance, incorrectly implies that governments in nations with institutionalized entitlements to universal, low-cost health care could indeed give market forces enough freedom to release powerful incentives. In fact, such action would be political suicide: replacing publicly controlled health systems by vigorous markets is likely to lead to escalating health costs, disruption of health services, unemployment, less equal access to care, and greater financial burdens on poorer and sicker citizens. In no nation with strong social democratic institutions and norms do voters knowingly endorse policies leading to these results.

Can health policymakers promote objectives like efficiency, enhancement of clinical quality, and responsiveness to patient concerns without foundering on the shoals of market restructuring or encountering barriers to highly centralized change, as some recent top-down reforms in the UK risk doing? It does indeed seem possible for policymakers to chart such a course. The following guidelines for a decentralized, learning-focused approach to implementing health system change derive from reflection on implementation of health system reforms and planned change in other types of systems and organizations (Harrison and Shirom, 1999).

Decentralize budgets and devolve authority to local or regional agencies and providers, while maintaining national health insurance and finance arrangements that assure universal coverage and solidarity.
Many governmental agencies and complex business operations successfully decentralize their operations. Effective decentralization allows for experimentation, learning, and adjustment to local conditions by sub-units, while still requiring attainment of centrally established performance targets.[19]

Enhance accountability and integration through valid and comprehensive management information systems. To decentralize successfully, managers of systems and organizations must develop and use information and control systems far more effectively than did officials and managers in the three health systems examined in this book. The countries studied here attempted to decentralize their hospital systems *before* they had developed adequate management information systems. Instead, national health system officials need to work closely with managers and providers at the regional and local levels to develop reporting systems that reflect the most important dimensions of service provision and finance. For example, Britain's Commission for Health Improvement has recently made substantial progress toward developing indicators that cover many important features of hospital quality and organization, which were previously neglected in performance assessments. In like manner, experts in the all three countries are developing clinical guidelines that will eventually provide a basis for reporting on clinical practices and evaluating their quality. Improvements in recording and reporting of hospital finance and management are also occurring. As such systems become operational, national or regional authorities (e.g., the county councils in Sweden) can appropriately delegate responsibility to local managers and health professionals and still continue to monitor the performance of these local actors.

Help health managers and professionals develop *independent* systems for gathering confidential data on clinical outcomes, medical errors, and gaps in quality of care and learning to improve quality.

Data on clinical practices can only enhance professional and organizational learning if data-gathering and reporting processes are nonpunitive and do not create threats of organizational sanctions or malpractice claims. For example, the Veteran's Association in the United States hired an independent agency to gather data and provide feedback to hospital staff on 'close-calls' – situations where an error almost occurred or an error did occur but was corrected *before* it led to a negative outcome (Bagian, 2001). This type of feedback gives practitioners opportunities to examine sources of problems and find ways to overcome them (Helmreich, 2000). In addition, local managers and practitioners should be encouraged to examine entire treatment chains and ways to improve links between hospitals and communities. Attention to these issues can be greatly facilitated by computer systems that allow for recording of activities and assessments by *all* of a patient's caregivers, in and out of hospital.[20]

While enforcing global budget ceilings, use targeted budget allocations and financial incentives to encourage productivity, responsiveness to clients, and coordination among units and organizations.

Budget ceilings helped hold down costs and foster hospital efficiency in all three countries studied here, as well in many other countries (OECD, 1992; Bishop et al., 1994). As the experiences of Sweden and the Netherlands show, targeted funding can reduce shortages of specific services. Similarly, redesign of reward systems can create incentives for providers to become more responsive to patients or provide particular services, such as the health promotion tasks specified in the UK's 1990 GP Contract.[21]

To facilitate policy implementation, allocate extra resources, allow sufficient time, and assign responsibilities for supporting and managing program implementation. Too often in the past, governments announced major changes and expected local managers and practitioners to implement them without training, guidance, or resources. Moreover, they expected changes to occur quickly. When one program did not yield demonstrable results, the governments quickly launched another. Experience with implementing planned change shows that successful organizational transitions can take years, require guidance by facilitators and change managers, and absorb considerable additional resources (Beckhard and Harris, 1977).

Carefully diagnose the needs for system change, plan programs, and assess their feasibility.[22] By diagnosing the root causes of system problems and assessing the feasibility of proposed programs, policymakers can plan and implement programs that genuinely fit system needs. Otherwise they risk introducing programs that are unlikely to solve problems and can even aggravate them. When possible, planners of complex change should consult with the people who will be responsible for implementing change and empower them to initiate new programs and fit existing ones to local needs. If deep resistance by some groups rules out cooperation of this sort, decisionmakers should at least obtain information about the concerns and practices of the groups on whom successful implementation depends and seek the most feasible ways of mobilizing their support or overcoming their resistance. By following this approach, policymakers and program planners are more likely to develop programs that are compatible with prevailing practices and orientations among user groups or contain incentives for users to change their practices. Rather than consulting extensively with users in advance, policymakers can sometimes facilitate implementation by allowing participants to 'reinvent' them to fit local conditions (Rogers, 1995, p. 177). Dutch officials successfully applied elements of this approach when they led medical specialty associations to develop and implement quality assessment standards and processes, in cooperation with insurers and representatives of patient associations.

Develop procedures for periodic assessment of implementation, so as to provide feedback to decisionmakers and guide reassessment of change targets and programs. Frequent follow-up and feedback during implementation help decisionmakers at all system levels adapt programs to unfolding realities of implementation. For instance, by observing events in Stockholm, officials in western Sweden were able to learn quickly that productivity-related payments to hospitals could lead to cost over-runs unless tight budget ceilings were enforced.

Application of these principles may produce less dramatic and fashionable policies and programs than the market reforms of the 1990s. Nonetheless, the more incremental and iterative approach sketched here seems likely to produce system benefits at lower cost and less risk to social solidarity and universal access than quasi-market restructuring. Moreover, the decentralized approach proposed here creates more opportunities than highly centralized reforms for local experimentation, organizational learning, and mobilization of health professionals on behalf of change. While investigating the policy issues discussed thus far, I also sought to advance research and theorizing about the implementation of public policies and their impacts on system change. To this end, I developed the model of public policy fashions presented above. I also created the analytic framework that combines current thinking about policy implementation into the administrative, bargaining, interpretive, and institutional frames. It is my hope that this framework helped illuminate the complexities of policy implementation and brought to light system changes that might not otherwise have been as evident.

Finally, what does this study imply about the current direction of health policy in the countries studied and others like them? Past experience suggests that there will be further waves of fashion in health finance and delivery, as in other areas of public policy and management. Many of these waves of reform leave imprints on the health system by altering administrative procedures and structures; shifting power relations; and redirecting behavior, beliefs, norms, and rhetoric.

Popular ideas about government administration and health care, along with the precedents of the last two decades, make it unlikely that governments in any of the countries studied will try to manage their health systems from the top as closely as they did before the market reforms. Instead, these countries are evolving a complicated mix of private and public systems, that use both market and conventional regulatory mechanisms. At the same time increasing numbers of citizens are becoming active consumers of health care. They will shop for the best available care and try to pay for it out of pocket or with supplementary insurance. Initiatives by these younger and more consumer-oriented patients, along with drives by private practitioners, insurers, entrepreneurs, and drug manufacturers may contribute to the further marketization of health care. Yet in all three countries, as in most industrial nations, the majority of the public want to sustain social solidarity and universal entitlements to a broad basket of services. Without moderation of the trend toward privatization of health finance and inequality in access to health services, the governments of countries with strong traditions of solidarity and universal access to care will fail to meet the expectations of their constituents. There are yet additional dangers to expanding quasi-markets in health and encouraging for-profit insurance and practice: These trends may threaten the clinical quality of care, create barriers to integrated care networks, and handicap promotion of individual wellness and public health.

NOTES

1 The term payer is used here to include public purchasers in the UK (Health Authorities and GP fundholders) and Sweden (purchasing boards in county councils) and statutory insurers in the Netherlands (sickness funds).

2 There was considerable irony in this choice of business models, since hospitals and some other health organizations contain many features in common with knowledge-based firms and companies that customize products and services to fit client needs. While health providers were busy trying to imitate practices from older, more bureaucratic businesses and industries, many for-profit firms were developing new management systems. These were based on expertise, interdisciplinary teams, and customization of production – much like the systems that prevail in modern hospitals.

3 Decentralization formed part of the market policies and occurred in conjunction with the introduction of quasi-markets. Nonetheless, it could have been achieved without introducing competition among providers and payers.

4 If decisionmakers raise this question in advance in relation to proposed change programs, they may assess whether they and other system actors have the political, managerial, organizational, financial, and technical capacities needed to sustain

program implementation. Implementation plans can then be modified to include steps toward developing critical capacities and dealing with likely implementation barriers and limitations (Harrison and Shirom, 1999). In practice, as shown in part three of this chapter, decisionmakers often decide on new policies and sweeping changes without much forethought and only later examine the feasibility and likely results of change programs.

5 Much of the research literature of relevance to this chapter is cited in Chapter 1.

6 The British government exercised less centralized control over the health systems of Scotland and Wales. As a result, those health systems introduced some variations in the internal market policies.

7 See Appleby et al. (1994) on the application of the concept of contestability to the internal market.

8 See Chapter 1, p. 4–5 and compare Table 1.3 and C.1 in Appendix C.

9 See Chapter 1, p. 19 on these types of control.

10 This definition may fit firms with standard products and services, but assessment of the efficiency of health services – like other human services – also requires attention to substantive features of the services and their quality (see Chapter 1 and Harrison and Shirom, 1999).

11 The British government boosted total health budgets during the market reforms but continued trying to curtail hospital expenditures.

12 Enthoven (1993), suggests that, in addition to government, employers or purchasing cooperatives, which represent large groups of consumers, can act as sponsors. Sponsors contract with health maintenance organizations, manage enrollment, and assure freedom of choice and movement among insurers.

13 My analysis builds on Abrahamson's (1996; Abrahamson and Fairchild, 1999) important research on fashion setting and demand for fashionable management techniques. To apply these ideas to the field of public policy, I focus on processes of formation and adoption of policy fashions, including agenda setting and coalition building, which are not as relevant to management fashions. Another difference from Abrahamson, is that I examine closely how implementation of fashionable policies leads to disaffection with them. Furthermore, I examine political forces that encourage decisionmakers to search for new fashions, as well as the normative and rhetorical ones discussed by Abrahamson.

14 In contrast, Mossberger (2000) provides an illustration of critical and informed decisionmaking in the early stages of policy adoption at the state level.

15 Staw and Epstein (2000) document analogous outcomes for organizations adopting fashionable managerial techniques.

16 In a similar fashion, Cole (1999) shows how adoption of successive mini-fads in manufacturing quality gradually led to fundamental transformations of the ways that American firms understand and deal with quality.

17 Mid-level variations also play a major role in health policy in other nations, including Germany, Canada, and the United States.

18 See, for example, Light (2000); Saltman and Figueras (1997), and the references in Chapter 1.

19 Structures and processes supporting effective decentralization are widely treated in the literature on management (e.g., Daft, 1995; Mintzberg, 1979).

20 See Chapter 5, p. 120.

21 Like the NHS, American health plans are now experimenting in using financial incentives to encourage physicians to provide preventive care and effective disease measurement (Greene, 2002). Some employers and public purchasers in the United States now use purchasing to reward quality measurement and assurance (Lee et al., 1999). Systematic evaluations of programs may point to procedures that can be adapted to other health systems.

22 Many approaches and techniques for diagnosing and assessing complex organizations can be applied to systems like health care (Harrison and Shirom, 1999).

Appendix A: Abbreviations

AWBZ	Exceptional Medical Expenses Act (6–7)
BMA	British Medical Association (2–3)
CC	County Council (4–5)
CHI	Commission for Health Improvement
DOH	Department of Health (2–3)
DRG	diagnosis related group (4–7)
FCE	finished consultant episode (2–3)
Federation of CCs	Federation of Swedish County Councils (4–5)
GDP	gross domestic product (1–7)
GP	general practitioner (2–7)
GPFH	general practitioner fundholder (2–3)
HA	health authority (2–3)
HMO	health maintenance organization (1)
Int./Ints.	Interview/s (1–8)
LOS	length of stay (1–8)
LSV	National Association of Medical Specialists (7)
NHS	National Health Service (1–3)
OECD	Organization for Economic Cooperation and Development (1–8)
PCG	Primary Care Group (3)
PCT	Primary Care Trust
PPP	Purchasing Power Parity (1–8)
SMA	Swedish Medical Association (4–5)
WHO	World Health Authority (1–8)

The numbers in brackets refer to the chapters to which the abbreviation is relevant.

Appendix B: Research Methods

Interviews

I conducted all the interviews face to face, except for three phone interviews. A small group of interviews took place in 1994, while most were conducted in 1996 and 1997. All interviews were held in English, except for one in Swedish, where a translator was used. The interviews usually took place in the respondent's office or in a meeting room and typically lasted from 45 minutes to an hour. Following conventional fieldwork procedures, I made notes during the interviews (usually totaling five or more pages), edited them subsequently, and then analyzed them.

I used an interview guide tailored to the person's role and organizational affiliation. The questions focused on the nature of recent reforms, mandated changes in regulations and work arrangements, implementation within the organization where the person worked, developments at other levels about which he or she was knowledgeable, and effects of reforms on physicians and other health professionals. I also encouraged the people interviewed to raise other issues that they thought would help me understand recent developments.

Except where paraphrased, statements from the interviews appear in the text of this book as recorded during the interview. Occasionally I have added or changed a word or two to render the statements more idiomatic. Any changes or additions that might affect the original meaning are enclosed in square brackets. I cite an anonymous interview as a source (e.g., 'Int.') when the interview provides the chief source of support for a statement in the text. The plural, 'Ints.' shows that two or more interviews support a statement.

The interviews are not cited as sources on topics about which there was widespread knowledge and agreement (e.g., the contents of a government proposal for reform). Unattributed quotations are from interviews except for jargon and terms that were in wide usage, such as 'value for money' (UK) and 'buy-sell system' (Sweden). Such terms are only enclosed in quotations when first used. Where it is appropriate to refer to specific interviews or organizations, I provide fictitious names and initials. There are occasional bibliographic references to people who made 'on the record' statements as experts or spokespersons.

Documentary materials included many unpublished materials and local press coverage, some of which were translated from the original language. These documents were suggested by people interviewed, by colleagues in each country, and located through library and web searches. In addition, I examined national statistical data on the country's health services, along with the data published by the OECD (2001, 2002).

207

Validity

Many opportunities arose for triangulation among interviews, documents, and statistics (Jick, 1979), which helped compensate for some of the limitations in the three types of data. In addition I was often able to check for consistency and plausibility through comparisons within data types and within individual sources of data (e.g., a single statistical report or a single interview).

I checked the validity of my country analyses by soliciting comments from local experts on the chapters in my earlier monograph (Harrison, 1995a) and in this book. Collaboration with local scholars (Harrison and Calltorp, 2000; Harrison and Lieverdink, 2000) also contributed to the validity of my findings and interpretations. I also received helpful feedback and suggestions from many local scholars, all of whom are listed in the references, footnotes, or Preface.

Appendix C: Health Expenditures, Resources, and Utilization, 1998[1]

	U.K.	Sweden	Netherlands	OECD[2]	USA
Expenditures					
Total as % GDP	6.8	7.9	8.1	7.8	12.9
Per capita in $, PPP[3]	1527	1748	2172	1835	4178
Resources					
Practicing physicians/1000	1.8	3.1	2.9	2.7	2.7
Acute beds/ 1000 (2000)	3.3	2.4	3.5	4.3	3.0
Utilization					
Acute, in-patient admissions/ yr./1000[4]	214	159	98.8	115.2	117.8
Physician consultations per capita[5] (1996)	6.1	2.9	5.4	5.8	6.6
Avg. length of stay, acute hospitals (1999)	6	5.0	9.5	7.1	5.9

1 1998 was the last year for which data were available for all countries, unless otherwise noted. Source: OECD (2001, 2002).

2 The number of countries on which the OECD averages are based varies from 14 through to 30.

3 Purchasing power parities, see Chapter 1, footnote 24.

4 Includes day patients in UK (1996); data for Sweden are from 1996.

5 Ambulatory visits; excludes private visits for UK, excludes maternal and child care for Sweden and Netherlands.

References

Abbott, A. (1988) *The system of professions: An essay on the division of expert labor.* Chicago: University of Chicago Press.

Abel-Smith, B. (1992) 'Cost containment and new priorities in the European Community', *Milbank Quarterly*, 70: 393–422.

Abrahamson, E. (1996) 'Management fashion', *Academy of Management Review*, 21: 254–85.

Abrahamson, E. and Fairchild, G. (1999) 'Management fashion: Lifecycles, triggers, and collective learning processes', *Administrative Science Quarterly*, 44 (4): 653–863.

Alford, R. (1975) *Health care politics: Ideological and interest group barriers to reform.* Chicago: University of Chicago Press.

Allsop, J. (1998) *Identity maintenance in conditions of change: The medical profession in the UK in the late 20th century.* Paper presented at a Conference on Professional Identities in Transition. International Sociological Association Working Group 2, Gothenburg, Sweden, April 1998.

Altenstetter, C. and Haywood, S.C. (1991) 'Introduction', in C. Altenstetter and S. Haywood (eds.) *Comparative health policy and the new right: From rhetoric to reality.* New York: St. Martin's Press. pp. 1–22.

Andersen, R., Smedby, B. and Vågerö, D. (2001) 'Cost containment, solidarity, and cautious experimentation: Swedish dilemmas', *Social Science and Medicine*, 52: 1195–1204.

Anderson, G. and Hussey, P. (2001) 'Comparing health system performance in OECD countries', *Health Affairs*, 20 (3): 219–232.

Andersson, G. and Karlberg, I. (2000) 'Integrated care for the elderly: The background and effects of the reform of Swedish care of the elderly', *International Journal of Integrated Care*, 1. Retrieved from www.ijic.org.

Anell, A. (1995) 'Implementing planned markets in health services: The Swedish case', in R. Saltman and C. Von Otter (eds) *Implementing planned markets in health care: Balancing social and economic responsibility.* Buckingham: Open University Press. pp. 209–236.

Anell, A. and Jendteg, S. (1993) 'Free choices in health care – what effects will they have'. *IHE Information*, No. 1, 1–3. Swedish Institute for Health Economics.

Anell, A., Rosen, P. and Hjortsberg, C. (1997) 'Choice and participation in the health services: A survey of preferences among Swedish residents', *Health Policy*, 40: 157–168.

Anell, A. and Svarvar, P. (1999) 'Health care reforms and cost containment in Sweden', in E. Mossialos and J. Le Grand (eds) *Health care and cost containment in the European Union.* Aldersoot, UK: Ashgate. pp. 701–731.

Appleby, J. (1995, 21 September) 'Managers in the ascendancy', *Health Service Journal*, 105: 32–33.

Appleby, J. (1999a) 'Government funding of the UK National Health Service: What does the national record reveal?' *Journal of Health Service Research Policy*, 4: 79–89.

Appleby, J. (1999b) 'The modernisation fund', in J. Appleby and A. Harrison (eds) *Health Care UK*. London: King's Fund. pp. 152–158.

Appleby, J. and Coote, A. (eds) (2002) 'Introduction', *Five-year health check: A review of health policy, 1997–2002*. London: King's Fund. Retrieved from http://194.66.253.160/eKingsFund/assets/applets/FiveYearHealthCheckIntro.pdf

Appleby, J., Smith, P., Ranade, W. and Little, V. (1994) 'Monitoring managed competition', in R. Robinson and J. Le Grand (eds) *Evaluating the NHS reforms*. London: King's Fund Institute. pp. 24–53.

Ashburner, L. Cairncross, L. (1993) 'Membership of the "new style" health authorities: Continuity or change', *Public Administration*, 71: 357–375.

Association of British Insurers (2000) *The private medical insurance market*. Retrieved from www.abi.org.uk

Association of British Insurers (2002) *The UK insurance industry – key facts*. Retrieved from http://www.abi.org.uk

Astley, W. and Zammuto, R. (1992) 'Organization science, managers, and language games', *Organization Science*, 3: 443–460.

Audit Commission (1995) *The doctors' tale: The work of hospital doctors in England and Wales*. London: HMSO (Her Majesty's Stationery Office).

Audit Commission (1996a) *The doctors' tale continued – the audits of hospital medical staffing*. London: HMSO.

Audit Commission (1996b) *What the doctor ordered: A study of fundholding in England and Wales*. London: HMSO.

Baakman, N., van der Made, J. and Mur-Veeman, I. (1989) 'Controlling Dutch health care', in G. Freddi and J. W. Bjorkman (eds) *Controlling medical professionals: The comparative politics of health governance*. London: Sage. pp. 99–115.

Baeza, J. and Calnan, M. (1997) 'Implementing quality: A study of the adoption and implementation of quality standards in the contracting process in a general practitioner multifund', *Journal of Health Service Research Policy*, 2: 206–211.

Bagian, J. (2001, October) 'Promoting patient safety at VA: Learning from close calls'. *Forum* [Veterans Association Office of Research and Development in conjunction with Academy for Health Services Research and Health Policy], 1–2: 8.

Banta, D. (2000/01, Winter) 'Quality of healthcare in Europe: An introduction', *Eurohealth*, 6: 18–19.

Barrett, S. and Fudge, C. (1981) *Policy and action: Essays on the implementation of public policy*. London: Methuen.

Bartlett, W. and Le Grand, J. (1994) 'The performance of trusts', in R. Robinson and J. Le Grand (eds) *Evaluating the NHS reforms*. London: King's Fund. pp. 54–73.

Bartlett, W., Roberts, J. and Le Grand, J. (1998a) 'The development of quasi-markets in the 1990s', in W. Bartlett, J. Roberts and J. Le Grand (eds) *A revolution in social policy: Quasi-market reforms in the 1990s*. Bristol: Policy Press. pp. 1–16.

Bartlett, W., Roberts, J. and Le Grand, J. (1998b) *A revolution in social policy: Quasi-market reforms in the 1990s*. Bristol, UK.

Becher, E. and Chassin, Mark. (2001) 'Improving the quality of health care: Who will lead?', *Health Affairs*, 20 (5): 164–179.

Beckhard, R. and Harris, R. (1977) *Organizational transitions: Managing complex change*. Reading, MA: Addison-Wesley.

Beecham, L. (1998a) 'GPs are angry over pay for primary care groups', *British Medical Journal*, 317: 1104.

Beecham, L. (1998b) 'GPs have continuing concern over primary care groups', *British Medical Journal*, 316: 1477.

Beecham, L. (1999a) 'NHS Direct will cover England by end of 2000', *British Medical Journal*, 318: 1097.

Beecham, L. (1999b) 'NHS doctors in England face audit and annual appraisals', *British Medical Journal*, 319: 1319.

Beecham, L. (1999c) 'Primary care trusts will have wide powers', *British Medical Journal*, 318: 555.

Bennett, C. and Ferlie, E. (1996) 'Contracting in theory and in practice: Some evidence **211** from the NHS', *Public Administration*, 74: 49–66.

Berg, M. (1996) 'Problems and promises of the protocol', *Social Science and Medicine*, 44: 1081–1088.

Berger, P. and Luckman, T. (1967) *The social construction of reality.* Garden City, NY: Doubleday.

Bergman, S.-E. (1993) 'Purchaser-provider systems in Sweden'. Paper presented to the Scottish Comparative Study Tour. September 1, Gavle, Sweden.

Bergman, S.-E. (1997) 'Swedish models of health care reform: A review and assessment', *International Journal of Health Planning and Management*, 13: 91–106.

Bergman, S.-E. (1999) Personal communication.

Bergman, S.-E. (2002, 22 November) Personal communication reporting findings from unpublished survey of payment systems in county councils.

Bergman, S.-E. and Dahlbäck, U. (1995) *Att beställa Häslo-och sjukvård erfarenheter från landsting med beställarstyrning* [Commissioning health care: Experiences from county councils with commissioner steering]. Trosa: Landstingsförbundet.

Birnbaum, R. (2000) *Management fads in higher education: Where they come from, what they do, why they fail.* San Francisco: Jossey-Bass.

Bishop, C., Wallack, S., Cohen, A., Hendricks, A., Tompkins, C., Skwara, K. et al. (1994) *Evaluation of global budgeting strategies* (June 1994) (Final Report under Health Care Financing Administration Contract No. 500-92-0020). Waltham, MA: The Collaborative for Health Care Financing Research.

Bjorkman, J.W. and Okma, K.G. (1997) 'Restructuring health care systems in the Netherlands: The institutional heritage of Dutch health policy reforms', in C. Altenstetter and J.W. Bjorkman (eds) *Health policy reform, national variations and globalization.* London: Macmillan. pp. 79–108.

Blaauwbroek, H.G. (1997) 'Patient organizations and patients' rights', in A. Schrijvers and L.D. Kodner (eds) *Health and health care in the Netherlands.* Utrecht: De Tijdstroom. pp. 223–237.

Blomqvist, A. G. (1992) 'The Swedish health care system', – an economist's view. *Health Policy*, 21: 113–128.

'BMA favors mergers as best way forward' (1997, 30 October) *Health Service Journal*: 9.

Bolman, L. and Deal, T. (1991) *Reframing organizations: Artistry, choice, and leadership.* San Francisco: Jossey-Bass.

Boot, J.M. (1997) 'Hospital planning', in A. Schrijvers and L. Kodner (eds) *Health and health care in the Netherlands.* Utrecht: De Tijdstroom, pp. 171–177.

Bordieu, P. (1989) 'Social space and symbolic power', *Sociological Theory*, 7: 14–25.

Borgert, L. (1993) 'The model is a process: A case of management rhetoric in Swedish health care'. Paper presented at the European Group for Organizational Studies. Paris, July 6–8.

Borgert, L. (1994, August 3) Personal communication.

Borst-Eilers, E. (1997) 'Health policy in the Netherlands: A balance between containment and expansion', in A. Schrijvers and L.D. Kodner (eds) *Health and health care in the Netherlands.* Utrecht: De Tijdstroom. pp. 15–19.

Boyce, J. and Lamont, T. (1998) 'The new health authorities: Moving forward, moving back?', *British Medical Journal*, 316: 215.

Brazier, M., Lovecy, J., Moran, M. and Potton, M. (1993) 'Falling from a tightrope: Doctors and lawyers between the market and the state', *Political Studies*, 61: 197–213.

Broadbent, J. (1998) 'Practice nurses and effects of the new general practitioner contract in the British NHS: The advent of a professional project?', *Social Science and Medicine*, 4: 497–506.

Brommels, M. (1997) Personal communication.

Brouwer, W. and Schut., F.T. (1999) 'Priority care for employees: A blessing in disguise?', *Health Economics*, 8: 65–73.

Brown, D. (1995, May 15) 'Republican budget proposals put cost-cutting initiatives at risk: House panel would kill agency that compares medical treatments', *Washington Post*, p. A17.

Brown, L. and Amelung, V. (1999) '"Manacled competition": Market reforms in German health care', *Health Affairs*, 18 (1): 76–91.

Bruce, A. and Jönsson, E. (1996) *Competition in the provision of health care – the experience of the United States, Sweden and Britain*. Brookfield, VT: Ashgate.

Buckland, R.W. (1994) 'Healthcare resource groups', *British Medical Journal*, 308: 1056.

Burke, K. (2001) 'GMC chief retires as council votes for revalidation', *British Medical Journal*, 322: 1323.

Burström, B. (2002) 'Increasing income inequalities in health care utilisation across income groups in Sweden during the 1990s?', *Health Policy*, 62: 117–129.

Butler, J. (1994) 'Origins and early development', in R. Robinson and J. Le Grand (eds) *Evaluating the NHS reforms*. London: King's Fund. pp. 13–23.

Butler, P. (1994, December 15) 'Hospitals' fate could rest on "popularity with the public"', *Health Service Journal*, p. 4.

Butler, P. (1995, April 20) 'Give GPs buying power, says BMA', *Health Service Journal*, 20: 4.

Butler, P. (1995, December 7) 'Audit commission slates standards of care in A&E', *Health Service Journal*, p. 3.

Butler, P. (1996, January 4) 'New-look HAs get familiar old faces', *Health Service Journal*, p. 3.

Butler, P. (1996, May 12) 'Against the grain', *Health Science Journal*, p. 12.

Butler, P. (1997, June 12) 'Private investigations', *Health Service Journal*, 107: 20.

Cabiedes, L. and Guillen, A. (2001) 'Adopting and adapting managed competition: Health care reform in Southern Europe', *Social Science and Medicine*, 52: 1205–1217.

Calhoun, E. and Joyce, B. (1998) '"Inside-out" and "outside-in": Learning from past and present school improvement paradigms', in A. Hargreaves, A. Lieberman, M. Fullan and D. Hopkins (eds) *International handbook of educational change*. Dordrecht, Netherlands: Kluwer. pp. 1286–1298.

Calltrop J. (1993) *Management development for doctors*. Position paper from Sweden for European Health Care Management Association.

Calltorp, J. (1995) 'Swedish experience with fixed regional budgets', in F. Schwartz, H. Glennerster and R. Saltman (eds) *Fixing health budgets: Experience from Europe and North America*. Chichester, England: John Wiley and Sons Ltd. pp. 155–164.

Calltorp, J. (1999a) 'Market forces project – report from Sweden'. Draft submitted to European Health Management Association project for European Commission Contract No. SOC 98201309 05FI (98 PRVF 1-001-0), Stockholm, March 28.

Calltorp, J. (1999b) *Strukturförändringar tro och vetande* [Structural changes – Belief and Knowledge]. Paper presented to the Swedish Federation of County Councils, Stockholm, March.

Calnan, M., Halik, J. and Sabbat, J. (1998) 'Citizen participation and patient choice in health reform', in R. Saltman, J. Figueras and C. Sakellarides (eds), *Critical challenges for health care reform in Europe*. Buckingham: Open University press. pp. 325–338.

Calnan, M. and Williams, S. (1995) 'Challenges to professional autonomy in the United Kingdom? The perceptions of general practitioners', *International Journal of Health Services*, 25: 219–241.

'Care review on the way' (1997, 24 October) *Faxed from Sweden*. Stockholm, Swedish Institute.

Case C-157/99, No. Case C-157/99 (European Court 12 July, 2001).

Cauthen, N. & Amenta, E. (1996) 'Not for widows only: Institutional politics and the formative years of Aid to Dependent Children', *American Sociological Review*, 61: 427–448.

Cervi, B. (1996, March 21) 'DOH has failed to monitor audit, admits Langland', *Health Service Journal*, p. 7.

Chadda, D. (1993, October 21) 'Mac for life', *Health Service Journal*, pp. 12–13.

Chadda, D. (1997, January 23) 'Crisis point as emergency admissions go on soaring', *Health Service Journal*, 107: 3.

Chadda, D. (1998, July 2) 'BMA backs calls to close A&Es', *Health Service Journal*, p. 8.

Chadda, D. (1998) 'Future of Guy's Hospital finalised', *British Medical Journal*, 317: 702.

Chadda, D. and Crail, M. (1996, December 5) 'Labour proposes GP-led "mini-Has."', *Health Service Journal*, 106: 3.

Charpentier, C. and Samuelson, L.A. (1996) 'Effects of new control systems in Swedish health care organizations', *Financial Accountability and Management*, 12 (2): 157–171.

Chia, R. (1995) 'From modern to postmodern organizational analysis', *Organization Studies*, 16: 579–603.

Clarke, A., Mckee, M., Appleby, J. and Sheldon, T. (1993) 'Efficient purchasing', *British Medical Journal*, 307: 1436–37.

Cohen, M. D., March, J. and Olsen, J. (1972) 'A garbage can model of organizational choice', *Administrative Science Quarterly*, 17: 1–25.

Cole, A. (1995, February 16) 'Mixed blessings', *Health Service Journal*, p. 18.

Cole, R. (1999) *Managing quality fads: How American business learned to play the quality game*. New York: Oxford.

Commission for Health Improvement (2001a) *Holding a mirror up to ourselves: CHI's combined annual report and accounts, 2000–2001*. Retrieved from London: CHI: http://www.chi.nhs.uk/eng/about/chi_annual_report_00-01.pdf

Commission for Health Improvement (2001b) *Corporate plan, 2001–2004*. Retrieved from London: CHI: http://www.chi.nhs.uk/eng/about/corporate_plan.pdf

Committee on Quality of Health Care in America – Institute of Medicine (2001) *Crossing the quality chasm*. Washington, D.C.: National Academy Press.

Common, R. (1998) 'Convergence and transfer: A review of the globalisation of new public management', *International Journal of Public Sector Management*, 11 (6): 440–450.

Coulter, A. (1998) 'Managing demand at the interface between primary and secondary care', *British Medical Journal*, 316: 1974–1976.

Coulter, A. and Mays, N. (1997) 'Primary care: Opportunities and threats: Delegating primary care', *British Medical Journal*, 314: 506.

Court of Justice of the European Community (2001, July 12) Case C-157/99 B.S.M. Geraets-Smits v Stichting Ziekenfonds VGZ and H.T.M. Peerbooms v. Stichting CZ Groep Zorgverzekeringen. Retrieved from http://www.curia.eu.int/en/act/0120en.htm.

Crail, M. (1994, December 1) 'It's not always fair weather' [Budget Special], *Health Service Journal*, p. 6.

Crail, M. (1995, January 19) 'How far can you go?', *Health Service Journal*, p. 16.

Crail, M. (1997, March 13) 'Office politics', *Health Service Journal*, p. 13.

Crail, M. (1998, October 15) Crossing the flaw – report on The Health of a Nation – a policy assessed, *Health Service Journal*, pp. 14–15.

'Crisis in welfare care for elderly creates headache for politicians' (1997, November 11). *Faxed from Sweden* (Stockholm: Swedish Institute), No. 38, p. 2.

Cross, M. (1998, March 12) 'Read all about it', *Health Service Journal*, p. 9.

'Crumbs from Blair's table' (1999, June 12) *Economist*, pp. 38–39.

Culyer, A., Evans, R.G., Graf van der Schulenburg, M.J., van de Ven, W.P. and Weisbrod, B.A. (1991, November) *International review of the Swedish health care system* (34) Occasional paper. Stockholm, Sweden: SNS.

Cumbers, B. and Donald., A. (1999, April 15) 'Evidence-based practice: Data day', *Health Service Journal*, pp. 30–31.

Czarniawska-Joerges, B. (1989) 'The wonderland of public administration reforms', *Organization Studies*, 10 (4): 531–548.

213

Daft, R. (1995) *Organization theory and design.* 5th ed. Minneapolis, MN: West.

Day, P. and Klein, R. (1989) 'The politics of modernization: Britain's national health service in the 1980s', *The Milbank Quarterly*, 67: 1–34.

de Folter, R. (1997) 'The services of medical specialists and hospitals', in A. Schrijvers and L. Kodner (eds) *Health and health care in the Netherlands.* Utrecht: De Tijdstroom. pp. 90–100.

de Melker, R.A. (1997) 'The family doctor', in A. Schrijvers and L. Kodner (eds) *Health and health care in the Netherlands.* Utrechet: De Tijdstroom. pp. 60–72.

de Roo, A. (1988) 'Netherlands', in R.B. Saltman (ed.) *The international handbook of health care systems.* New York: Greenwood Press. pp. 215–228.

de Roo, A. (1995) 'Contracting and solidarity: Market-oriented chances in Dutch health insurance schemes', in R. Saltman and C. von Otter (eds) *Implementing planned markets in health care.* Buckingham, UK: Open University Press. pp. 45–64.

de Roo, A. (1997a, May) 'Business rules', *European Health Reform*, 5: 6–7.

de Roo, A. (1997b, November 12) Email message, Nov 12, 1997 (Health-Israel Digest [email discussion group] VI #47).

de Roo, A. (1999, December) *Care for the elderly in Israel: A Dutch view.* Presentation to Workshop on Long-term care of the elderly, Tel Ha Shomer, Israel: Israel National Institute for Health Policy and Health Services Research.

de Roo, A. (2001, March 10) Personal communication.

de Roo, A. and Boonekamp, L. (1994) Some notes on the structure and dynamics of the Dutch health care market. Unpublished memorandum, Tilburg University.

de Roo, A. and Maarse, H. (1990) 'Understanding the central-local relationship in health care: A new approach', *International Journal of Health Planning and Management*, 5: 15–25.

Dean, M. (1997, August 23) 'Government starts to tackle inequalities in Britain', *The Lancet*, 350: 571.

Decker, D. (1995, January 19) 'Market testing – does it bring home the bacon?', *Health Service Journal*, pp. 26–28.

Dent, M. (1995) 'Doctors, peer review and quality assurance', in T. Johnson, G. Larkin, and Mike Saks (eds) *Health professions and the state in Europe.* London: Routledge. pp. 86–102.

Dent, M. (1998) *Clinical judgment and the role of protocols, guidelines and EBM: Britain, Netherlands and Sweden.* Paper presented at the 14th World Congress of Sociology, (International Sociological Association, Working Group 02).

Department of Health (1998) *The Health of the nation – a policy assessed.* London: HMSO.

Department of Health, Expert Advisory Group on Cancer (1995) *A Policy Framework for Commissioning Cancer Services* (Report to the Chief Medical Officers of England and Wales. Guidance for Purchasers and Providers of Cancer Services). London: HMSO.

Diderichsen, F. (1993) Why Sweden copied the NHS reforms. Health care and the common market. Proceedings of the 8th International Association for Health Policy (Europe) Conference.

Diderichsen, F. (1995) 'Market reforms in health care and sustainability of the welfare state', *Health Policy*, 32: 141–153.

DiMaggio, P. and Powell, W.W. (1983) 'The iron cage revisited: Institutional isomorphism and collective rationality in organizational fields', *American Sociological Review*, 48: 147–160.

Directorate-General for Health (1993) *Health care reform in the Netherlands – fact sheet* V-5-E. Rikswijk: Ministry of Welfare, Health and Cultural Affairs.

Dixon, J. (1997) 'Funding the NHS: A little local difficulty', *British Medical Journal*, 314: 216.

Dixon, J., Boyle, S. and Harrrison, A. (1996) 'Financial meltdown for the NHS?', *British Medical Journal*, 312: 1432–1433.

Dixon, J. and Dewar, S. (2000) 'The NHS plan: As good as it gets', *British Medical Journal*, 321: 315–316.

Dixon, J., Holland, P. and Mays, N. (1998) 'Developing primary care: Gatekeeping, commissioning and managed care', *British Medical Journal*, 317: 125–128.

Dixon, J., Inglis, S. and Klein, R. (1999) 'Is the English NHS underfunded?', *British Medical Journal*, 318: 522–526.

Dobson, F. (1999) 'Modernizing Britain's National Health Service', *Health Affairs*, 18 (3): 40–41.

Dohler, M. (1991) 'Policy networks, opportunity structures and neo-Conservative reform strategies in health policy', in B. Marin and R. Mayntz (eds) *Policy networks: Empirical evidence and theoretical considerations*. Boulder, Colorado: Westview Press. pp. 235–296.

Dopson, S., Locock, L. and Stewart, R. (1999) 'Regional offices in the new NHS: An analysis of the effects and significance of recent changes', *Public Administration*, 77: 91–110.

Dowding K. (1995) 'Model or metaphor? A critical review of the policy network approach', *Political Studies*, 43: 136–158.

Dowling, B. (1997) 'Effect of fundholding on waiting times: Database study', *British Medical Journal*, 315: 290–292.

Dowswell, G., Harrison, S. Wright, J. (2002) 'The early days of primary care groups: general practitioner perceptions', *Health and Social Care in the Community*, 10: 46–54.

Drummond, M., Cooke, J. and Walley, T. (1997) 'Economic evaluation under managed competition: Evidence from the UK', *Social Science and Medicine*, 45: 583–595.

Duffy, D. (1989) 'The effect of Sweden's corporatist structure on health policy and outcomes', *Scandinavian Studies*, 61: 128–145.

Dyer, C. (1995) 'Bristol doctors found guilty of serious misconduct', *British Medical Journal*, 316: 1924.

Dyer, C. (2001) 'Bristol inquiry: Bristol inquiry condemns hospital's club culture', *British Medical Journal*, 323: 181.

Dyke, R. (1998) *The new Patient's Charter: A different approach: Report on the new NHS charter*. London: Department of Health.

Eaton, L. (2002) 'Government proposes licensing system for doctors', *British Medical Journal*, 324: 1235.

Edelman, M. (1964) *The symbolic uses of politics*. Urbana: University of Illinois Press.

Edelman, M. (1988) *Constructing the political spectacle*. Chicago: University of Illinois Press.

Ellwood, P. (1972) 'Models for organizing health services and implications of legislative proposals', *Milbank Memorial Fund Quarterly*, 50 (part 2): 73–101.

Elmore, R. (1979–80) 'Backward mapping: Implementation research and policy decisions', *Political Science Quarterly*, 94: 601–616.

Elmore, R. and Sykes, G. (1992) 'Curriculum policy', in Phillip Jackson (ed.) *Handbook of research on curriculum*. New York: Macmillan. pp. 185–215.

Elsinga, E. (1989) 'Political decision-making in health care: The Dutch case'. *Health Policy*, 11: 243–255.

Enthoven, A. (1978) 'Consumer-choice health plan: A national health insurance proposal based on regulated competition in the private sector', *New England Journal of Medicine*, 298: 709–720.

Enthoven, A. (1985) *Reflections on the management of the National Health Service: An American looks at incentives to efficiency in health services management in the UK*. London: Nuffield Provincial Hospitals Trust.

Enthoven, A. (1993) 'The history and principles of managed competition', *Health Affairs*, 12 (supplement): 24–48.

Enthoven, A. (2000) 'In pursuit of an improving National Health Service', *Health Affairs*, 19 (3): 102–119.

Epsing-Andersen, G. (1994) 'Welfare states and the economy', in N. Smelser, and Richard Swedberg (eds) *Handbook of economic sociology* Princeton: Princeton University Press. pp. 711–732.

Ericson, T. Melin, L. (2000, August) *Strategic change in hospital organizations – the role of the actors' way of thinking.* Presented at annual meeting. Academy of Management.

Etzioni, A. (1975, September) 'Deinstituionalization: A public policy fashion', *Human Behavior,* 4: 12–13.

Evans, Robert (1997) 'Going for the gold: The redistributive agenda behind market-based health care reform', *Journal of Health Politics, Policy and Law,* 22 (2): 427–465.

Evans, Roger (1983).'Health care technology and the inevitability of resource allocation and rationing decisions', Part 1. *Journal of the American Medical Association,* 249: 2047–2053.

Expert Group (HSU 2000) (1994) Three models for health care reform in Sweden Report to the committee on funding and organization of health services and medical care. Sweden.

Fairfield, G., Hunter, D., Mechank, D., David, and Rosleff, F. (1997) 'Managed care: Origins, principles, and evolution', *British Medical Journal,* 314: 1823.

Farmer, A. (1993) 'The changing role of general practice in the British National Health Service', in D. Light and A. May (eds) *Britain's health system: From welfare state to managed care.* New York: Faulkner and Gray. pp. 57–66.

Feachem, R., Sekhri, N., and White, K. (2002) 'Getting more for their dollar: A comparison of the NHS with California's Kaiser Permanente', *British Medical Journal,* 321: 135–143.

Federation of Swedish County Councils (1990) *Some innovation projects at Swedish county councils.* Brochure. Stockholm: Author.

Federation of Swedish County Councils (1993) *Health care utilization and resources in Sweden, 1980–1992.* Stockholm: Author.

Federation of Swedish County Councils (2002) *Swedish health care in the 1990s: Trends 1992–2000.* Stockholm: Author.

Ferlie, E., Pettigrew, A., Ashburner, L., and Fitzgerald, L. (1996) *The new public management in action.* Oxford: Oxford University Press.

Ferriman, A. (2000) 'Health spending in UK to rise to 7.6% of GDP', *British Medical Journal,* 320: 889.

Fisher, P. (1999) 'The reform of the British National Health Service', *Journal of Public Health Policy,* 20: 138–148.

Fitzgerald, L. and Dufour, Y. (1997) 'Clinical management as boundary management: A comparative analysis of Canadian and UK health care institutions', *International Journal of Public Sector Management,* 10: 5–20.

Flynn, R. (1992) *Structures of control in health management* (J. Urry, ed.). London: Routledge.

Flynn, R. and Williams, G. (eds) (1997) *Contracting for health: Quasi-markets and the National Health Service.* Oxford: Oxford University Press.

Forsberg, E. and Calltorp, J. (1993) *Ekonomiska incitament och medicinskt handlande – Forsta året av Stockholmsmodellen* [Economic incentives and medical action – first year of the Stockholm model]. Fou-rapport 2, Samhallsmedicinska enheten. Huddinge, Sweden.

Forsberg, E. and Calltorp, J. (1994) *Nya styrformer, Forändrat medicinskt handlande – Attiyd och beteendeforandringar efter två år med Stockholmsmodellen* [New forms of steering, changed medical action – changes of attitudes and action after two years with the Stockholm model]. Stockholm, unpublished manuscript.

Fougere, G. (2001) 'Transforming health sectors: New logics of organizing in the New Zealand health system', *Social Science and Medicine,* 52: 1233–1242.

Francome, C. and Marks, D. (1996) *Improving the health of the nation – The failure of the government's health reforms.* London: Middlesex University Press.

Freeman, T., Latham, L., Walshe, K., Spurgeon, P. and Wallace, L. (1999) *The early development of clinical governance: A survey of NHS trusts in the South West Region.* Birmingham: Health Services Management Centre.

216

Freidson, E. (1985) 'The reorganization of the medical profession', *Medical Care Review*, 42: 11–35.

'From Bedlam to bedsit' (1995, September 2) *The Economist*, pp. 31–32.

Gaffney, D., Pollock, A., Price, D. and Shaoul, J. (1999a) 'NHS capital expenditure and the private finance initiative – expansion or contraction', *British Medical Journal*, 319: 48–51.

Gaffney, D., Pollock, A., Price, D. and Shaoul, J. (1999b) 'PFI in the NHS – is there an economic case?', *British Medical Journal*, 319: 116–118.

Gaffney, D., Pollock, A., Price, D. and Shaoul, J. (1999c) 'The politics of the private finance initiative and the new NHS', *British Medical Journal*, 319: 249–253.

Gamson, W. (1989) 'Media discourse and public opinion on nuclear power: A constructionist approach', *American Journal of Sociology*, 95: 1–37.

Gamson, W. and Lasch, K. (1983) 'The political culture of social welfare policy', in S. Spiro and E. Yaar-Yuchtman (eds) *Evaluating the welfare state: Social and political.* New York: Academic Press.

Garpenby, P. (1995) 'Health care reform in Sweden in the 1990s: Local pluralism versus national coordination', *Journal of Health Politics, Policy and Law*, 20 (3): 695–717.

Garpenby, P. (1997) 'Implementing quality programmes in three Swedish county councils: The views of politicians, managers, and doctors', *Health Policy*, 39: 195–206.

Garpenby, P. and Carlsson, P. (1994) 'The role of national quality registers in the Swedish health services', *Health Policy*, 29: 183–195.

Garside, P. (1999) 'Evidence based mergers?', *British Medical Journal*, 318 (7180): 345–346.

Gertham, U.-G. and Jonsson, B. (1994) 'Health care expenditure in the Nordic countries', *Health Policy*, 26: 207–220.

Giamo, S. and Manow, P. (1997) 'Institutions and ideas into politics: Health care reform in Britain and Germany', in C. Altenstetter and J.W. Bjorkman (eds) *Health Policy Reform, national variations and globalization.* London: Macmillan. pp. 175–202.

Gibson, J.W. and Tesone, D. (2001) 'Management fads: Emergence, evolution, and implications for managers', *Academy of Management Executive*, 15 (4): 122–133.

Gilley, J. (1999) 'Meeting the information and budgetary requirements of primary care groups', *British Medical Journal*, 318: 168–170.

Glaser, W. (1987) *Paying the hospital: The organization dynamics and effects of differing financial arrangements.* San Francisco: Jossey-Bass.

Glennerster, H., Matsaganis, M., Owens, P. and Hancock, S. (1994) 'GP Fundholding: Wild card or winning hand?', in R. Robinson and J. Le Grand (eds) *Evaluating the NHS reforms.* London: King's Fund Institute. pp. 74–107.

Godsen, T. and Torgerson, D. (1997) 'The effect of fundholding on prescribing and referral costs: A review of evidence', *Health Policy*, 40: 103–114.

Gold, M., Hurley, R., Lake, T., Ensor, T., Berenson, R. (1995) 'A national survey of the arrangements managed-care plans make with physicians', *New England Journal of Medicine*, 333: 1678–1683.

Goodwin, Neil (2000) 'Implementing PCGs: The implications for the NHS', *British Journal of Health Care Management*, 6: 316–319.

Goodwin, Neil (2000, May 15) Personal communication. email [CEO Greater Manchester Health Authority].

Goodwin, Nicholas (1998) 'GP fundholding', in J. Le Grand, N. Mays and J.-A. Mulligan (eds) *Learning from the NHS internal market: A review of the evidence.* London: King's Fund. pp. 43–68.

Goodwin, Nicholas, Mays, N., McLeod, H., Malboh, G., Rafterty Mays, N., Griffiths, J. and Posnett, J. (1998) 'Evaluation of total purchasing pilots in England and Scotland and implications for primary care groups in England: Personal interviews and analysis of routine data' *British Medical Journal*, 317: 256–259.

Goodwin, Nick (2000) 'The long term importance of English primary care groups for integration in primary health care and deinstitutionalisation of hospital care', *International Journal of Integrated Care*, 1 (1). Retrieved from http://roquade. library.uu.nl

Gould, M. (1998, November 19) 'Longer waits at three in four A&E departments compared to 1996', *Health Service Journal*, 108: 4–5.

Greene, J. (2002) 'Paying for performance', *Healthplan*, 43 (5): 4–18.

Gres, S., Groenewegen P.P., Kerssens, J., Braud, B. and Wasem, J. (2002) 'Free choice of sickness funds in regulated competition: Evidence from Germany and the Netherlands', *Health Policy*, 60: 235–254.

Grin, J. and van de Graaf, H. (1996) 'Implementation as communicative action – an interpretive understanding of interactions between policy actors and target groups', *Policy Sciences*, 29: 291–319.

Groenewegen, P.P. (1993) 'Primary health care in the Netherlands: From imperfect planning to an imperfect market?', in D.P. Chinitz and M.A. Cohen (eds) *The changing roles of government and the market in health care systems*. Jerusalem: JDC-Brookdale Institute of Gerontology and Human Development and State of Israel, The Ministry of Health. pp. 41–64.

Gross, R. and Harrison, M. (2001) 'Implementing managed competition in Israel', *Social Science and Medicine*, 52: 1219–1231.

Groves, T. (1997) 'Primary care: Opportunities and threats: What the changes mean', *British Journal of Medicine*, 314: 436–438.

Haas, P. (1992) 'Introduction: Epistemic communities and international policy coordination', *International Organization*, 46: 1–36.

Hafferty, F. and McKinley, J. (1993) *The changing character of the medical profession: An international perspective*. New York: Oxford University Press.

Håkansson, S. (1993) *New ways of financing and organizing health care in Sweden*. Paper presented at the 1993 European Healthcare Management Association annual conference, Warsaw.

Hall, R. (1968) 'Professionalism and bureaucratization', *American Sociological Review*, 33: 92–104.

Hall, R. (1991) *Organizations: Structures, processes, and outcomes*. Englewood Cliffs, NJ: Prentice Hall.

Halligan, A. and Donaldson, L. (2001) 'Implementing clinical governance: Turning vision into reality', *British Medical Journal*, 322: 1413–1417.

Ham, C. (1987) *Steering the oil tanker: Power and policy making in the Swedish health service*. London: King's Fund Institute.

Ham, C. (1992) *Health policy in Britain: The politics and organisation of the National Health service* (3rd ed.). London: Macmillan.

Ham, C. (1996) 'Population-centered and patient-focused purchasing: The UK experience', *Milbank Quarterly*, 74: 191–214.

Hamblin, R. (1998) 'Trusts', in J. Le Grand, N. Mays and J.A. Mulligan (eds) *Learning from the NHS internal market: A review of the evidence*. London: King's Fund. pp. 100–116.

Hanning, M. (1996) 'Maximum waiting-time guarantee – an attempt to reduce waiting lists in Sweden', *Health Policy*, 36: 17–35.

Hardy, B., Mur-Veeman, I., Steenbergen, M. and Wistow, G. (1999) 'Inter-agency services in England and the Netherlands: A comparative study of integrated care development and delivery', *Health Policy*, 48: 87–105.

Harris, C. and Scrivener, G. (1996) 'Fundholders' prescription costs: The first five years', *British Medical Journal*, 313: 1531–1534.

Harrison, A. (1998) 'National service frameworks', in R. Klein (ed.) *Implementing the white paper: Pitfalls and opportunities*. London: King's Fund. pp. 33–44.

Harrison, A. and New, B. (1996) 'Health Policy review', in A. Harrison (ed.) *Health care UK 1995/6*. London: King's Fund. pp. 1–99.

Harrison, A. and New, B. (1997) 'Health policy review', in A. Harrison (ed.) *Health care UK 1996/7*. London: King's Fund. pp. 1–122.

Harrison, M. (1994) 'Professional control as process: Beyond structural theories', *Human Relations*, 47: 1201–1231.

Harrison, M. (1995a) *Implementation of reform in the hospital sector: Physicians and health systems in four countries*. Tel Hashomer: Israel: Israel National Institute for Health Policy and Health Services Research.

Harrison, M. (1995b) 'Organizational rhetoric and collective action in a medical association', *Studies in Cultures, Organizations, and Societies*, 1: 209–230.

Harrison, M. (1999) 'Health professionals and the right to health care', in A. den Exter and H. Hermans (eds) *The right to health care in several European countries*. London: Klewer Law International. pp. 81–99.

Harrison, M. (2002) 'Professional autonomy under managed care: Physicians and health system reform in Germany and the Netherlands', in D. Chinitz (ed) *The changing face of health systems*. Jerusalem: Israel National Institute for Health Policy and Health Services Research and Gefen Publishing House. pp. 225–251.

Harrison, M. and Lieverdink, H. (2000) 'Controlling medical specialists: Hospital reform in the Netherlands', *Research in the Sociology of Health Care*, 17: 61–77.

Harrison, M. and Shalom, N. (2002) *Strategic changes in Israeli hospitals since passage of the National Health Insurance Act*. Tel Hashomer, Israel: Israel National Institute for Health Policy and Health Services Research (in Hebrew with English Executive Summary).

Harrison, M. and Shirom, A. (1999) *Organizational diagnosis and assessment: Bridging theory and practice*. Thousand Oaks, CA: Sage.

Harrison, S. (1998) 'The politics of evidence-based medicine in the United Kingdom', *Policy & Politics*, 26 (1): 15–31.

Harrison, S. and Choudry, N. (1996) 'General practice fundholding in the UK National Health Service: Evidence to date', *Journal of Public Health Policy*, 17: 331–346.

Harrison, S. and Dowswell, G. (2002) 'Autonomy and bureaucratic accountability in primary care: What English general practitioners say', *Sociology of Health and Illness*, 24: 208–226.

Harrison, S., Dowswell, G. and Wright, J. (2002) 'Practice nurses and clinical guidelines in a changing primary care context: An empirical study', *Journal of Advanced Nursing*, 39: 299–307.

Harrison, S., Hunter, D., Marnoch, G. and Pollitt, C. (1992) *Just managing: Power and culture in the National Health Service*. London: Macmillan.

Harrison, S. and Lachmann, J. (1996) *Towards a high-trust NHS: Proposals for minimally-invasive reform*. London: Institute for Public Policy Research.

Harrison, S., Moran, M. and Wood, B. (2002) 'Policy emergence and policy convergence: The case of "scientific-bureaucratic medicine" in the United States and United Kingdom', *British Journal of Politics and International Relations*, 4: 1–24.

Harrison, S. and Mort, M. (1998) 'Which champions, which people? Public and user involvement in health care as a technology of legitimation', *Social Policy & Administration*, 32: 60–70.

Harrison, S. and Pollitt, C. (1994) *Controlling health professionals: The future of work and organization in the NHS*. Buckingham: Open University Press.

Harrison, S. and Wood, B. (1999) 'Designing health service organization in the UK, 1968 to 1998: From blueprint to bright idea and "manipulated emergence"', *Public Administration*, 77: 751–768.

Hawkes, N. (2002, Febuary 12) 'Milburn replaces chiefs of failing health trusts', *London Times*, News, p. 8.

'Health action zones receive boost' (1999) *British Medical Journal*, 318: 335.

HealthScope (2003) An independent source of information to help you select the best quality care in California. Retrieved from http://www.healthscope.org/

Heath, I. (1994) 'The creeping privatisation of NHS prescribing', *British Medical Journal*, 309: 623–624.

Heclo, H. (1974) *Modern social politics in Britain and Sweden*. New Haven: Yale.

Heidenheimer, A. and Elvander, N. (eds) (1980) *The shaping of the Swedish medical system*. London: Croom Helm.

Helmreich, R. (2000) 'On error management: Lessons from aviation', *British Medical Journal*, 320: 781–785.

Hensher, M. and Edwards, N. (1999) 'Hospital provision, activity, and productivity in England since the 1980s', *British Medical Journal*, 319: 911–914.

Hermans, B. (2001, December 24) Personal communication.

Hibble, A., Kanka, D., Pencheon, D. and Pooles, F. (1998) 'Guidelines in general practice: The new Tower of Babel', *British Medical Journal*, 317: 862–863.

Hill, M. (1981) 'The policy-implementation distinction: A quest for rational control?', in S. Barrett and C. Fudge (eds) *Policy and action: Essays on the implementation of public policy*. London: Methuen. pp. 207–223.

Hill, M. (1995) 'Implementation theory: Yesterday's issue', *Policy and Politics*, 25: 375–385.

Hirschman, A. (1970) *Exit, voice, and loyalty: Responses to decline in firms, organizations, and states*. Cambridge: Harvard University Press.

Holm, S. (1998) 'Goodbye to the simple solutions: The second phase of priority setting in health care', *British Medical Journal*, 317: 1000–1007.

Honigsbaum, F., Calltorp, J., Ham, C. and Holmstrom, S. (1995) *Priority setting processes for healthcare*. Oxford: Radcliffe Medical Press.

Hood, C. (1991) 'A public management for all seasons?', *Public Administration*, 69: 3–19.

Hopton, J. and Heaney, D. (1999) 'The development of local healthcare cooperatives in Scotland', *British Medical Journal*, 318: 1185–1187.

Hsaio, W.C. (1994) 'Marketization: The illusory magic pill', *Health Economics*, 3: 351–357.

Hughes, D., Griffiths, L. and McHale, J.V. (1997) 'Do quasi-markets evolve? Institutional analysis and the NHS' *Cambridge Journal of Economics*, 21: 259–276.

Hunter, D. (1999, March 18) 'Pick and mix at the policy store'. Review of J. Le Grand, N. Mays and J-A. Mulligan. *Learning from the NHS internal market: A review of the evidence. Health Service Journal*, p. 109.

Immergut, E. (1989) 'Procedures for conciliation: The institutional basis of Swedish national health insurance', *Scandinavian Studies*, 62 (2–3): 146–168.

Immergut, E. (1992) *Health politics: Interests and institutions in Western Europe*. New York: Cambridge University Press.

Immergut, E. (1998) 'The theoretical core of the new institutionalism', *Politics and Society*, 26: 5–34.

In brief. (1995, February 9) *Health Service Journal*, p. 10.

In brief. (1995, February 16) *Health Service Journal*, p. 10.

in t'Veld, R. (1999) *Allocating responsibilities between the public and the private sectors*. Keynote address, European Healthcare Management Association. Parma, Italy.

Irvine, D. (1997a) 'The performance of doctors I: Professionalism and self regulation in a changing world', *British Medical Journal*, 314: 1540–1542.

Irvine, D. (1997b) 'The performance of doctors II: Maintaining good practice, protecting patients from poor performance', *British Medical Journal*, 314: 1613–1615.

Irvine, D. (1999) GMC's reply [Letter]. *British Medical Journal*, 319: 322 1613–1615.

Jacobs, A. (1998) 'Seeing difference: Market health reform in Europe', *Journal of Health Politics, Policy and Law*, 23: 1–33.

James, J. (1995) 'Reforming the British National Health Service: Implementation problems in London', *Journal of Health Politics, Policy, and Law*, 20: 191–210.

Jenkins, C. (1983) 'Resource mobilization theory and the study of social movements', *Annual Review of Sociology*, 9: 527–553.

Jenkins, S. (1995) *Accountable to none: The Tory nationalization of Britain*. London: Penguin Books.

Jones, C. and Dewing, I. (1997) 'The attitudes of NHS clinicians and medical managers towards changes in accounting controls', *Financial Accountability and Management*, 13: 261–280.

Jones, L., Schedler, K., Wade, S. (eds) (1997) *International perspectives on the new public management*. Greenwich, CONN: JAI.

Jones, R. (1997, March 27) 'Admissions of difficulty', *Health Service Journal*, 107: 28–31.

Jordan, J., Dowswell, T., Harrison, S., Liford, R. and Mort, M. (1998) 'Health needs assessment: Whose priorities? Listening to users and the public', *British Medical Journal*, 316: 1668–1670.

Kahn, P. S. (1997) 'On triangles and marriages: Considerations on the integration of medical specialist care act' [original in Dutch], *Zorg en verzekering*, 5: 561–569.

Kalo, I. (2000/2001, Winter) 'Development of quality of health systems in Europe', *Eurohealth*, 6 (5): 20–16.

Kavanagh, D. and Seldon, A. (eds) (1989) *The Thatcher effect*. Oxford: Clarendon Press.

Kendrick, S. (1995, May 4) 'Emergency admissions: What is driving the increase?', *Health Service Journal*, pp. 26–27.

Kenis, P. and Schneider, V. (1991) 'Policy networks and policy analysis: Scrutinizing a new analytical toolbox', in B. Marin and R. Mayntz (eds) *Policy networks: Empirical evidence and theoretical considerations*. Boulder, Colorado pp. 25–59.

Kerrison, S., Packwood, T. and Buxton, M. (1994) 'Monitoring medical audit', in R. Robinson and J. Le Grand (eds) *Evaluating the NHS reforms*. London: King's Fund Institute. pp. 155–177.

Killoran, A., Mays, N., Griffiths, J. and Posnett, J. (1998, 5 November) 'Growing pains', *Health Service Journal*, 108: 32–35.

Kimberly, J., Pouvourville, G. and Associates (1993) *The migration of managerial innovation: Diagnosis-related groups and health care administration in Western Europe*. San Francisco: Jossey-Boss.

Kingdon, J.W. (1984) *Agendas, alternatives, and public policies*. Boston: Little Brown.

King's Fund (2001, February 28) *Still no primary-care NHS under New Labour, says King's Fund* (Information – News). Retrieved from www.kingsfund.org.uk/pr010228.html

Kirkman-Liff, B.L. (1989) 'Cost containment and physician payment methods in the Netherlands', *Inquiry*, 26: 468–482.

Kirkman-Liff, B.L., Lapre, R. and Kirkman-Liff, T. (1988) 'The metamorphosis of health planning in the Netherlands and the USA', *Health Planning and Management*, 3: 89–109.

Kitchener, M. (1998) 'Quasi-market transformation: An institutionalist approach to change in UK hospitals', *Public Administration*, 76: 73–95.

Klazinga, N. (1994) 'Compliance with practical guidelines: Clinical autonomy revisited', *Health Policy*, 28: 51–66.

Klazinga, N., Lombarts, K. and van Everdingen, J. (1998) 'Quality management in medical specialties: The use of channels and dikes in improving health care in the Netherlands', *Joint Commission Journal on Quality Improvement*, 24: 240–250.

Klein, R. (1989) *The politics of the National Health Service* (2nd ed.) London: Longman.

Klein, R. (1995) *The new politics of the NHS*. London: Longman.

Klein, R. (ed.) (1998a) *Implementing the white paper – pitfalls and opportunities*. London: King's Fund.

Klein, R. (1998b) 'Puzzling out priorities: Why we must acknowledge that rationing is a political process', *British Medical Journal*, 317: 959–960.

Klein, R. (1998c) 'Why Britain is reorganizing its national health service – yet again', *Health Affairs*, 17 (4): 111–125.

Klein, R., Day, P. and Redmayne, S. (1996) *Managing scarcity: Priority setting and rationing in the National Health Service*. Buckingham: Open University Press.

Klein, R. and Dixon, J. (2000) 'Cash bonanza for NHS: The price is centralisation', *British Medical Journal*, 320: 883–884.

221

Knoke, D., Pappi, F., Broadbent, J. and Tsujinaka, Y. (1996) *Comparing political networks: Labor policy in the United States, Germany, and Japan.* Cambridge: Cambridge University Press.

Kohn, M. (1987) 'Cross-national research as an analytical strategy' (American Sociological Association, 1987 Presidential Address). *American Sociological Review*, 52: 713–731.

Konnen, E. and Koning, R. (1998) *How to charm integrated care.* Paper presented at European Health Management Association annual conference, Dublin.

Labour's health policy: 'Improvising' (1995, March 25) *Economist*, pp. 62–63.

Laing, A. and Galbraith, A. (1996) 'Developing a market orientation in the health service: NHS trusts in Scotland', *Journal of Management in Medicine*, 10: 24–35.

Lamers, L. (1999) 'Risk-adjusted capitation based on the diagnostic cost group mode: An empirical evaluation with health survey information', *Health Services Research*, 33: 1727–1744.

Latham, L., Freeman, T., Walshe, K., Spurgeon, P. and Wallace, L. (1999) *The early development of clinical governance: A survey of NHS trusts in the West Midlands.* Birmingham: Health Services Management Centre.

Lawton, R. and Parker D. (1999) 'Procedures and the professional: The case of the British NHS', *Social Science & Medicine*, 48: 353–361.

Lazin, F. (1995) 'Lessons for the study of policy implementation: Project renewal in Israel', *Governance: An International Journal of Policy and Administration*, 8: 261–279.

Le Grand, J. (1999) 'Competition, cooperation, or control? Tales from the British National Health Service', Health Affairs 18 (3): 27–39.

Le Grand, J. and Bartlett, W. (eds) (1993) *Quasi markets and social policy.* London: Macmillan.

Le Grand, J., Mays, N. and Dixon, J. (1998) 'The reforms: Success or failure or neither?', in J. Le Grand, N. Mays and J.-A. Mulligan (eds) *Learning from the NHS internal market: A review of the evidence.* London: King's Fund. pp. 117–143.

Lee, C., Rogal, D. and Kemp, K. (1999) *Purchasing pathfinders: On their way, but still wrestling with the realities of containing costs and promoting quality.* Washington, D.C.: Alpha Center.

Leichter, H. (1984) 'Controlling health care costs: A cross-national perspective', in H. Rodgers (ed.) *Public policy and social institutions.* Greenwich, Conn: JAI. pp. 99–126.

Leichter , H. (1989) 'United Kingdom', in J.P. DeSario (ed.) *International public policy sourcebook: Health and social welfare.* New York: Greenwood Press. Vol. 1, pp. 141–161

Levin, M. and Ferman, B. (1985) *The political hand: Policy implementation and youth employment programs.* New York: Pergamon.

Lieverdink, H. (2001a) 'The marginal success of regulated competition policy in the Netherlands', *Social Science and Medicine*, 52: 1183–1194.

Lieverdink, H. (2001b, August 1) Personal communication.

Lieverdink, H. (2002, December 20) Personal communication.

Lieverdink, H. and van der Made, J. (1997) 'The reform of health insurance systems in the Netherlands and Germany: Dutch gold and German silver?', in C. Altenstetter and J.W. Bjorkman (eds) *Health policy reform, national variations and globalization.* London: Macmillan. pp. 109–135.

Light, D. (1988) 'Turf battles and the theory of professional dominance', *Research in the Sociology of Health Care*, 7: 203–225.

Light, D. (1990, October 11) 'Bending the rules', *Health Service Journal*, 100: 1513–1514.

Light, D. (1991) 'Professionalism as a countervailing power', *Journal of Health Politics, Policy and Law*, 16: 499–506.

Light, D.W. (1997a) 'From managed competition to managed cooperation: Theory and lessons from the British experience', *The Milbank Quarterly*, 75: 297–341.

Light, D. (1997b, October 16) 'Poor bets on the pools', *Health Service Journal*, p. 22.

Light, D. (1999) 'Here we go again: Repeating implementation errors', *British Medical Journal*, 319: 616–618.

Light, D. W. (2000) 'The sociological character of health care markets', in G.L. Albrecht, R. Fitzpatrick and S. Scrimshaw (eds) *Handbook of social studies in health and medicine*. London: Sage.

Light, D. (2001) 'Comparative institutional response to economic policy: Managed competition and governability', *Social Science and Medicine*, 52: 1151–1166.

Limb, M. (1996, March 14) 'Flavour of the month', *Health Service Journal*, p. 18.

Limb, M. (1996, August 15) 'Health of the nation failing key targets, says NAO', *Health Service Journal*, p. 5.

Limb, M. (1997, November 6) 'Destination unknown', *Health Service Journal*, p. 11.

Limb, M. and Chadda, D. (1996, February 2) 'Managers and doctors dismiss Redwood "dogma"', *Health Science Journal*, 106: 7.

Lindkvist, L. (1996) 'Performance based compensation in health care – a Swedish experience', *Financial Accountability and Management*, 12: 89–105.

Lipsky, M. (1980) *Street-level bureaucracy*. New York: Russel Sage.

Ljungkvist, M.-O., Andersson, D. and Gunnarsson, B. (1997) 'Cost and utilisation of pharmaceuticals in Sweden', *Health Policy*, 41 (Supplement): s55–s69.

Locock, L. (2000) 'The changing nature of rationing in the UK National Health Service', *Public Administration*, 78: 91–109.

Loveridge, R. (1992) 'The future of health care delivery – markets or hierarchies?', in R. Loveridge and K. Starkey (eds) *Continuity and crisis in the NHS: The politics of design and innovation in health care*. Buckingham: Open University Press. pp. 216–225.

Lukes, S. (1974) *Power – a radical view*. London: Macmillan.

Lunt, N., Atkin, K. and Hirst, M. (1997) 'Staying single in the 1990s: Single-handed practitioners in the new National Health Service', *Social Science Medical*, 45 (3): 341–349.

Lyall, J. (1995 February 16) 'Gains and pains', *Health Service Journal*, p. 1.

Maarse, J. (1993a) *Hospital finance in the Netherlands* Report. Office of Technology Assessment, Organization of Economic Development and Coordination (OECD).

Maarse, J. (1993b) 'The insurer-provider relationship in health care', *European Journal of Public Health*, 3: 72–76.

Maarse, H. (1996) 'Fixed budgets in the inpatient sector: The case of the Netherlands', in F. Schwartz, H. Glennerster and R.B. Saltman (eds) *Fixing health budgets: Experience from Europe and North America*. Chichester, England: Wiley. pp. 75–92.

Maarse, H. (1997) 'Change of heart', *European Health Reform* (May): 7–9.

Maarse, H. (1999) *The changing public-private mix in Dutch health care*. Presented at the annual conference, European Health Management Association: Parma, Italy.

Macpherson, D. and Mann, T. (1992) 'Medical audit and quality of care – a new English initiative', *Quality Assurance in Health Care*, 4 (2): 89–95.

Maddox, G. (1999) 'General practice fundholding in the British National Health Service Reform, 1991–1997: GP accounts of the dynamics of change', *Journal of Health Politics, Policy, and Law*, 24: 815–834.

Mahon, A., Wilkin, D. and Whitehouse, C. (1994) 'Choice of hospital for elective surgery referrals: GP's and patients' views', in R. Robinson and J. Le Grand (eds) *Evaluating the NHS reforms*. London: King's Fund Institute. pp. 108–129.

Mailly, R. (1997, January 23) 'Less than was bargained for', *Health Service Journal*, pp. 24–25.

Majeed, A. (1999) 'Commentary: Accurate information may be difficult to produce', *British Medical Journal*, 318: 168.

'The making of NHS Ltd' (1995, January 21) *Economist*, pp. 57–58.

'Management growth figures "misleading"' (1994, November 10) *Health Service Journal*, p. 6.

223

Maniadakis, N., Hollingsworth, B. and Thanassoulis, E. (1999) 'The impact of the internal market on hospital efficiency, productivity, and service quality', *Health Care Management Science*, 2: 75–85.

March, J. and Olsen, J. (1983) 'Organizing political life: What administrative reorganization teaches us about government', *American Political Science Review*, 77: 281–296.

March, J. and Olsen, J. (1989) *Rediscovering institutions*. New York: Free Press.

Marin, B. and Mayntz, R. (eds) (1991) *Policy networks: Empirical evidence and theoretical considerations*. Boulder, Colorado: Westview.

Marmot, M. (1999) 'Acting on the evidence to reduce inequalities in health', *Health Affairs*, 18 (3): 42–44.

Marsh, D. and Rhodes, R. (1992) 'Policy communities and issue networks', in Marsh, D. and Rhodes, R. (eds) *Policy networks in British politics*. Oxford: Clarendon Press. pp. 248–268.

Marshall, M. (1999) 'How well do GPs and hospital consultants work together? A survey of professional relationships', *Family Practice*, 16: 33–38.

Martin, J. (1992) *Cultures in organizations: Three perspectives*. New York: Oxford.

Maynard, A. (1993) 'Market reforms and the funding of the NHS', in D. Light and A. May (eds) *Britain's health system: From welfare state to managed markets*. New York: Faulkner and Gray. pp. 29–38.

Mayntz, R. (1979) 'Public bureaucracies and policy implementation', *International Social Science Journal*, 31: 663–645.

Mays, N. and Dixon, J. (1996) *Purchaser plurality in UK health care – is a consensus emerging and is it the right one?* London: King's Fund Publishing.

Mays, N.and Keen, J. (1998) 'Will the fudge on equity sustain the NHS into the next millennium?', *British Medical Journal*, 317: 66–69.

Mays, N. and Mulligan, J.A. (1998) 'Total purchasing', in J. Le Grand, N. Mays and J.-A. Mulligan (eds) *Learning from the NHS internal market: A review of the evidence*. London: King's Fund. pp. 84–100.

Mc Cormick, B. (1998) 'Community care for the elderly', *British Medical Journal* 317: 552–553.

McIver, S. and Martin, G. (1996, September 19) 'Uncharted territory', *Health Service Journal*, 106: 24–26.

McMaster, R. (1998) 'The X-efficiency properties of competitive tendering', in W. Bartlett, J. A. Roberts and J. Le Grand (eds) *A Revolution in social policy: Quasi-market reforms in the 1990s*. Bristol, UK: Policy Press. pp. 43–60.

McNulty, T., Whittington, R. and Whipp, R. (1995) 'Practices' and market-control: Work experiences of doctors, scientists and engineers', in J. Leopold, M. Hughes and I. Glover (eds) *Beyond reason? The National Health Service and the limits of management*. London: Avebury Press.

McNulty, T., Whittington, R., Whipp, R., and Kitchener, M. (1994) 'Implementing marketing in NHS hospitals', *Public money and management*, 14 (July–September) 51–59.

Meyer, J. and Rowan, B. (1977) 'Institutionalized organizations: Formal structure as myth and ceremony', *American Journal of Sociology*, 83: 340–363.

Milewa, T., Valentine, J. and Calnan, M. (1998) 'Managerialism and active citizenship in Britain's reformed health service: Power and community in an era of decentralisation', *Social Science and Medicine*, 47: 507–517.

Millar, B. (1994, November 17) 'Out of the bunker', *Health Service Journal*, Vol. 13.

Millar, B. (1996, December 5) 'Putting the knife in', *Health Service Journal*, 106: 13.

Millar, B. (1997, March 27) 'Falling between the cracks', *Health Service Journal*, 107: 13.

Ministry of Welfare, Health and Cultural Affairs (1988a) 'Change assured', in *Changing healthcare in the Netherlands*. Rijswijk: Ministry of Welfare, Health and Cultural Affairs. pp. 65–90.

Ministry of Welfare, Health and Cultural Affairs (1988b) 'Changing health care', in *Changing healthcare in the Netherlands*. Rijswijk: Ministry of Welfare, Health, and Cultural Affairs. pp. 7–26.

Ministry of Welfare, Health and Cultural Affairs (1988c) 'Willingness to change' [Summary of Dekker Committee report], in *Changing health care in the Netherlands* Booklet. Rijswijk: Ministry of Health, Welfare and Cultural Affairs.

Mintzberg, H. (1979) *The structuring of organizations*. Englewood-Cliffs, NJ: Prentice Hall.

Mitchell, P. (1998, May 28) 'Two cheers for HISS' [IT Update], *Health Service Journal*, p. 10.

Moore, W. (1995, November 9) 'Is doctors' power shrinking?', *Health Service Journal*, 105: 24–27.

Moore, W. (1999, January 13) 'On the line', *Health Service Journal*, pp. 20–23.

Moore, W. (2002) 'NHS to receive an extra £40bn over next five years', *British Medical Journal*, 324: 993.

Morgan, G. (1986) *Images of organization*. Thousand Oaks, CA: Sage.

Morgan, K., Prothero, D. and Frankel, S. (1999, July 17) 'The rise in emergency admissions – crisis or artifact? Temporal analysis of health services data', *British Medical Journal*, 319: 158–159.

Morrione, T. (1985) 'Situated interaction', in H. Farberman and R. Perinbanayagam (eds) *Studies in symbolic interaction foundations of interpretive sociology: Original essays in symbolic interaction*, Supplement 1. Greenwich, CONN: JAI. pp. 161–192.

Mossberger, K. (2000) *The politics of ideas and the spread of enterprise zones*. Washington, DC: Georgetown University Press.

Muijen, M. and Ford, R. (1996) 'The market and mental health: Intentional and unintentional incentives', *Journal of Interprofessional Care*, 10: 13–22.

Mulligan, J.-A. (1998a) 'Health authority purchasing', in J. Le Grand, N. Mays and J.-A. Mulligan (eds) *Learning from the NHS internal market: A review of the evidence*. London: King's Fund. pp. 20–23.

Mulligan, J.-A. (1998b) 'Locality and GP commissioning', in J. Le Grand, N. Mays and J.-A. Mulligan (eds) *Learning from the internal market; A review of the evidence*. London: King's Fund. pp. 69–83.

Mulligan, J.-A. and Judge, K. (1997) 'Public opinion and the NHS', in *Health care UK 1996/7*. London: King's Fund. pp. 123–137.

Mur-Veeman, I., van Raak, A. and Paulus, A. (1999) 'Integrated care: The impact of governmental behavior on collaborative networks', *Health Policy*, 49: 149–159.

National Audit Office (1996) *The NHS Executive: The hospital information support systems initiative* (Report by the Comptroller and Auditor General). London: HMSO.

Nelson, J., Megill, A. and McCloskey, D. (eds) (1987) *The rhetoric of the human sciences – language and argument in scholarship and public affairs*. Madison, Wisconsin: University of Wisconsin Press.

Newhouse, J. (1993) 'An iconoclastic view of health cost containment', *Health Affairs*, 12 (Supplement): 152–171.

NHS Executive (1996) *Priorities and planning: Guidance for the NHS 1996/97*. Leeds, UK: HMSO.

NHS Executive (1998) *A first class service – quality in the new NHS*. London: HMSO

Nicholls, R. (1997, Autumn) *Seismic shift or noisy tremor?* King's Fund London News, 1: 6–12.

Ninerood-Bare, T.C.S. (1997, June 26) Interview. Utrecht: National Hospital Institute.

Obermann, K. and Tolley, K. (1997) *The state of health care priority setting and public participation*. Discussion Paper 154. York: The University of York.

OECD (Organization for Economic Cooperation and Development) (1992) *The reform of health care: A comparative analysis of seven OECD countries*, in Health policy studies No. 2. Paris: Author.

OECD (Organization for Economic Cooperation and Development) (1994) *The reform of health care systems: A review of seventeen OECD countries*, in Health Policy Studies No. 5. Paris: Author.

OECD (Organization for Economic Cooperation and Development) (1995) *New directions in health care policy*, in Health Policy Studies No. 7. Paris: Author.

225

OECD (Organization for Economic Cooperation and Development) (2001) *OECD Health Data 2001*. Data base. Paris: Author

OECD (Organization for Economic Cooperation and Development) (2002) *OECD Health Statistics*. Retrieved from http://www.oecd.org/oecd/pages/home/displaygeneral/0,3380,EN-statistics

Oldham, J. and Rutter, I. (1999) 'Independence days', *British Medical Journal*, 318: 748–749.

Ong, B. N. and Schepers, R. (1999) 'Variations on a theme: Clinicians in management in England and the Netherlands', in A.L. Mark and S. Dopson (eds) *Organisational behaviour in health care: The research agenda*. London: Macmillan. pp. 117–133.

Orchard, C. (1993, December 9) 'Mind your language', *Health Service Journal*, p. 24–25.

Osborne, D. and Gaebler, T. (1992) *Reinventing government – how the entrepreneurial spirit is transforming the public sector*. Reading, MA: Addison-Wesley.

Osborne, D. and Plastrik, P. (2000) *The reinventor's fieldbook: Tools for transforming your government*. San Francisco: Jossey-Bass.

Ovretveit, J. (1994) 'A comparison of approaches to health service quality in the UK, USA & Sweden and of the use of organizational audit frameworks', *European Journal of Public Health*, 4 (1): 46–54.

O'Toole, L. (1986) 'Policy recommendations for multi-actor implementation', *Journal of Public Policy*, 6: 181–210.

Packwood, T., Keen, J., Buxton, M. (1991) *Hospitals in transition: The resource management experiment*. Milton Keynes: Open University Press.

Packwood, T., Kerrison, S., and Buxton, M. (1994) 'The implementation of medical audit', *Social Policy and Administration*, 28: 299–316.

Paice, E., Aitken, M., Cowan, G. and Heard, S. (2000) 'Trainee satisfaction before and after the Calman reforms of training specialist training: A questionnaire survey', *British Medical Journal*, 320: 832–836.

'Pains, strains, and automobiles' (1998, April 30) *Health Service Journal*, p. 17.

Parry, G., Gould, C., McCabe, C. and Tarnow-Mordi, W. (1998) 'Annual league tables of mortality in neonatal intensive care units: Longitudinal study', *British Medical Journal*, 316: 1931–1935.

Paton, C. (2000) *Scientific evaluation of the effects of the introduction of market forces into health systems*. Dublin: European Health Management Association.

Paton, C., Birch, K., Hunt, K., Jordan, K. (1997, August 21) 'Counting the costs', *Health Service Journal*, pp. 24–27.

Paulson, E.M. (1993) 'Sweden: A health care model in transition', in J. Kimberly, G. Pouvouruille and Associates (eds) *The migration of managerial innovation: Diagnosis-related groups and health care administration in Western Europe*. San Francisco: Jossey-Bass Publishers. pp. 131–172.

Pen, J. (1987) 'Expanding budgets in a stagnating economy: The experience of the 1970s', in C. Maier (ed.) *Changing boundaries of the political*. Cambridge: Cambridge University Press. pp. 323–361.

Perleth, M., Jakubowski, E., and Busse, R. (2001) 'What is "best practice" in health care? State of the art perspectives in improving the effectiveness and efficiency of the European health care systems', *Health Policy*, 56: 235–250.

Pettigrew, A., Ferlie, E. and McKee, L. (1992) *Shaping strategic change*. London: Sage.

Pettiger, N. (1997, April 10) 'Measure for measure', Health Service Journal, pp. 26–27.

Pfeffer, J. (1981) *Power in organizations*. Marshfield, MA: Pitman.

Pollock, A. (2000) 'Will intermediate care be the undoing of the NHS?', *British Medical Journal*, 321: 393–394.

Pollock, A. (2001a) 'How private finance is moving primary care into corporate ownership', *British Medical Journal*, 322: 960–963.

Pollock, A. (2001b) 'Will primary care trusts lead to US-style health care?', *British Medical Journal*, 322: 964–967.

Pollock, A., Dunngan, M., Gaffney, D., Price, D. and Shaoul, J. (1999) 'Planning the "new" NHS: Downsizing for the 21st century', *British Journal of Medicine*, 319: 179–184.

Pool, J. (1992) 'Hospital management: Integrating the dual hierarchy?', *The International Journal of Health Planning and Management*, 6: 193–207.

Posnett, J. (1993) 'The political economy of health care reform in the United Kingdom', in R. Arnould, R. Rich and W. White (eds) *Competitive approaches to health care reform.* Washington: Urban Institute Press. pp. 293–312.

Pressman, J. and Wildavsky, A. (1973) *Implementation.* Berkeley, CA: University of California Press.

Prismat. (2000) *Statistics on general hospitals, 1994–1999.* Unpublished manuscript. Utrecht, Netherlands.

Proctor, S. and Campbell, L. (1999) 'Managing the future in Bradford', *British Medical Journal*, 318: 783–785.

Propper, C. and Bartlett, W. (1997) 'The impact of competition on the behaviour of National Health Service trusts', in R. Flynn and G. Williams, (eds) *Contracting for health: Quasi-markets and the National Health Service.* Oxford: Oxford University Press. pp. 14–29.

Prottas, J. (1979) *People processing: The street-level bureaucrat in public service bureaucracies.* Lexington, MA: Heath.

'Public inquiry sought in Britain's "Dr. Death" case', (2000, February 1). Retrieved from: http://www.nytimes.com/reuters/international/international-britain.htm

'Public softens stance on change', (1996, June 6) *Health Service Journal*, p. 7.

Pugner, K. and Glennerster, H. (1998, June 4) 'Called to accountability', *Health Service Journal*, pp. 28–29.

Radical Statistics Health Group (1995) 'NHS "indicators of success": What do they tell us?', *British Medical Journal*, 310: 1045–1050.

Ramström, D. and Dahlström, A. (1995) Interview [Summary of research findings].

Ranade, W. and Haywood, S.C. (1991) 'Privatising from within: The National Health Service under Thatcher', in C. Altenstetter and S.C. Haywood (eds) *Comparative health policy and the new right: From rhetoric to reality.* New York: St. Martin's Press. pp. 91–110.

Rappolt, S. (1997) 'Clinical guidelines and the fate of medical autonomy in Ontario', *Social Science and Medicine*, 44: 977–987.

Rathwell, T. (1998) 'Implementing health care reform: A review of current evidence', in R. Saltman, J. Figueras and C. Sakellarides (eds) *Critical challenges for health care reform in Europe.* Buckingham, UK: Open University Press. pp. 385–399.

Regen, E., Smith, J., Goodwin, N., McLeod, H. and Shapiro, J. (2001) *Passing on the baton: Final report of a national evaluation of primary care groups and trusts (Summary).* Birmingham: Health Services Management Centre.

Rehn, G. and Viklund, B. (1990) 'Changes in the Swedish model', in G. Baglioni and C. Crouch (eds) *European industrial relations: The challenge of flexibility.* London: Sage. (pp. 300–325).

Rehnberg, C. (1995) 'The Swedish experience with internal markets', in J. Jerome-Forget, J. White and J. Weiner (eds) *Health care reform through internal markets: Experience and proposals.* Montreal and Washington: Institute for Research on Public Policy and Brookings Institution. pp. 49–73.

Reinhardt, U. (1994) 'Germany's health care system: It's not the American way', *Health Affairs*, 13 (Fall): 22–24.

Rice, T. (1997) 'Can markets give us the health system we want?', *Journal of Health Politics, Policy and Law*, 22: 383–426.

Rice, T. (1998) *The economics of health reconsidered.* Chicago: Health Administration Press.

Rice, T., Biles, B., Brown, E.R., Diderichsen, F. and Kuehn, H. (2000) 'Reconsidering the role of competition in health care markets: Introduction' [to special issue], *Journal of Health Politics, Policy, and Law*, 25: 864–873.

Riska, E. (1993) 'The medical profession in the Nordic countries', in F. Hafferty and J. McKinlay (eds) *The changing character of the medical profession: An international perspective.* Oxford, England: Oxford University Press.

Robinson, J. (1993) 'Managed competition and the demise of nursing', in D. Light and A. May (eds) *Britain's health system: From welfare state to managed markets*. New York: Faulkner and Gray. pp. 149–160.

Robinson, J. and Poxton, R. (1998) 'Health and social care partnerships', in R. Klein (ed.) *Implementing the white paper – pitfalls and opportunities*. London: King's Fund. pp. 56–66.

Robinson, R. (2002) 'Gold for the NHS', *British Medical Journal*, 324: 987–988.

Rogers, E. (1995) *Diffusion of Innovations* (4th ed.). New York: Free Press.

Rosen, R. and Mays, N. (1998) 'The impact of the UK NHS purchaser–provider split on the "rational" introduction of new medical technologies', *Health Policy*, 43: 103–123.

Rosenthal, M. (1992) 'Growth of private medicine in Sweden: The new diversity and the new challenge', *Health Policy*, 21: 155–166.

Rosenthal, M.M. (1995) *The incompetent doctor – behind closed doors*. Buckingham: Open University Press.

Rutten, F.F. and Freens, R.J. (1986) 'Health care financing in the Netherlands: Recent changes and future options', *Health Policy*, 6: 313–320.

Sabatier, P. (1986) 'Top-down and bottom-up approaches to implementation research: A critical analysis and suggested synthesis', *Journal of Public Policy*, 6: 21–48.

Sabatier, P. (1988) 'An advocacy coalition framework of policy change and the role of policy-oriented learning', *Policy Sciences*, 21: 129–168.

Sabatier, P. (1991) 'Toward better theories of the policy process', *Political Science and Politics*, 24: 147–156.

Saint-Martin, D. (1998) 'Management consultants, the state, and the politics of reform in Britain and Canada', *Administration and Society*, 30: 533–568.

Salter, B. (1999) 'Change in the governance of medicine: The politics of self-regulation', *Policy and Politics*, 27 (2): 143–158.

Saltman, R. (1990) 'Competition and reform in the Swedish health system', *The Milbank Quarterly*, 68: 597–618.

Saltman, R. (1992) 'Recent health policy initiatives in Nordic countries', *Health Care Financing Review*, 13: 157–166.

Saltman, R. and de Roo, A. (1989) 'Hospital policy in the Netherlands: The parameters of structural stalemate', *Journal of Health Politics, Policy and Law*, 14: 773–795.

Saltman, R. and Figueras, J. (eds) (1997) *European health care reform: analysis of current strategies*. WHO Regional Publications, European series, No. 72. Copenhagen: World Health Organization.

Saltman, R. and von Otter, C. (1992) *Planned markets and public competition: Strategic reform in northern European health systems*. Buckingham: Open University Press.

Sarason, S. (1971) *The culture of the school and the problem of change*. Boston: Allyn and Bacon.

Savas, S., Sheiman, I., Tragakes, E. and Maarse, H. (1998) 'Contracting models and provider competition', in R. Saltman, J. Figueras and C. Sakellarides (eds) *Critical challenges for health care reform in Europe*. Buckingham, UK: Open University Press pp. 157–178.

Schon, D. and Rein, M. (1994) *Frame reflection: Toward the resolution of intractable controversies*. New York: Basic Books.

Schrijvers, A. and Kodner, L. (eds) (1997) *Health and health care in the Netherlands – a critical self-assessment of Dutch experts in medical and health sciences*. Utrecht: De Tijdstroom.

Schut, F. (1992) 'Workable competition in health care: Prospects for the Dutch design', *Social Science and Medicine*, 35: 1445–1455.

Schut, F. (1995) 'Health care reform in the Netherlands: Balancing corporatism, etatism, and market mechanisms', *Journal of Health Politics, Policy and Law*, 20: 615–652.

Schut, F. (1996) 'Health care systems in transition: The Netherlands. Part I: Health care reforms in the Netherlands: Miracle or mirage?', *Journal of Public Health Medicine*, 18: 278–284.

Scott, A. and Wordsworth, S. (1999) 'The effects of shifts in the balance of care on general practice workload', *Family Practice*, 16: 12–17.

Scott, W.R. (1995) *Institutions and organizations*. Thousand Oaks, CA: Sage Publications.

Scott, W.R., Reuf, M., Mendel, P. and Cronna, C. (2000) *Institutional change and health-care organizations: From professional dominance to managed care*. Chicago: University of Chicago Press.

Secretary of State for Health (1989) *Working for patients*. London: Her Majesty's Stationery Office.

Secretary of State for Health (1992) *The Health of the nation: A strategy for health in England*. London: HMSO.

Secretary of State for Health (1997) *The new NHS: Modern, dependable*. London: Her Majesty's Stationery Office.

Secretary of State for Health (1998) *Modernising social services*. London: Her Majesty's Stationery Office.

Secretary of State for Health (1999) *Saving lives: Our healthier nation*. London: Her Majesty's Stationery Office.

Secretary of State for Health – Bristol Royal Infirmary Inquiry (2001) *Learning from Bristol: The report of the public inquiry into children's heart surgery at the Bristol Royal Infirmary 1984 –1995*. London: HMSO.

Seng, C., Lessof, L. and McKee, M. (1993, January 7) 'Who's on the fiddle?', *Health Services Journal*, 103: 16–17.

Shadmi, H. (2002, November 25) '*A basket case and getting worse*'. Ha'aretz, English Edition. Retrieved from www.haaretz.com

Sheldon, T. (1998) 'Dutch coalition tackles waiting lists', *British Medical Journal*, 316: 955.

Sheldon, T. (2000a) 'Dutch waiting lists increase despite £36 million campaign', *British Medical Journal*, 321: 530.

Sheldon, T. (2000b) 'EU law makes Netherlands reconsider health system', *British Medical Journal*, 320: 206.

Sheldon, T. (2001a) 'Dutch government plans to reform health insurance system', *British Medical Journal*, 323: 70.

Sheldon, T. (2001b) 'Netherlands aims to tackle health divide', *British Medical Journal*, 323: 828.

Shortell, S., Morrison, E. and Friedman, B. (1990) *Strategic choices for America's hospitals: Managing change in turbulent times*. San Francisco: Jossey-Bass.

Sibbald, B., Wilkie, P., Raftery, J., Anderson, S. and Freeling, P. (1992) 'Prescribing at the hospital–general practice interface II: Impact of hospital outpatient dispensing policies in England on general practitioners and hospital consultants', *British Medical Journal* (London), 304: 31–34.

Silcock, J., and Ratcliffe, J. (1996) 'The 1990 GP contract – meeting needs?', *Health Policy*, 36: 199–207.

Silverman, D. (1970) *The theory of organizations: A sociological perspective*. London: Heinneman.

Smit, R.L. (2000) *Health care chains in the Netherlands* [English version of article originally published as "L'assistenza va a catena" in *Sanita & Management, supplement of Il Sole*, 24 Ore, 2/3 August/September]. Utrecht.

Smith, R. (1998) 'Regulation of doctors and the Bristol inquiry', *British Medical Journal*, 317: 1539–1540.

Smith, R. (1999a) 'NICE: A panacea for the NHS?', *British Medical Journal*, 318: 823–824.

Smith, R. (2001) 'GMC: Approaching the abyss?', *British Medical Journal*, 322: 1196.

Smith, R. (2002) 'Oh NHS, thou art sick', *British Medical Journal*, 324: 127–128.

Socialstyrelsen (1993) *Ädelreformen* [The Ädel Reform]. Stockholm: Author.

Socialstyrelsen (1995) *Den planerade marknaden: Om nya styrformer i Hälso-och sjukvården*. [The planned market: New forms of financing and organization]. Stockholm: Author.

229

Socialstyrelsen (1998) *Ädelparadoxen: sjukhemmen fore och efter Ädelreformen* [The Ädel paradox: nursing homes before and after the Ådel Reform]. Stockholm: Author.

Söderland, N., Csaba, I., Gray, A., Milne, R. and Raftery, J. (1997) 'Impact of the NHS reforms on English hospital productivity: An analysis of the first three years', *British Medical Journal*, 315: 1126–1129.

Somerset, M., Faulkner, A., Shaw, A., Dun, L. and Sharp, D. (1999) 'Obstacles on the path to a primary-care led National Health Service: Complexities of outpatient care', *Social Science and Medicine*, 48: 213–225.

Spillane, J. (1998) 'A cognitive perspective on the role of the local educational agency in implementing instructional policy: Accounting for local variability', *Educational Administration Quarterly*, 34: 31–57.

Stacey, M. (1992) 'For public or profession? The new GMC performance procedures', *British Medical Journal*, 305: 1085–1087.

Starr, P. (1982) *The social transformation of American medicine.* New York: Basic Books.

Starr, P. and Immergut, E. (1987) 'Health care and the boundaries of politics', in C. Maier (ed.) *Changing boundaries of the political: Essays on the evolving balance between the state and society, public and private in Europe.* Cambridge: Cambridge University Press. pp. 221–254.

Staw, B.M. and Epstein, L. (2000) 'What bandwagons bring: Effects of popular management techniques on corporate performance, reputation, and CEO pay', *Administrative Science Quarterly*, 45: 523–556.

Stewart, R. (1994, December 1) 'Compound interests', *Health Service Journal*, p. 30.

Stewart, R. (1996, 21 March) 'Divided loyalties', *Health Service Journal*, 106: 30–31.

Styrborn, K. and Thorslund, M. (1993) 'Bed blockers' delayed discharge of hospital patients in a nationwide perspective in Sweden', *Health Policy*, 26: 155–170.

Swedish Institute (1993) 'The health care system in Sweden', in *Fact sheets on Sweden.* Author.

Swinkels, J.A. (1999) 'Reregistration of medical specialists in the Netherlands', *British Medical Journal*, 319: 1191–1192.

Thomson, R. (1998) 'Quality to the fore in health policy – at last', *British Medical Journal*, 317: 95–96.

'Three quarters of HAs in the red last year' (1997, January 2) *Health Service Journal*, p. 3.

'Too good to be true' (1999, January 23) *Economist.*

'Top doctor joins NHS controversy' (1994, December 8) *Health Service Journal*, p. 4.

'Tougher than the Taliban' (2001, November 24) [Editorial]. *Economist*, p. 13.

Tuohy, C.H. (1999a) *Accidental logics: The dynamics of change in the health care arena in the United States, Britain, and Canada.* New York: Oxford.

Tuohy, C.H. (1999b) 'Dynamics of a changing health sphere: The United States, Britain, and Canada', *Health Policy*, 18: 114–134.

Twaddle, A. (1999) *Health care reform in Sweden, 1980–1994.* Westport, Conn: Auburn House. An unhealthy silence (1997, March 15) *Economist*, pp. 37–38.

U.S. Congress, Office of Technology Assessment (1995) *Health care technology and its assessment in eight countries*, in H. Banta, H. Gelband, R. Battista, and E. Jonsson (eds) OTA-BP-H-140. Washington, D.C.: U.S. Government Printing Office.

van Andel, F. and Brinkman, N. (1997) 'Government policy and cost containment of pharmaceuticals', in A. Schrijvers and L. Kodner (eds) *Health and health care in the Netherlands.* Utrecht: De Tijdstroom. pp. 152–162.

van de Ven, W.P. (1987) 'The key role of health insurance in a cost-effective health care system', *Health Policy*, 7: 253–272.

van de Ven, W.P. (1990) 'From regulated cartel to regulated competition in the Dutch health care system', *European Economic Review*, 34: 632–645.

van de Ven, W.P. (1991) 'Perestrojka in the Dutch health care system: A demonstration project for other European countries', *European Economic Review*, 35: 430–440.

van de Ven, W. P. (1993, June–July) *Regulated competition in health care: Lessons for Europe from the Dutch 'demonstration project'.* Key-note lecture at the annual conference of the European Healthcare Management Association. Warsaw, Poland.

230

van de Ven, W. (1997) 'The Netherlands', in C. Ham (ed.) *Health care reform: Learning from international experience*. Buckingham, England: Open University Press. pp. 87–103.

van de Ven, W., van Vliet, R., Barneveld, E. and Lamers, L. (1994) 'Risk-adjusted capitation: Recent experiences in the Netherlands', *Health Affairs*, 13 (Winter): 120–136.

van der Grinten, T. (1996) 'Scope for policy: Essence operation and reform of the policy of Dutch health care', in *Fundamental questions about the future of health care*. Netherlands Scientific Council for Government Policy. pp. 135–155.

van der Grinten, T., Kasdorp, J. (1999) 'Choices in Dutch health care: Mixing strategies and responsibilities', *Health Policy*, 50: 105–122.

van der Grinten, T., Meurs, P. and Putters, K. (1998) *Healthcare reform in the context of alliances: Social entrepreurship in Dutch health care*. Paper presented at the annual meeting of the European Healthcare Management Association, June 24–26, Dublin, Ireland.

van der Linden B., Spreeuwenberg, C. and Schrijvers, A. (2001) 'Integration of care in the Netherlands: The development of transmural care since 1994', *Health Policy*, 55: 111–120.

van Doorslaer, E. and Schut, F. (2000) 'Belgium and the Netherlands revisited', *Journal of Health Politics, Policy and Law*, 25: 875–888.

van Etten, G. and Okma, G. (1992) *Health care reforms in the Netherlands*. Rijswijk: Ministry of Welfare, Health and Cultural Affairs.

Van Herk, R., Klazinga, N., Schepers, R. and Casparie, A.F. (2001) 'Medical audit: Threat or opportunity for the medical profession? A comparative study of medical audit among medical specialists in general hospitals in the Netherlands and England, 1970–1990', *Social Science and Medicine*, 53: 1721–1732.

van Het Loo, M., Kahan, J.P. and Okma, K. (1999) 'Developments in health care cost containment in the Netherlands', in E. Mossialos and J. Le Grand (eds) *Health care and cost containment in the European Union*. Brookfield USA: Ashgate. pp. 573–603.

Vass, A. (2002) 'Performance of individual surgeons to be published', *British Medical Journal*, 324: 189.

Vektis (2002) *Zorgmonitor [Care monitor] 2002*. Zeist, Netherlands: Author.

Versluis, J. (1993) *Managementparticipatie van medisch specialisten in algemene ziekenhuizen* [Management participation of medical specialists in hospitals]. Utrecht, Netherlands: National Hospital Institute.

Vienonen, M. (1997) 'Health and the health care system in the Netherlands: An international comparison', in A. Schrijvers and L. Kodner (eds) *Health and health care in the Netherlands*. Utrecht: De Tijdstroom. pp. 20–32.

Visser, J. (1990) 'Continuity and change in Dutch industrial relations', in G. Baglioni and C. Crouch (eds) *European industrial relations: The challenge of flexibility*. New York: Sage. pp. 199–241.

von Montfort, J. (1994) Interview (Director, National Hospital Institute). Utrecht, Netherlands.

Walshe, K. (2000) 'NHS trusts make a start on clinical governance', *Focus on the NHS* (Health Services Management Centre Newsletter), 6 (1): 6.

Walshe, K., Deakin, N., Smith, P., Spurgeon, P. and Thomas, N. (1997) *Contracting for change: Contracts in health, social care, and other government services*. Oxford: Oxford University Press.

Walshe, K. and Ham, C. (1997, April 3) 'Evidence based care – who's acting on the evidence?', *Health Service Journal*, 107: 22–25.

Walt, G. (1998) 'Implementing health care reform: A framework for discussion', in R. Saltman, J. Figueras and C. Sakellarides (eds) *Critical challenges for health care reform in Europe*. Buckingham, UK: Open University Press. pp. 365–384.

Ward, S. (2002) 'PFI is here to stay', *British Medical Journal*, 324: 1178.

Warden, J. (1998a) 'NHS hospital doctors face compulsory audit', *British Medical Journal*, 316: 1851.

Warden, J. (1998b). 'NHS gets more cash to modernise', *British Medical Journal*, 317: (7153) 231.

231

Warden, J. (1998c) 'St. Bartholomew's saved in London plan *British Medical Journal*, 316: 493.

Warden, J. (1998d) 'UK waiting lists grow longer', *British Medical Journal*, 316: 1625.

Warner, M. (1993) 'Prevention and health gain: A declaration of interdependence', in D. Light and A. May (eds) *Britain's National Health Service: From welfare state to managed markets*. New York: Faulkner and Gray. pp. 101–118.

Watt, N. (2002, November 15) 'Dobson rounds on "two-tier" hospitals', Guardian, p. 15.

Webber, D. (1992) 'The politics of regulatory change in the German health sector', in K. Dyson (ed.) *The politics of German regulation*. Aldershot, England: Dartmouth. pp. 209–234.

Webster, C. (1989) 'The health service', in D. Kavanagh and A.Seldon (ed.) *The Thatcher effect*. Oxford: Clarendon Press. pp. 166–182.

Webster, C. (1993) 'The National Health Service: The first forty years', in D. Light and A. May (eds) *Britain's health system: From welfare state to managed markets*. New York: Faulkner and Gray. pp. 13–20.

Weick, K. (1979) *The social psychology of organizing* (2nd ed.) Reading, MA: Addision-Wesley.

Weir, M. and Skocpol, T. (1985) 'State structures and the possibilities for "Keynesian" responses to the great depression in Sweden, Britain, and the United States', in P. Evans, D. Rueschmeyer and T. Skocpol (eds) *Bringing the state back in*. Cambridge: Cambridge University Press. pp. 107–163.

White, C. (2002, April 27) 'Primary care trusts need local flexibility', *British Medical Journal*, 324: 996.

Whitehead, M., Evandrou, M., Haglund, B., and Diderichsen, F. (1997) 'As the health care divide widens in Sweden and Britain, what's happening to access to care', *British Medical Journal*, 315: 1006–1009.

Whitehead, M., Gustafsson, R. and Diderichsen, F. (1997, October 11) 'Why is Sweden rethinking its NHS style reforms?', *British Medical Journal*, 315: 935–939.

Whitfield. (1998, May 28). 'Groups dynamic', *Health Services Journal*, 108: 9–10.

Whynes, D.K. and Baines, D.L. (1998) 'Income-based incentives in UK general practice', *Health Policy*, 43: 15–31.

Wiggers, C. (1994) 'Moderne Revialidatie' (Modern rehabilitation), in *Handboek structur en Fianciering Gezondheidszorg* Utrecht: De Tijdstroom.

Wilhelmsson, S., Faresjö, T., Foldevi, M. and Åkerlind, I. (1998) 'The personal doctor reform in Sweden: Perceived changes in working conditions', *Family Practice*, 15: 192–198.

Wilkin, D., Gilliam, S. and Coleman, A. (2001) *National tracker survey of primary care groups and trusts 2000/2001: Modernising the NHS? 2001*. Retrieved from Manchester: University of Manchester, National Primary Care Research and Development Centre in collaboration with King's Fund: http://www.npcrdc.man.ac.uk/Pages/Publications/PDF/Trackrp2.pdf

Wilkin, D., Gillam, S. and Leese, B. (2000) *Progress and challenges 1999/2000 National tracker survey of primary care groups and trusts*, Executive briefing. Manchester and York: National Primary Care Research and Development Centre.

Wilsford, D. (1995) 'States facing interests: Struggles over health care policy in advanced, industrial democracies', *Journal of Health Politics, Policy and Law*, 20 (3): 571–613.

Wilson, C. (2000) 'Policy regimes and policy change', *Journal of Public Policy*, 20 (3): 247–274.

Wintour, P. (2002, June 16) 'Public to run new hospitals', *Guardian*, p. 1.

Wise, J. (1998, June 27) 'BMA wins guarantees on primary care groups', *British Medical Journal*, 316 (7149): 1927.

Wise, J. (2001, May 5) 'Milburn proposes to decentralise the NHS', *British Medical Journal*, 322: 1083.

Wistow, G. (1992) 'The health policy community: Professionals pre-eminent or under challenge?', in D. Marsh and R.Rhodes (eds) *Policy networks in British politics*. Oxford: Clarendon Press. pp. 51–74.

Wistow, G. (1995) 'Aspirations and realities: Community care at the crossroads. *Health and Social Care in the Community*, 3 (4): 227–240.

Wistow, G. (1997) 'Decentralisation from acute to home care settings in England', *Health Policy*, 41 Supplement, S91-S108.

Wistow, G., and Harrison, S. (1998) 'Rationality and rhetoric: The contribution to social care policy making of Sir Roy Griffths, 1986–1991', *Public Administration*, 76: 649–668.

Woolf, S., Grol, R., Hutchinson, A., Eccles, M. and Grimshaw, J. (1999) 'Clinical guidelines: Potential benefits, limitations, and harms of clinical guidelines', *British Medical Journal*, 318: 527–530.

World Health Organization (1985) *Targets for health for all.* Copenhagen: WHO Regional Office for Europe.

World Health Organization (1998) *Health21: An Introduction to the Health for All Policy Framework for the WHO European Region European Health for All Series*, No. 5. Copenhagen: WHO Regional Office for Europe.

Yamey, G. (1999) 'Primary care groups frustrated by variations in funding', *British Medical Journal*, 319: 1026.

Yanow, D. (1993) 'The communication of policy meanings: Implementation as interpretation', *Policy Sciences*, 26: 41–61.

Yates, J. (1995) *'Private eye, heart and hip – surgical consultants, the National Health Service and private medicine.* Edinburgh: Churchill Livingstone.

Yates, J., Harley, M. and Jayes, B. (2000, April 27) 'Blade runners', *Health Service Journal*, 110: 20–21.

Young, D. and Saltman, R. (1985) *The hospital power equilibrium: Physician behavior and cost control.* Baltimore, MD: Johns Hopkins University Press.

233

Index